Contents

Infection Control

Science, Management and Practice

Edited by

JANET McCULLOCH

Infection Control Nurse Specialist,
Wiltshire Health Authority

W

WHURR PUBLISHERS

LONDON AND PHILADELPHIA

© 2000 Whurr Publishers
First published 2000 by
Whurr Publishers Ltd
19b Compton Terrace, London N1 2UN, England and
325 Chestnut Street, Philadelphia PA 1906, USA

Reprinted 2001

British Library Cataloguing in Publication Data
A catalogue record for this book is available from the British
Library.

ISBN: 1 86156 053 2

Printed and bound in the UK by Athenacum Press Ltd,
Gateshead, Tyne & Wear

Contributors

Kath Banfield BSc, RGN, Senior Nurse Infection Control, Harrogate Healthcare NHS Trust

Jane Barnett MSc, RGN, Senior Nurse Infection Control, Southmead NHS Trust

Julie Bushell BSc, RGN, RHV, PGCEA, Senior Nurse Infection Control, Public Health Laboratory, Southampton PHL

Lesly Finn RGN, Dip N (Lond), Dip Infection Control (Glasgow), Public Health Nurse Communicable Disease, Dorset Health Authority

Neil Keyworth PhD, M Phil Medical Microbiology, Infection Control Officer, Winchester and Eastleigh Healthcare NHS Trust

Andrew Kingsley RGN, Clinical Nurse Specialist Infection Control and Tissue Viability, North Devon Healthcare NHS Trust

Janet McCulloch (Editor) MSc, BSc, RGN, Infection Control Nurse Specialist, Wiltshire Health Authority

Patricia Mills BSc, PG Dip HE, RGN, Dip Nursing (Lond), Health Adviser, Genito-Urinary Medicine, Royal United Hospital Bath NHS Trust

Christine Perry RGN, Senior Nurse Infection Control, United Bristol Healthcare NHS Trust

Lauren Tew PGDip(HE), RNT, BSc (Hons), DN (Lond), RGN, Infection Control Nurse Manager, Royal United Hospital Bath NHS Trust

Preface

Control of infection is an essential part not only of healthcare but also of everyday life. Stories of 'super-bugs' and exotic infections find their way into newspaper headlines, raising fears that infection is uncontrollable and inevitably devastating. Increasingly, healthcare is being given in community settings – care homes as well as in the home. Caregivers are frequently unqualified individuals such as home carers and members of the family.

This book attempts to place infection control within this context. Although much of the text must concentrate on the healthcare environment, where the risk of infection is increased through clinical interventions, I hope it will also be a resource for a wider readership than healthcare professionals.

The authors, who are all practising specialists, have considered hospital and community issues where possible, have incorporated current regulations and legislation, and included guides to good practice which should be of use to both the professional and layperson.

The book aims to explain how we can all play our part in control of infection, from ensuring that healthcare buildings are designed with infection control in mind, to practising good food hygiene in the kitchen. It is hoped that in addition to the usual readers of infection control books, others such as care managers, health visitors, etc. will also be able to use the book to inform their own practice and to educate their clients in safe infection control practice.

Chapters 1 and 2 provide an introduction to the underpinning science of infection control. Since the focus of book is the practice of infection control, readers with a need for more than this introduction will need to refer to a specialist textbook on microbiology and immunology.

Chapters 3 to 8 describe the management systems which must be in place to promote infection control, including: the roles of infection control specialists, systems for the management of outbreaks including case studies, the design of the buildings, management of waste and laundry services and the provision of safe food.

Chapters 9–20 describe the practice of infection control in a variety of settings. They include assessments of the risks of acquiring infection and also the risks of transmitting infection to others. Chapter 20 also contains details of the sources, methods of spread and control measures for a wide range of infections.

Acknowledgements

There are many people who should be thanked for their support and patience in the production of this book. Not least, the authors who worked so hard with such good spirits. I would particularly like to thank Janet Hooper, who did much of the transcription, Dr Susan Murray who offered technical advice, and Lesly Finn for keeping my eye on the ball. Thanks also to my partner, Bob, for not minding the evenings and weekends spent alone.

Finally, I would like to remember Betty Bowell who offered me the chance of a new career in infection control and who provided such inspiration to me and many others. Betty sadly died before she was able to complete her chapters on risk assessment and handwashing, subjects she had virtually made her own through her enthusiasm and her humorous presentations.

Chapter 1
Introduction to the immune system

NEIL KEYWORTH

Introduction

The term 'immunity' has its origin as 'exemption from military service or paying taxes'. It had been recognized from early times that those who had suffered and recovered from infectious disease, e.g. smallpox, measles or diphtheria, were exempt from further attacks of that disease. Such people had developed a specific immune response to the infecting organism. There is no such thing as generalized immunity to all infectious diseases. Immunity is specific, that is it indicates the ability of the individual (host) to resist one particular infectious agent.

The immune system includes a complex series of defences whose prime role is to protect the individual against infection. These include non-specific defence mechanisms, which act as the natural barriers to infection, and specific immune responses that come into force if non-specific mechanisms fail.

The specific immune response involves lymphocytes in the lymph nodes and spleen. In the immune individual, re-exposure to the organism results in rapid recognition and destruction of the organisms before they can cause disease. Immunity may result from either vaccination or previous infection.

Non-specific mechanisms are not dependent on previous exposure to the organism, but attempt to prevent the establishment of infection. These protective mechanisms include the skin, mucous surfaces, secretions and mechanical structures, the inflammatory process and phagocytosis (or the engulfing of organisms) and the complement system.

Non-specific defence mechanisms

There are several elements involved in the non-specific defence system. They can be affected by a wide range of factors which will vary from one individual to another and will affect that person's response to any invading organism. These factors include general health, any underlying disease, state of nutrition, metabolic activity, hormonal influences and genetic factors.

The elements which are involved in non-specific immunity include:

1. Prevention of invasion:
    (a) skin
    (b) mucous surfaces
    (c) secretions
    (d) mechanical arrangement of structures.

2. Mechanisms following invasion:
    (a) inflammation
    (b) phagocytosis
    (c) interferon production.

3. The complement system.

Prevention of invasion

The body is surrounded by organisms, both pathogenic and non-pathogenic, which are present on everything we touch and eat and in the air we breathe. Therefore the skin and mucous surfaces form the first line of defence.

The skin

Intact skin forms a barrier against many pathogenic bacteria and its secretions have antibacterial properties. It is dry and acidic and colonized with normal bacterial flora called commensals. The skin is a complex structure which contains hair follicles, sweat and sebaceous glands. It constantly renews itself. The hair follicles and sweat glands harbour many organisms which are impossible to remove. Pathogenic organisms frequently invade from these sites resulting in superficial infections such as axillary abscesses and beard infections which can be difficult to treat.

Mucous surfaces

At certain body sites where bacterial numbers are high the surfaces are moistened with a mucous secretion to entrap the organisms until they can be removed; the nose, mouth and vagina are good examples of these.

Secretions

All organs in the body which are in contact with the external environment produce secretions. These are most appreciable in places where there is potentially the greatest danger of bacterial invasion. These secretions act in two ways.

1. *Mechanical action* – the physical removal of organisms. For example, bronchial secretions entrap organisms and the action of the cilia on the bronchial walls moves the flow away from the alveoli. As they reach the upper respiratory tract they are expelled by coughing. Tears also wash organisms away from the conjunctivae.

2. *Chemical action of their constituents* – secretions may be acid (sweat, adult vaginal secretion and gastric juice); strongly alkaline (bile); or contain fatty acids (sweat). Abrupt changes from an acid to an alkaline environment are known to keep the bacterial flora, for example in the alimentary canal in check. Tears and certain other mucosal secretions, for example nasal mucus and saliva, contain an active antibacterial substance, lysozyme.

The mechanical arrangement of structures

Certain physical structures of the body can play a part in reducing infection. For example, during respiration, air, which may contain many pathogenic organisms, is inhaled at high velocity. The arrangement of the mucus-covered turbinate bones in the nose is such that the air impinges upon the lining and bacteria stick to the mucous surfaces. The airflow is considerably reduced, due to the increasing area of bronchial passages, with the result that by the time air reaches the alveoli it is travelling very slowly and contains very few organisms. The mucus, swept by the cilia up the air passages into the pharynx, is subsequently swallowed and many of the organisms are killed by the acid in the gastric juice, or expelled by coughing.

In the urinary tract, other physical structures help to prevent urinary tract infection by preventing urinary stasis. These include the continuous flow of urine from the kidneys to the bladder; the prevention of backflow of urine by the structure of the ureters; and the complete periodic voiding of the bladder.

However, in some instances body structure can contribute to the development of infection, for example the direction of the bronchi may have something to do with the localization of lung infections and the short straight auditory tubes in infants may play a part in the greater frequency of middle-ear infections in comparison with infections in adults. Also, the shortness of the female urethra compared with that of the male accounts for the ease with which organisms can ascend to the bladder and cause cystitis.

Non-specific defence mechanisms following invasion

If organisms succeed in getting through the non-specific barriers described above and enter the tissues, further non-specific defence mechanisms are activated. Although not dependent on the specific immune response, their efficiency is greatly enhanced by it, as will be described later.

Inflammation

Once they have entered the tissues, most organisms will cause inflammation. The signs of inflammation are heat, redness, swelling and tenderness or pain. These signs are similar whether the tissue irritant is a micro-organism, a foreign body or a chemical.

Capillary dilation results in an outpouring of fluid, white cells and some red cells from the blood vessels into the tissues. This outpouring of neutrophils, phagocytes and serum is important, since it brings them into contact with the organisms. Serum contains substances which attach non-specifically to the surfaces of many organisms.

Should the bacteria manage to reach the bloodstream, lymph nodes or organs, they will meet other phagocytic cells including circulating neutrophils, monocytes and macrophages. Phagocytosis is enhanced by activation of the 'complement system'; both of these are described below.

Phagocytosis

Phagocytic white blood cells engulf invading organisms and destroy them with enzymes. Two types of white cell are involved, both arising in stem cells of the bone marrow.

1. *Neutrophils* – these circulate in the blood for only a few hours and are attracted to the scene of infection by chemicals released in the inflammatory process, called chemotactic substances.

2. *Mononuclear phagocytes* – these pass into the blood as monocytes and are then integrated into tissue as fixed macrophages, or wander as free macrophages. They can maintain their activity for a considerable period of time. They also process antigens and secrete interleukin-2, which is responsible for activating T- and B-lymphocytes, which in turn are involved in specific immunity.

Interferon

Interferons are a family of natural proteins produced by cells in response to viral infection. When cells are infected by viruses they may release interferon, which increases the resistance of neighbouring cells to the infection. It is now clear that there are many related types of interferon which play a complex regulatory role in cellular processes, which need not involve viruses. They appear to be the first line of defence against viral infection, appearing within 48 hours of infection, several days before antibody production. They do not act as antiviral agents themselves, but stimulate proteins to be synthesized in cells which inhibit replication of the virus.

The complement system

The complement system (abbreviated as 'C') consists of numerous enzymes and co-factors that interact with each other in an orderly sequence, often called an 'enzyme cascade'. When the complement system is activated, there are several important consequences which help in the destruction of invading organisms.

Activation of the complement system

The complement system can be activated by contact with some organisms. This type of complement activation is called the 'alternative pathway'. The other type of complement activation, called the 'classical pathway' because it was the first to be described, involves antibody and will be considered later with the 'specific' immune response. The two pathways lead, via enzyme cascades, to activation of the most important complement component, known as C3 (see Figure 1.1).

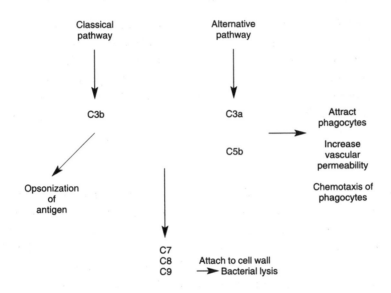

Figure 1.1 The complement pathway

Antimicrobial effects of the complement system

Complement components from the blood leak out at a site of inflammation and infection. Once activated at such a site the following things may happen:

1. They enhance phagocytosis when the organisms may become coated with derivatives of one of the complement components known as C3. This is known as 'opsonization'. It causes the organisms to adhere strongly to the membranes of phagocytic cells which have a binding site or 'receptor' for C3. This attachment of the organisms to phagocytes greatly increases the efficiency with which they are engulfed. Indeed C3 is so important

that congenital absence of it leads rapidly to death from infection.

2. They can increase vascular permeability and attract more phagocytic cells to the site by acting as chemotaxins.

3. Another group of complement components can lyse cell membranes (the lytic pathway). These are the factors which lyse red blood cells when an unmatched blood transfusion has been given. A few species of bacteria and viruses can be killed by the lytic pathway, but this function of complement, although the most well known, is not as important as the binding to membranes via C3 and congenital absence of one of the factors involved can be symptomless.

Destruction of engulfed organisms

Once engulfed by phagocytes (neutrophils or macrophages) with the help of the alternative complement pathway and C3, the organisms are contained within membrane-bound vacuoles called 'phagosomes', where they are exposed to a variety of microbiocidal mechanisms. Then the contents of the lysosomes are emptied into the phagosomes. Lysosomes contain a number of digestive enzymes that help to eliminate the organisms (see Figure 1.2). Occasionally the situation is reversed and the organisms kill the phagocytes.

The specific immune response

Whilst the struggle outlined above is going on, the lymphocytes in the lymphoid system are beginning to mount the specific immune response, which then comes to the aid of the non-specific mechanisms. Specific immune responses include:

1. Induction of the immune response.
2. Mechanisms of the specific immune response:
    (a) humoral immunity (B-lymphocytes and antibody production)
    (b) cell-mediated immunity (T-lymphocytes).

The induction of the immune response

Stage 1

Every organism is made up of a unique mixture of cell wall components,

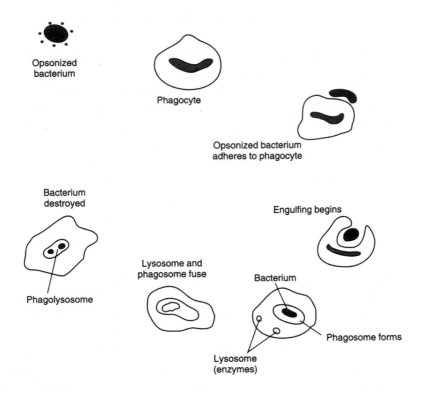

Figure 1.2 The process of phagocytosis

cytoplasm, enzymes and perhaps toxins. Most of these molecules are unlike anything present in the host's own tissues and so are recognized as 'foreign'. They are known as 'antigens'. Antigens from the infecting organism pass along the lymphatics, free or in macrophages, to the draining lymph nodes.

Stage 2

In the draining lymph node, the antigens come into contact with the surfaces of lymphocytes. Each lymphocyte carries on its surface receptors that enable it to recognize one particular type of antigen. When an antigen attaches to lymphocytes with receptors of the right specificity the lymphocytes begin to proliferate. This proliferation leads to a great increase in the number of lymphocytes which are able to recognize the antigen in question.

Stage 3

The lymphocytes leave the lymph node via the efferent lymphatics and travel to the site of the infection via the bloodstream. Here they assist in the struggle against the infection in a number of ways.

Table 1.1 Sites responsible for production of lymphocytes

- Tonsils
- Lymph nodes
- Thymus
- Bone marrow
- Spleen
- Kupffer cells (liver)
- Peyers patches (gut)
- Blood

Mechanisms of the specific immune response

The lymphocytes discussed above are of two kinds: B-lymphocytes and T-lymphocytes (see Table 1.1).

B-lymphocytes (B-cells) are derived from bone marrow. They protect the host from bacterial infection and are involved with *humoral immunity*.

T-lymphocytes (T-cells) are also derived from bone marrow but become thymus-dependent, requiring the thymus gland for development. T-cells are concerned with *cell-mediated immunity*, protecting the host from viral infection, tumours, tuberculosis and have a role in organ transplant rejection.

Humoral immunity

The B-lymphocytes are the basis of humoral immunity and they are the precursors of antibody-producing cells (plasma cells). Plasma cells release molecules similar to the antigen-recognizing receptors already described. These molecules, which are referred to as antibody, accumulate in the serum and may be present in very large quantities.

Antibodies are subdivided into several classes, each of which has different properties; they are referred to collectively as 'immunoglobulins'. They are proteins that are produced in response to infection.

The immunoglobulins are Y-shaped and parts have the combining sites for specific antigens. Antibody and antigen are constructed so that they fit like pieces of a jigsaw puzzle (see Figure 1.3). One fragment of immunoglobulin has the complement attachment site. Each antibody molecule has the ability to combine specifically with more antigen of the kind which induced the proliferative lymphocyte response in the draining lymph node. In fact, since each antibody molecule may have several antigen-specific combining sites, it may be able to attach to several antigen molecules.

Other B-cells develop into memory cells which respond quickly to any further invasion by the same antigen. They spread through the lymphatic system, to be 'on guard'. They may take several weeks to form an immunological memory, but that memory then lasts for life. Second exposure to the antigen will lead to a much more rapid and powerful production of antibody. This is seen clearly when giving a booster immunization many years after the initial course.

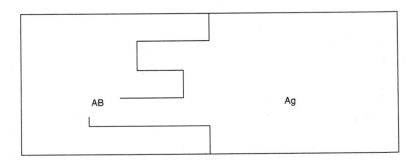

Figure 1.3 Antibody-antigen binding

The major classes of antibody

IgG

The most abundant class of antibody in the serum is immunoglobulin G (IgG). IgG crosses the placenta and is present in babies at birth. It appears in an individual 1–2 weeks after infection and lasts for a considerable time.

IgM

The other major class of antibody in serum is IgM. It is the first immunoglobulin to appear, about 1 week after the onset of an acute infection, and lasts for 4–6 weeks. Small amounts of IgM may be produced in chronic infections.

Other antibodies

Other classes of antibody are usually present only in small quantities in serum and have rather special properties.

IgA is actively secreted into the gut, bronchi, tears and saliva. It helps to block adherence of bacteria and viruses to mucous surfaces.

IgE is the immunoglobulin class responsible for hayfever because, rather than circulating in the blood, it attaches itself to mast cells and basophils. These are triggered to release compounds such as histamine in the presence of the antigen to which the IgE binds. IgE is also found in high serum levels in worm infections.

Antibody (mainly IgM and IgG) can protect the host in a number of ways:

1. Antibody can combine with the active parts of toxins, such as those released in diphtheria or tetanus, to neutralize their effects.
2. Antibody can cover viral cells and block their ability to attach to tissues.
3. Antibody can cause clumping (agglutination) of antigens or antigen-carrying organisms making them more easily engulfed by phagocytic cells.
4. Some organisms become coated with complement by means of a direct interaction with various serum factors. Other organisms do not activate complement until antibody molecules have attached to their surfaces. After this has occurred, the antigen-bound antibody itself can activate the complement system (classical pathway), which leads to attachment of complement to the surface of the organism. Some organisms are lysed by these complement components (lytic pathway).
5. Receptors for complement (C3 receptors) are found on the membranes of phagocytic cells. There are also receptors for the free end of antibody molecules, and the 'opsonized' organism thus sticks firmly to macrophages and polymorphs which can

then phagocytose the organism very efficiently.

6. Antibody (IgA) is secreted into the bronchi, the gut and tears and so can reinforce the non-specific barriers such as mucus and cilia. Antibody is also secreted in maternal milk and some subclasses (IgG) can cross the placenta so that babies are protected for the first few months of life by the mother's antibody. Meanwhile they begin to develop their own immune responses.

Cell-mediated immunity

T-lymphocytes (T-cells) are the cells responsible for cell-mediated immunity, which protects an individual from intracellular bacterial infections, viral and some fungal infections. It is also the major element of defence against parasites and tumours and is involved in transplant rejection.

Several types of cell are involved in this system but the primary effector cells are the T-lymphocytes, which are so called because they are dependent, particularly in early life, on the thymus gland where these cells mature. Lymphocytes are absent in children with congenital absence of the thymus and such children have very low resistance to infection, due primarily to loss of cell-mediated immunity. As the name implies, this involves the direct interaction of T-cells with antigen.

T-lymphocyte-mediated immunity protects the host in two important ways.

1. When a T-cell encounters the antigen which its receptors recognize, it may release mediators known collectively as 'lymphokines'. Alpha interferon is an example of a lymphokine. The lymphokines cause macrophages in the vicinity to become activated. This involves a number of complex metabolic changes, the most important of which is an increased ability to destroy micro-organisms. For example, tubercle bacilli, even when coated with antibody and complement, appear not to be killed by normal macrophages but activated macrophages can destroy them. This is also the mechanism of defence against leprosy.
2. T-cells and their 'assistants', the activated macrophages, are also

able to recognize and damage cells which have become foreign to the host. For instance, virus-infected cells may express viral antigens on to their surface. The cell-mediated response can recognize these antigens and help to localize the infection by attacking such cells and interrupting the virus replication cycle (the attacking cells are known as cytotoxic cells). This mechanism is of particular importance for defence against viruses such as varicella-zoster which can pass directly from cell to cell without being released into the body fluids where they would be exposed to antibody. This is why it is common to see an exacerbation of varicella-zoster when T-cell function is compromised, e.g. in patients undergoing cytotoxic therapy.

When T-cells proliferate they differentiate into two main types of cell: helper T-cells and suppressor T-cells.

Helper T-cells (CD4) activate or encourage B-cell proliferation and so encourage antibody production (humoral immunity) by the new plasma cells.

Suppressor T-cells (CD8) counteract the action of the helper cells, preventing excessive reaction and damage to tissues.

Within this population there are further subgroups including cytotoxic T-cells, which destroy foreign cells, tumour cells and infected cells; and lymphokine-producing cells, which stimulate phagocytosis (see Figure 1.4).

The interaction between the main population and the subpopulations is extremely complex but, in summary, the balance between the two is crucial: if the helpers are in excess this will lead to autoimmune disease, whilst if the helpers are decreased this will result in immune deficiency disease.

Memory T-cells are also formed at each new meeting with an invader cell and this immunological memory will last for many years. They can then produce a rapid response to any future contact with a particular antigen in the same way as memory B-cells (see Figure 1.5).

Imbalance in the immune system

In some genetic diseases, either or both B- and T-cells can be absent. T-cells are necessary for stimulation of B-cells, leading to antibody

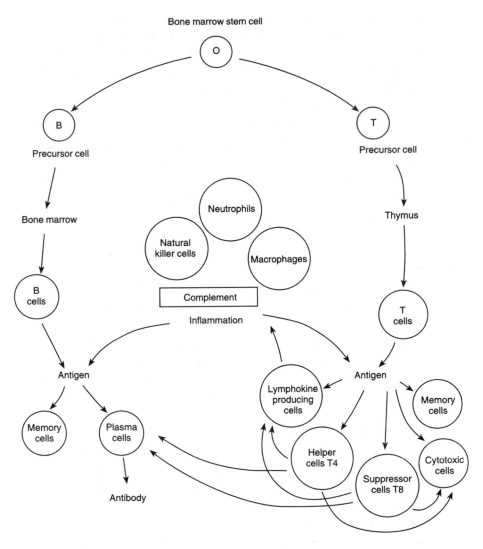

Figure 1.4 The role of the lymphyocytes in acquired immunity

production. Lack of B-cells and antibodies leads to agammaglobuli-
naemia (relative or total lack of one class of antibody), which can
leave the individual susceptible to overwhelming infection.

Autoimmune diseases, such as rheumatoid arthritis and systemic
lupus erythematosus, are thought to be connected with some failure
of balance in the immune system, a possible failure of suppressor T-
cells leading to the body's defences attacking itself.

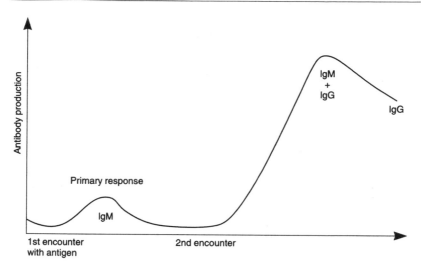

Figure 1.5 Antibody response

The action of T-cells and macrophages in controlling cancers has already been mentioned. The increased incidence of malignancies in old age may be connected with the decreasing influence of the thymus gland itself. T-cell numbers in the blood fall progressively with age. In treatment of infection with HIV, measurement of the ratio of CD4 to CD8 cells is used to define the progression of the disease and the need for therapy.

Vaccination and immunization

The aim of immunization is to stimulate a positive immune response in an individual to specific pathogenic micro-organisms so as to confer protection against their harmful effects.

Immunization can occur naturally or may be induced artificially. Both natural and artificially induced immunity may be passive or active (see Figure 1.6).

Active natural immunity

Active natural immunity results from natural exposure to an antigen, for example, a disease-producing micro-organism that causes an individual's immune system to respond against the antigen. During the first exposure symptoms of infection may not develop because the individual is not yet immune.

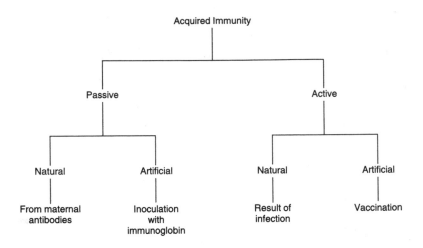

Figure 1.6 Acquired immunity

Active artificial immunity

In active artificial immunity an antigen is deliberately introduced into an individual to stimulate the immune system. This process is called vaccination, and the introduced antigen is a vaccine. Injection of the vaccine is the most usual mode of administration. Sometimes the vaccine is ingested, as in the oral poliomyelitis vaccine. The vaccine usually consists of some part of a micro-organism, a dead micro-organism or a live altered micro-organism. The antigen has been changed so that it will stimulate the immune system but will not cause the symptoms of the disease.

Passive natural immunity

Passive natural immunity results from the transfer of antibodies from a mother to her foetus across the placenta before birth. The mother, having been exposed to many antigens during her life, has antibodies to many infections. Following birth these antibodies provide protection for the first few months of the baby's life. Eventually the baby will come to rely on its own immune system.

Passive artificial immunity

Achieving passive artificial immunity involves the vaccination of antibodies contained in serum. This substance termed 'antiserum' can be derived from the serum of a vaccinated animal, such as a horse, or may be genetically engineered. Antisera are available against micro-organisms that cause diseases such as hepatitis, measles, diphtheria and rabies.

Factors reducing immunity

There are many factors that may diminish the ability of the immune system to protect against infection.

Hospital and long-term care patients are at risk of developing infection because they are often elderly, poorly nourished and may have difficulties with personal hygiene. In addition, underlying medical disorders such as malignancies, diabetes, renal failure, human immunodeficiency virus and cirrhosis decrease T- and B-cell mediated immune function.

Breaches of the body's integrity by devices such as intravascular cannulae and urinary catheters impair the body's non-specific defence mechanisms. Medical treatments such as the use of broad-spectrum antibiotics increase the risk of *Clostridium difficile* diarrhoea. Immunosuppressive agents and oral corticosteroids decrease the ability of the body to resist infection.

The immunocompromised patient

Patients who have a compromised immune system are at great risk of acquiring an infection, especially whilst in hospital. There are a number of ways that an individual's immune system may be compromised. These include: medical conditions such as HIV infection and diabetes, or chemical or radiological suppression as in the treatment of malignancies or organ transplantation protocols.

These patients are very susceptible to any form of infection, even those caused by opportunistic micro-organisms that are not ordinarily harmful to other individuals, such as environmental fungi. They are also at risk from their own commensal flora including *Staphylococcus epidermidis*, particularly in the presence of invasive devices. They may also suffer from re-activation of previous infection due to reduced antibody levels. Protective isolation of immunosuppressed patients may involve barrier nursing in purpose-built single rooms which are ventilated with filtered air under positive pressure.

Care must also be taken to prevent exposure to potential pathogens in food and via invasive devices.

Conclusion

The human body is constantly fighting a battle with the organisms that surround us. This battle continues without us being aware that it is being fought. Without a functioning immune system we will all quickly succumb to infection, which may be overwhelming.

Yet it is very easy for parts of the immune system to be temporarily damaged or bypassed, putting the individual at risk. Every invasive device that is inserted increases the risk of infection. Dependent or sick patients who cannot manage their own hygiene, brush their teeth, blink their eyes, cough or swallow are at an increased risk. We must ensure that these basic needs are met, and where possible restore the patient to good health. If we do not, we must recognize our own responsibility when the patient develops an infection (such as pneumonia) which may finally end their life.

Further reading

Cooke E Hare's Bacteriology and Immunity for Nurses. London: Churchill Livingstone, 1991.

Department of Health Immunisation Against Infectious Disease. London: HMSO, 1996.

Elliot T, Hastings M, Desselberger U Lecture Notes on Medical Microbiology, 3rd Edition. Oxford: Blackwell Science, 1997.

Kirkwood E, Lewis C Understanding Medical Immunology, 2nd Edition. Chichester: John Wiley and Sons Ltd, 1989.

Reeves G Lecture Notes on Immunology. London: Blackwell Scientific Publications, 1987.

Wilson G, Dick H (eds) Topley and Wilson's Principles of Bacteriology, Virology and Immunity, 7th Edition, vol. 1. London: Edward Arnold, 1983.

Zuckerman A, Banatrala J, Patterson J Principles and Practice of Clinical Virology, 3rd Edition. Chichester: John Wiley and Sons, 1994.

Chapter 2
Introduction to microbiology and virology

NEIL KEYWORTH

Introduction

Microbiology is the study of micro-organisms, or microbes, which are terms used to describe any living organism that is too small to be seen by the naked eye. Micro-organisms were first seen about 1675 by the Dutchman Antony Van Leeuwenhoek. He found many micro-organisms in materials such as water, mud, saliva and the intestinal contents of healthy subjects, and he recognized them as 'animalcules' because they swam about actively. Microbiology related to medicine includes the study of bacteria, viruses, fungi and protozoa. Some organisms benefit man, others can cause disease and death. An understanding of the ways they behave and their effects enables the application of the principles of safe patient care.

Micro-organisms are part of the ecological chain, performing functions that range from acting as food for other higher organisms, to helping with the breakdown of dead organic matter into simple materials that can be used by others. A variety of foodstuffs such as bread, beer, vinegar, wine and yoghurt are the products of the activities of micro-organisms.

Only a small proportion of the micro-organisms that abound in nature are disease-producing or 'pathogenic' for man. Most are free-living in soil, water and similar habitats, and are unable to invade the living body.

Micro-organisms capable of causing disease are referred to as 'pathogens'. Infection results when pathogens gain access to the body's tissues and, having established themselves, multiply and cause an adverse reaction in the individual 'host'. Most areas of the body have a natural flora or 'commensal' population of microbes. Commensals are harmless in the area where they normally live but if transmitted to other parts of the body may cause infection. Some organisms will only cause an infection when the body's defence system is impaired. These are referred to as 'opportunistic' pathogens. An example of such an organism is *Pneumocystis carinii*, which causes the respiratory infection often seen in patients with acquired immune deficiency syndrome (AIDS).

Classification of micro-organisms

Living creatures are composed of one of two cell types: prokaryotic or eukaryotic cells. Prokaryotic cells have a simpler structure and the nuclear material is free in the cytoplasm; they include bacteria. In contrast eukaryotic cells have their DNA enclosed within a nuclear membrane and a clear nucleus can be seen under the microscope. The simplest single-cell eukaryocytes are protozoa, fungi and some algae. Viruses are prokaryotic, obligate intracellular parasites – that is, they require other living cells in order to reproduce.

The shape of the bacterium is maintained by a rigid cell wall. There may be additional layers of material and a protective coat or capsule outside the cell wall. Reproduction is by binary fission, during which the cell divides, the DNA replicates and the daughter chromosomes are drawn apart. Despite the fact that prokaryotic cells are much simpler than eukaryotic cells they can still contain all the components necessary for an independent existence.

Bacteria

Bacteria are microscopic organisms that range from 0.3 to 14 microns in length and therefore need a microscope to observe them. They are classified according to three main properties: Gram stain, shape (morphology), and oxygen requirement.

Gram staining

In their natural state bacteria are small colourless organisms when seen under the microscope. To make them more easily visible they can be stained with a dye, usually crystal violet. Gram-positive organisms retain this dye following decolourization with acetone and appear deep violet in colour. Gram-negative organisms lose the violet stain in the decolourization process but take up a red counter-stain and appear pink.

Staphylococcus aureus, which can cause skin infections, is a typical Gram-positive organism. *Escherichia coli*, part of the normal flora of the bowel and a common cause of urinary tract infection, is a typical Gram-negative organism.

The Gram stain is useful as it can distinguish structural differences between Gram-positive and Gram-negative micro-organisms, and help to give an understanding of the disease-causing capabilities of Gram-positive and Gram-negative bacteria. Gram-positive bacteria have a much thicker cell wall (mucopeptide layer) than Gram-negatives.

Outside the cell wall Gram-negative bacteria have a layer of lipopolysaccharide (LPS), which is a complex of sugars, fatty acids and phosphate, whereas Gram-positive bacteria have a layer of teichoic acid, which is a complex of sugar and phosphate. Both types of bacteria may be enclosed in a capsule composed of a layer of gelatinous material, produced by the bacterium itself, which adheres to the outside of the cell and shields the bacterium from the host's defence mechanisms.

Morphology

Bacteria are classified into four main groups by their shape:

1) Cocci – which are round
2) Bacilli – which are rod-shaped
3) Coccobacilli – which are very short rods and may resemble cocci
4) Spirochaetes – which are spiral.

Under the microscope the manner in which the bacterial cells are arranged can also be seen. Some grow in chains (streptococci), some in pairs (diplococci) and some in clusters (staphylococci). An important structure seen in Gram-negative bacteria and some Gram-positive bacilli is the flagellum, which is capable of inducing movement in the bacterium in a liquid environment.

Under adverse conditions two groups of Gram-positive bacteria, the genera *Clostridium* and *Bacillus*, produce structures called endospores (commonly referred to as spores). A mature spore can survive in a dormant state in dust, vegetation or soil for weeks, months or even years until it finds itself in an environment which is suitable for its germination. As a spore the organism is significantly more resistant to heat, cold and disinfectants than the original organism.

Oxygen requirement

Some bacteria require oxygen in their environment in order to grow. These are classified as obligate aerobes. Others cannot tolerate the presence of oxygen and these are classified as obligate anaerobes. Some, facultative anaerobes, are able to grow with or without oxygen.

Bacterial growth

Bacteria reproduce through binary fission, which is a simple process by which one cell divides into two smaller 'daughter' cells. The rate of growth, or the time it takes for a cell population to divide, varies between different types of bacteria. Some species such as *Escherichia coli* divide every 20 minutes or so. Under ideal conditions a single cell can multiply into a million cells in under eight hours. The rapid growth of some organisms can cause considerable infection control hazards.

Common organisms

Gram-positive cocci

Staphylococci

Staphylococci are identified or distinguished by their ability to clot plasma by means of the enzyme coagulase. *Staphylococcus aureus* is coagulase positive (that is it has the ability to clot plasma) whereas *Staphylococcus epidermidis* and other species are coagulase negative. *Staph. aureus* is an important pathogen causing superficial and deep infections e.g. boils, impetigo and surgical wound infections. It is found in approximately 20–30% of healthy individuals.

Staph. epidermidis is present as part of the normal skin flora and rarely causes infections although it may cause opportunistic infections at the sites of prostheses and intravascular cannulae, particularly in people who are immunocompromised.

Streptococci

Streptococci inhabit the mucous membranes of man and animals including the mouth, upper respiratory tract and the intestinal tract. Some strains destroy red blood cells and are termed haemolytic streptococci. Bacteria that produce complete lysis of red blood cells on blood agar growth medium are called beta-haemolytic streptococci. They are the commonest cause of streptococcal infections and are classified into Lancefield groups A to S. The most important human pathogen in this group is the beta-haemolytic streptococcus of Lancefield group A (*Streptococcus pyogenes*). This organism can cause common infections of the throat and skin. It also produces a toxin that can result in the systemic rash of scarlet fever.

Lancefield group B streptococcus is present in the normal vaginal flora of about 30% of all women and can cause infections in neonates if it is acquired from the mother's vagina during delivery.

Alpha-haemolytic streptococci such as *Streptococcus viridans* produce incomplete haemolysis of red cells giving a greenish appearance around the colony on blood agar. *Strep. viridans* is present as normal flora of the mouth but can cause bacterial endocarditis in patients with already damaged heart valves. *Streptococcus pneumoniae* is part of the normal respiratory tract but classically causes lobar pneumonia.

Gram-positive bacilli

Clostridium tetani, *Clostridium perfringens* and *Clostridium difficile* are spore-forming anaerobes which are Gram-positive rods.

The natural habitat of *Cl. tetani* is soil, and the usual means of infection is contamination of a wound with soil or manure. Although now relatively rare in the UK because of immunization programmes and prophylactic treatment at the time of injury, tetanus remains a serious problem in many developing countries.

Cl. perfringens lives as a commensal in human faeces. When contaminating a wound involving poor blood supply, the organism produces a toxin and the subsequent infection is known as gas gangrene.

Cl. difficile is sometimes present in normal faeces but its numbers are kept in check by other bacterial flora. However if certain antibiotics are given *Cl. difficile* may proliferate, and with its toxin may result in a severe bowel infection known as pseudomembranous colitis. This condition can prove fatal in the elderly if untreated. Outbreaks may occur in wards and nursing homes where susceptible patients are nursed.

Other Gram-positive bacilli include *Corynebacterium diphtheriae*, which may cause diphtheria in humans, and *Listeria monocytogenes*. This organism is widely found in the environment and may contaminate foodstuffs such as soft cheeses, causing food poisoning. It may also cause meningitis and septicaemia in neonates and in the immunosuppressed.

Gram-negative cocci

Neisseria are found in the mucous membranes of the upper respiratory and genital tract. Most are harmless but *Neisseria gonorrhoeae* and *Neisseria meningitidis* are important pathogens. *N. meningitidis* is often carried in the upper respiratory tract of healthy people but can become pathogenic and cause meningitis. Transmission is by close contact, especially kissing contact, and epidemics can occur where there is overcrowding, for instance in dormitory conditions.

N. gonorrhoeae is transmitted by sexual intercourse and causes urethritis and cervicitis. It can also be transmitted from mother to baby during birth, causing the eye infection ophthalmia neonatorum.

Gram-negative aerobic bacilli

Pseudomonas

Pseudomonas aeruginosa can colonize the lower intestinal tract of hospitalized patients. Because it may cause an infection when the host's defence mechanisms are impaired, it is often considered an opportunistic pathogen. Most pseudomonas species can be isolated from moist environmental sites in the hospital. It sometimes produces blue-green pus which has a distinctive smell.

Enterobacteriacae

Enterobacteriacae are Gram-negative bacilli which may inhabit the human intestine.

Salmonellae are important intestinal pathogens causing gastroenteritis. Inadequately cooked poultry is often the source of these organisms.

Shigellae cause mild dysentery infections and outbreaks are common amongst children.

Klebsiellae are non-motile Gram-negative bacilli often carried in the intestine and are capable of causing urinary tract, chest and wound infections.

Escherichia coli is a normal inhabitant of the human intestine. It is the most frequent cause of urinary tract infection. Some strains, e.g. *E. coli* 0157, are known as enteropathogenic types and can produce gastroenteritis in infants, sometimes with devastating consequences.

Proteus and **Serratia** are common in the hospital environment and are capable of causing urinary tract and wound infections.

Vibrios

Campylobacter jejuni frequently contaminates poultry and results in severe diarrhoea and abdominal pain if transferred to humans. Although person to person spread of this organism is rare, it has a small infectious dose so this should not be discounted.

Gram-negative anaerobic bacilli

Bacteroides is a non-sporing Gram-negative anaerobe found in the gut. *Bacteroides fragilis* can cause abdominal and gynaecological infections.

Fusobacteria colonizes the mouth and may cause oral infections including acute gingivitis.

Acid-fast bacilli

Mycobacteria are slender rods enveloped in a wax coat that makes it difficult to stain them with the Gram stain. After staining with hot carbol fuchsin the organisms are stain fast and cannot be decolourized with alcohol or strong acids. *Mycobacterium bovis* and *Mycobacterium tuberculosis* both cause human infection, the former being acquired from ingestion of infected milk. Tuberculosis is a slow, progressive, chronic infection of the lung, although many organs and tissues may be affected.

Mycoplasma

Mycoplasma may be aerobic or facultatively aerobic. They lack a cell wall so have no fixed shape. A few species cause disease, for example *Mycoplasma pneumoniae*.

Rickettsia and Chlamydia

Rickettsia and Chlamydia are prokaryotic cells that are unable to grow outside a host cell. They are therefore referred to as obligate intracellular parasites. Both Rickettsia and Chlamydia require factors from the host cell to support their growth.

Rickettsia are fragile and not viable when removed from the host cell (with the exception of the organism that causes Q fever) and transfer to humans often involves arthropods, such as ticks.

Chlamydia are round and slightly smaller than Rickettsia. *Chlamydia trachomatis* is responsible for sexually transmitted disease such as non-specific urethritis and pelvic inflammatory disease. *Chlamydia psittaci* and *Chlamydia pneumoniae* can cause chest infections.

Fungi

Fungi, which include mushrooms, yeasts and moulds, are eukaryotic cells and are more complex than bacteria. They consist of a nucleus containing chromosomes inside a membrane. The surrounding cytoplasm contains mitochondria and ribosomes. Few cause disease in humans.

Fungi reproduce sexually or by spore formation and are divided into four groups:

1   **Yeasts** – round/oval cells which reproduce by budding, for example *Cryptococcus neoformans*
2   **Yeast-like fungi** – most of these will reproduce by budding but some form filaments, e.g. *Candida albicans*
3   **Filamentous fungi** – these fungi grow as filaments (hyphae) which interweave into a mesh (mycelium), e.g. ringworm
4   **Dimorphic fungi** – grow in two forms according to their situation: as yeasts in the body or as mycelia in the environment or in culture, for example *Blastomyces* and *Histoplasma*.

Fungal disease (mycoses) can be divided into those affecting the skin only, e.g. ringworm (superficial) and those affecting the whole system, e.g. histoplasmosis (deep). The latter, such as *Aspergillus fumigatus*, are usually only pathogenic as opportunists, taking advantage of a lowered host resistance.

Protozoa

These are eukaryotic micro-organisms. They are the smallest single-cell animals and are much larger than most bacteria. They possess a nucleus surrounded by a limiting membrane lying within the cytoplasm, which in turn is divided into endoplasm (concerned with nutrition) and ectoplasm (which obtains the food). The ectoplasm may actively flow into pseudopodia to allow movement or the cell may have flagella or cilia.

Protozoa may cause human disease, including *Plasmodium* spp. (causing malaria), *Entamoeba histolytica* (amoebic dysentery), *Giardia lamblia* and *Cryptosporidium parvum* (diarrhoeal diseases), *Toxoplasma gondii* (congenital infection) and *Pneumocystis carinii* (opportunistic lung infection).

Viruses

Viruses are obligate, intracellular parasites and differ from other micro-organisms in several important ways. They are unable to grow in artificial growth media growing only within living cells. They are much smaller than other micro-organisms (20–300 nanometers in diameter) and most can only be seen using an electron microscope. They possess DNA or RNA, but never both.

Structure

Virus particles consist of a core of nucleic acid (DNA or RNA) surrounded by a protein coat (capsid). Some viruses, e.g. herpes viruses, are enclosed by a further layer or envelope. Viruses without envelopes are called naked viruses. The capsid protects the nucleic acid and facilitates the attachment of the virus to the target cell; it also contains antigenic material which is specific for each virus type. The capsid and the enclosed nucleic acid make up the nucleocapsid and the entire virus particle (including the envelope if there is one) is called a virion.

Replication

The virus recognizes protein receptors on the host (target) cell to which it attaches. It injects its nucleic acids into the host where they attach to the host nuclear DNA and take over the host cell protein and DNA synthesis so that new virus particles can be made. The protein of the outer coat is responsible for much of the immunological response to the virus as it is antigenic. Enveloped viruses are released from the cell by budding. The envelope is part of the parent cell membrane and these viruses are not infectious without the envelope. Viruses are true parasites, i.e. they cannot reproduce outside living cells, and many viruses do not survive long outside living cells.

Viruses are everywhere: many cause us no harm but, like bacteria, they are responsible for a wide range of diseases. These include influenza, colds, polio, herpes, glandular fever, gastro-enteritis, many childhood infections such as measles and chickenpox, several types of hepatitis and the more recently discovered acquired immune deficiency syndrome (AIDS), caused by human immuno-deficiency virus (HIV). The effect on the host cell may be manifest in several ways:

1) Cytopathic effect (CPE) – the infection kills the cell, e.g. adenovirus and respiratory syncytial virus
2) Latency – there is no obvious effect but cell remains potentially infectious e.g. varicella-zoster virus
3) Transformation – the host cell is transformed into a malignant form, e.g. Hepatitis B and C associated with liver carcinoma, and Epstein-Barr virus with Burkitt's lymphoma.

Therapeutic agents

Strictly speaking, the term 'antibiotic' refers to a substance produced by one micro-organism that is capable of destroying another micro-organism. Agents available nowadays are more likely to be man-made and engineered than derived solely from a bacterial culture. Any chemical substance inhibiting the growth or causing the death of a micro-organism is known as an antimicrobial agent. Whatever the agent is called it may act in one of two ways. The effect may result in the death of the organisms (bactericidal) or may prevent the replication of the organism and allow the host's immune system to destroy the pathogen (bacteriostatic).

Mechanisms of action

Antibiotic activity depends on a number of different mechanisms. There are four main mechanisms involved in the action of antimicrobial drugs:

1) inhibition of cell-wall synthesis
2) alteration of the cell membrane
3) inhibition of nucleic acid synthesis
4) inhibition of protein synthesis.

Inhibition of cell-wall synthesis

Bacterial cells differ from mammalian cells in that most have a cell wall. Certain antibiotics act by inhibiting the synthesis of the cell wall as the cell divides, leading to death of the cell without harm to the host cells, e.g. penicillins (flucloxacillin, benzyl penicillin), glycopeptides (vancomycin, teicoplanin) and cephalosporins (cefuroxime).

Alteration of cell membrane

The cell membrane of both fungi and bacteria have a different structure to mammalian cells and can be disrupted allowing the cytoplasm contents to escape. For example, polymixins affect Gram-negative bacteria cell membranes, amphotericin B and nystatin affect fungal cell membranes.

Inhibition of nucleic acid synthesis

This may occur by inhibiting RNA synthesis (e.g. rifampicin) or, more commonly, by inhibiting some stage of DNA synthesis e.g. metronidazole, quinolones (such as nalidixic acid or ciprofloxacin), sulphonamides (mistaken by bacterial enzymes for an essential metabolite in some DNA or RNA synthesis); also antifungal agents including 5-flucytosine, griseofulvin; and antiviral agents such as acyclovir and zidovudine.

Inhibition of protein synthesis

The ribosomes of bacterial cells appear to have sufficient differences in structure and function from mammalian cells to allow antimicrobial drugs to inhibit bacterial protein synthesis whilst leaving the host cells relatively undamaged. Examples of drugs that work in this way are aminoglycosides (gentamicin, neomycin, etc.), tetracycline, macrolides (erythromycin), chloramphenicol, lincomycin and fusidic acid.

Indications for use

In the ideal situation, the infecting organism should be identified and its antibacterial sensitivity determined in the laboratory before the single optimum therapy is initiated. In practice any patient with a life-threatening illness requires immediate 'blind' treatment. This treatment, usually with more than one antibacterial, will reflect the most likely cause of infection. To avoid the diagnosis being completely obscured, treatment must be preceded by sample-taking for bacteriological testing. Combination therapy in specific circumstances can prevent or delay the emergence of bacterial resistance. This type of protocol is virtually mandatory in the treatment of tuberculosis, where antimicrobials are given over extended periods of time.

Resistance to antimicrobial agents

There are a variety of mechanisms by which bacteria may become resistant to antibiotic agents. Antibiotic resistance may be coded for on chromosomes or on plasmids (extrachromosomal fragments of DNA). Resistance may be divided into natural and acquired resistance.

Natural resistance occurs irrespective of antibiotic usage. This may be due to:

(a) the production of drug-destroying enzymes
(b) the resistance of cell membranes (e.g. Gram-negative bacteria) which prevents the access of antibiotics to the organism
(c) bacteria that may lack a target site for the antimicrobial to act upon.

Acquired resistance is often associated with inappropriate or excessive use of antibiotics, the mechanisms by which this occurs are as follows:

(a) Chromosomal resistance occurs when mutant strains of a bacterium survive in the presence of an antibiotic and eventually multiply and predominate if exposure to the antibiotic persists

(b) Plasmid-mediated resistance occurs when plasmid transference takes place between strains involving genes coding for antibiotic resistance (R- factors), even crossing species in some Gram-negative organisms.

Significance of antibiotic resistance

Resistance is a problem because it limits the choice of antibiotics that can be used to treat infection. Methicillin-resistant *Staphylococcus aureus* (MRSA) is a prime example of acquired resistance. It was initially always sensitive to penicillin, but few if any strains of staphylococci isolated in hospitals are now sensitive because of the production of beta-lactamase, an enzyme that inactivates penicillin. Methicillin was designed to be a beta-lactamase resistant antibiotic. However shortly after its introduction resistance to methicillin began to emerge. The incidence of MRSA continued to increase and was highlighted by many serious outbreaks in the 1970s and 1980s.

Hospital strains of various bacteria show a greater tendency to develop resistance because of the extent of antibiotic use. Resistant bacteria are now found in many intensive care units where antibiotics are used extensively. To date our ingenuity in designing new antibiotics has remained one step ahead of the bacteria, but we cannot continue to rely on coming up with another alternative when resistance develops to the current treatment.

Antifungal agents

Most important antibiotics are produced by fungi, and it is not surprising that fungi should be resistant to their effects. There are, however, a few substances that are effective in the treatment of certain human fungal infections and they specifically interfere with cell wall lipid structure based on cholesterol peculiar to fungi. Substances currently in use include amphotericin B, nystatin, clotrimazole, econazole, miconazole, ketoconazole and fluconazole.

Antiviral agents

The main reason for the slow and limited development of antiviral agents is the nature of virus replication. As virus particles live within the host's cells and require cell metabolic processes to replicate, any agent must be able to target viral replication without damaging the host cell.

The first agent found to affect viruses was interferon, but this substance is not much use in the treatment of acute infections. Idoxuridine was the first specific antiviral drug used against herpes virus. More recently acyclovir, ganciclovir, vidarabine and inosine pranobex have been used. The advent of HIV infection and treatment has stimulated tremendous research into antiviral agents. Zidovudine (AZT) was the first antiviral agent to be developed for use against HIV and further drugs are currently being used. Others will surely follow.

Specimen collection

The collection of specimens for microbiological investigation will enable the diagnosis of infection, the identification of the causative organism and provide guidance on which antimicrobial agents will be effective. It is important that specimens sent to the laboratory are accompanied by essential clinical information. This will enable the laboratory to select the appropriate tests according to the information provided.

Examples of the information routinely required include:

- Demographic details: age, unit number, address or ward, date of birth, etc.
- Sample details: nature of sample (e.g. blood, swab) and sample site
- Clinical details: signs and symptoms, date of onset, underlying condition, co-existing illness, recent events such as surgery, information about others with the same symptoms suspected to be part of an outbreak
- Antibiotic history: recent, current or planned
- Other relevant history: recent travel abroad, occupation, hobbies, etc.

Collection of good quality specimens

The production of useful results is entirely dependent on the quality of the specimens provided. This depends on a number of factors such as the optimal time of collection, the correct type of specimen, the avoidance of contamination of the sample with normal flora, adequate quantities of specimen and in some cases appropriate numbers of samples, and the skill of the person obtaining the sample. It is vital that specimens for culture of bacteria are collected before the start of antibiotic treatment. Even single doses of an antibiotic may reduce or eliminate the causative organism.

Specimens should be collected which are most appropriate to the clinical condition. For example a sample of pus is always preferable to a swab. Pernasal swabs, rather than throat or ordinary nasal swabs, should always be collected from children who are suspected to have pertussis. Cervical and urethral swabs, rather than high vaginal swabs, should be collected from female patients with suspected gonorrhoea. Patients with possible bacterial meningitis should have blood cultures taken, as well as cerebrospinal fluid (CSF).

Handwashing must be carried out before the collection of specimens, and appropriate personal protective clothing worn. This may include disposable gloves, eye protection and/or face mask depending upon the type of sample collected (MacLeod, 1992). Decontamination of the site may also be required, for example disinfection of the skin before collecting blood or CSF samples. Good quality specimens will exclude or minimize the amount of normal flora present in the sample.

Details of the techniques of specimen collection are provided by many microbiology laboratories, and should be sought for best results. Specimens should be clearly labelled, contained in a leak-proof container and placed within a plastic bag or transport box. The laboratory form must not be in contact with the specimen container to prevent contamination of the laboratory staff.

Specimens should be as fresh as possible to optimize conditions for the isolation of micro-organisms. Urine and sputum samples should reach the laboratory within two hours of collection whenever possible. If delays are expected urine samples should be refrigerated at <4 °C. Inoculated transport media should be sent to the laboratory as soon as possible, and no more than 4 hours after their inoculation. It is possible for micro-organisms to multiply even in transport media after a few hours at room temperature, causing significant change in the results of the culture. Faeces for culture must be kept at room temperature.

It is important that when transporting specimens to the laboratory the correct labelling and packaging is used to protect others under the Duty of Care. Specimens which are, or are thought to be, infected with Hazard Category 3 pathogens (such as HIV, hepatitis B, salmonella, etc.) must be labelled 'inoculation risk' (ACDP, 1995).

Wound swabs

The detection and treatment of wound infection is based upon clinical signs. Wound swabs are not a reliable indicator of infection. The swab should be taken before the wound is cleaned, although excessive exudate and adhering debris should be gently removed. Care should be taken to sample any pus or exudate whilst not contaminating the specimen with commensal flora from the wound margins. As stated previously, a sample of pus is preferable. This can be aspirated by syringe and sent to the laboratory in a sterile universal container. Swabs should be taken using a close zig-zag movement of the swab across the surface of the wound.

Positive cultures do not indicate that treatment is needed. Only a positive result in conjunction with clinical signs of infection, such as localized pain, inflammation, swelling, pyrexia and purulent exudate should indicate that the patient should be treated. The old adage applies – treat the patient, not the swab. It is important to label the pathology form with the site from which the sample was taken to guide laboratory staff in deciding which organisms may be expected to be present.

Faeces samples

Faeces samples may be used to identify bacteria, viruses or toxin-producing organisms. Because faeces normally contain many millions of micro-organisms, the detection of pathogenic bacteria and viruses is complicated. Pathogens need to be distinguished from normal flora and this may take three to four days before a result is available. If a viral infection is suspected the faeces sample will need to be taken whilst the patient still has diarrhoea and as soon as possible after the onset of symptoms. It must then be examined using an electron microscope. The number of viral particles present in faeces is dramatically reduced after 24 hours. If *Clostridium difficile* infection is suspected, toxin tests in kit form can be used and results will be available within a few hours.

Faeces specimen pots should be one-third full, or 5–10 ml if liquid. Identification of threadworm can be achieved by pressing a length of sticky tape to the affected person's anus before washing.

The tape is then placed sticky side downwards onto a glass slide. An alternative method is to swab the perianal region and send the swab to the laboratory in normal saline.

Sputum samples

The mouth and upper respiratory tract are colonized by large numbers of commensal flora. It is therefore important to ensure that the specimen is mucoid or mucu-purulent. Specimens of saliva are of no value and will not be examined by the laboratory. The patient should not have eaten, drunk or cleaned their teeth recently. A physiotherapist may be needed to help the patient who has difficulty producing a sputum specimen. A diagnosis of respiratory tract infection does not rest solely on a positive sputum result, but is made by a combination of clinical symptoms, chest X-ray and microbiological examination.

Nasopharyngeal aspirate may be required for the identification of respiratory syncytial virus. Samples are obtained using a mucus extractor which is passed through the nostril into the nasopharynx. Gentle suction is applied to obtain epithelial cells. The extractor is sent to the laboratory with the tubing attached.

Tuberculosis

Tubercle bacillus are often present in low numbers in the sputum and therefore three separate samples taken on three consecutive days will increase the likelihood of detection. The organism *Mycobacterium tuberculosis* grows very slowly and extended culture times of up to eight weeks are needed before the final result can be given. Additional time is required to perform antibiotic sensitivity testing. In advanced cases where large numbers of bacilli are present in the sputum, a microscopic examination may be diagnostic. Special staining techniques are used which enable the mycobacterium to be detected under the microscope. The stain used cannot be removed by acid or alcohol, hence the term 'acid fast bacilli' or AFB.

Urine samples

Bacteria multiply readily in urine and therefore a strict aseptic technique should be used when collecting samples of urine for culture. If the patient has a urinary catheter, the sample must be collected from the sampling port in an aseptic manner. The port must be disinfected with an alcohol swab and the urine collected using a sterile needle and syringe. Catheter specimens of urine must not be collected from the drainage tap of the catheter bag. Contamination of urine in patients who do not have a catheter can be avoided by collecting a midstream specimen in a sterile receiver. A midstream specimen is collected after a small volume of urine has been voided. In women the genital area should be washed and dried prior to voiding; in men the foreskin should be retracted where possible.

The specimen must be examined as soon as possible, preferably within two hours of collection. Refrigeration allows storage for up to 24 hours before investigation. Urinary tract infection is strongly indicated by the presence of clinical symptoms (dysuria, pyrexia, frequency of micturition, and sometimes haematuria), more than 10^5 colony forming units and the presence of white cells.

Blood cultures

To identify the presence of bacteria in the bloodstream a strict aseptic technique is required when taking blood samples. This will avoid contamination of the sample with bacteria from the skin of the patient or the practitioner. Blood is inoculated into two bottles, one supporting the growth of aerobic organisms, the other supporting anaerobic organisms. 20 ml of blood is taken and 10 ml added to each bottle. Intravenous lines must not be used for this purpose.

The culture bottles are incubated for up to a week and checked for signs of growth. Increasingly automated blood culture machines are being used by laboratories. These automatically monitor the growth of micro-organisms biochemically at frequent intervals throughout the day. They enable results to be obtained quickly and facilitate efficient management of a potentially life-threatening infection.

Cerebrospinal fluid samples

Samples must be taken aseptically by lumbar puncture and preferably before antibiotics have been commenced. If the first sample is blood stained, it should be sent to the laboratory together with the third sample. Specimens are placed in a sterile container and examined immediately because fragile organisms such as *Neisseria meningitidis* may die in transit.

Other samples

The nose and throat can be swabbed using standard swabs that have been moistened in the transport media or sterile saline. Swabs of skin sites such as the perineum or axillae may also be taken in this way. A single swab can be used to sample both nostrils. The throat should be swabbed on the posterior pharynx, tonsillar area, sites of ulceration, exudate or membrane. For best results the site should be swabbed vigorously.

Specialists are required to obtain certain samples such as pernasal swabs, conjunctival swabs and swabs of the inner ear. A vaginal speculum should be used when taking vaginal swabs to prevent contamination and to help obtain a good quality sample.

Conclusion

A knowledge and understanding of microbiology and virology can greatly contribute to patient care in general and infection control in particular. Knowing what conditions micro-organisms require for survival can help to eliminate those conditions in the environment. Recognizing the early signs of infection will help us to decide the type of specimen that needs to be taken to identify the organism, and also the type of precautions we need to take to prevent transmission of infection to others. It can also help to inform our practice so that the precautions we take are relevant and not based on myth, ritual or fear.

The application of the information in this chapter is incorporated in many of the following sections.

Further reading

Advisory Committee on Dangerous Pathogens (ACDP). Protection Against Blood-borne Infections in the Workplace: HIV and hepatitis. London: HMSO, 1995.

Benenson AS (ed.) Control of Communicable Diseases Manual, 16th Edition. Washington: American Public Health Association, 1995.

Caddow P Applied Microbiology. Middlesex: Scutari Press, 1989.

Cooke EM Hare's Bacteriology and Immunity for Nurses. London: Churchill Livingstone, 1991.

Cooper R, Laurence JC The isolation and identification of bacteria from wounds. Journal of Wound Care 1996; 15 (7): 335–40.

Douglas Sleigh J, Timbury MC Notes on Medical Bacteriology, 4th Edition. London: Churchill Livingstone, 1994.

Duerden BL, Reid TMS, Jewsbury JM, Turk DC A New Short Textbook of Microbial and Parasite Infection. London: Hodder and Stoughton, 1987.

Elliot T, Hastings M, Dessleberger U Lecture Notes on Medical Microbiology, 3rd Edition. Oxford: Blackwell Science, 1997.

Horton R, Parker L Informed Infection Control Practice. London: Churchill Livingstone, 1997.

Lawrence JC, Ameen H Swabs and other sampling techniques. Journal of Wound Care 1998; 7 (5): 232–3.

MacLeod JA Collecting specimens for laboratory tests. Nursing Standard February 5 1992; 6 (20): 36–7.

Meers P, Sedgwick J, Worsley M The Microbiology and Epidemiology of Infection for Health Science Students. London: Chapman & Hall, 1995.

Morella JA, Minzer HE, Wilson ME, Grenata PA Microbiology in Patient Care, 6th Edition. Boston: WCB McGraw-Hill 1994.

Mayet FM An Introduction to Microbiology: A Resource Pack. Johnson and Johnson, 1997.

Shanson DC Microbiology in Clinical Practice, 2nd Edition. London: Wright, 1989.

Stillwell B Taking swabs. Community Outlook August 1991; 18–19.

Thomas CEA Medical Microbiology, 6th Edition. London: Balliere Tindall, 1988.

Chapter 3
The role of the infection control team

Kath Banfield

Introduction

Maintenance of high standards of infection control practice is the responsibility of *all* healthcare personnel. Under legislation, including the Health and Safety at Work Act and COSHH Regulations, (Health & Safety Executive, 1974, 1994), healthcare managers and employees alike are accountable for their part in ensuring a safe environment for staff, patients, and visitors. Under their Professional Code of Conduct (UKCC, 1992) all nurses are responsible for protecting both patients and colleagues from the dangers of cross-infection. Hence, infection control needs to be regarded as everyone's concern, rather than a specialist area of practice.

The 'speciality' of infection control has evolved over the past 40 years in response to ever-increasing challenges that threaten the safety of healthcare environments. In 1959 the first infection control nurse (ICN) was appointed in response to an outbreak of staphylococcal sepsis (Infection Control Nurse Association, 1996). Other posts gradually developed and the Department of Health and Social Security (1988) responded to increasing recognition of infection control problems by recommending that all acute hospitals should have access to an infection control service. More recently, as the emphasis of healthcare moves from secondary to primary care provision, and improved medical care has resulted in shorter hospital stays, infection control is being recognized as a problem that affects the wider community as well as hospitals. In response to this, an increasing number of community ICN posts are being developed (Hateley, 1996).

Despite the ever-extending knowledge and expertise required by infection control personnel and the developing scope of specialist practice, their prime concern remains the facilitation of high standards of infection control practice to prevent cross-infection. To achieve this, they use their specialist knowledge to influence the everyday practices of all healthcare workers. Only by 'getting the message across' to colleagues can the spread of infection be minimized. The remainder of this chapter outlines the roles and responsibilities of the infection control team (ICT) which are used to convey the need for good infection control practice.

Hospital infection control

The hospital infection control team

Updated guidelines issued by the Department of Health and NHS Executive (2000) (1995) reiterate the requirement for a co-ordinated infection control service within acute hospital settings. The overall responsibility for ensuring effective arrangements are in place lies with the Chief Executive. However, the day-to-day management of hospital infection control is the responsibility of the infection control team (ICT). This is made up of an infection control doctor, usually a consultant microbiologist, one or more infection control nurses, and occasionally a medical laboratory scientific officer from the microbiology department.

The Controls Assurance Standard (NHS Executive, 1999) stresses that to sustain the effective management and control of hospital infection, the ICT requires appropriate support, from secretarial, information technology and audit staff. It requires the commitment of senior managers through forums such as the Risk Management and Clinical Governance Committees. However, the extent to which this support and commitment is provided has been shown to be inconsistent (National Audit Offfice, 2000).

Functions of the ICT

The functions of the team are many and vary between establishments. However, certain core activities are included within the remit of all infection control teams. These can be broadly classified as:

Policy formulation and implementation

The production of written infection control policies which are evidence-based and regularly reviewed and updated. Consultation with relevant staff during policy formulation helps to ensure they are achievable and assists with implementation in practice.

Education

To facilitate the implementation of infection control policies all grades of staff need educational input. This may be in the format of presentations or teaching sessions to particular staff groups, but most often takes the form of giving timely advice regarding a particular situation or problem. Horton (1993) describes the Quality Infection Control (QIC) approach to education. This offers instruction on various aspects of infection prevention and control to all healthcare workers of all grades and disciplines to facilitate informed infection control practice. Underlying this important concept is the belief that if staff understand how infection is transmitted, and the role everyone plays in its prevention, then quality infection control practices at the bedside will be achieved.

Surveillance

The early identification and control of infection outbreaks has always been a priority for any ICT. More recently, many areas also use surveillance as a more proactive approach to the control of the spread of infection. Various surveillance methods can be used (Glenister et al., 1992; Public Health Laboratory Service, 1999) to identify patients at particular risk from infection and to identify the need for changes in practice as well as monitoring local infection trends.

Monitoring / audit

ICTs have an important role in the audit of infection control practices to monitor adherence to policies. A set of standards and audit criteria for various wards and departments are essential for this process (West Midlands Infection Control Nurse Association, 1998). To complete the audit cycle, any findings and recommendations need to be fed back to staff and discussed with them to identify ways of improving the quality of infection control practices (Shaw, 1990).

If the required changes have cost implications then they need to be discussed by the hospital infection control committee and with the appropriate budget holder(s). Audit reviews are necessary to monitor whether recommendations have been implemented or not.

Advice / liaison

An ICT can only be successful if it enables staff to carry out and correct practices. To achieve this, it needs to encourage all grades of staff to use their ICT as a resource for advice and information. This may cover many different aspects of healthcare ranging from the care of an individual patient, or the correct decontamination of a piece of equipment, to the development of new buildings or facilities. In order to offer sound advice the ICT must understand the problems encountered by staff and therefore close liaison is required. Many day-to-day decisions are based on an assessment of the degree of infection risk and this is only possible when the infection risk is seen as part of the total situation. Without good communication a thorough risk assessment will be unachievable.

The hospital infection control committee

Under the Department of Health Guidelines, (1995), every hospital should have an established infection control committee. This should meet at least twice a year and is usually chaired by the infection

Table 3.1 Membership of the hospital infection control committee

	Infection Control Team
Core membership	Chief Executive or representative
	Director of Nursing or representative
	Consultant in Communicable Disease Control
	Occupational Health Physician or Nurse
	Infectious Diseases Physician
	Senior clinical medical staff
Possible member	Pharmacist
	Domestic Manager
	Catering Manager
	Engineering Manager
	Sterile Supplies Manager
	Supplies Officer
	A representative from other hospitals covered

control doctor. Its membership is made up of a broad range of senior clinical and managerial staff (Table 3.1). The committee serves two main purposes. Firstly, it acts as a communication network. Feedback is given on current infection control issues and problems to increase the awareness of senior staff. Secondly, members of the committee are consulted regarding the content of infection control policies and activities to secure their endorsement and support.

Community infection control

The community infection control team

The need for infection control input in community care environments is now being recognized and addressed with the development of services in many areas.

Since the early 1990s Health Authorities have employed Consultants in Communicable Disease Control (CCDCs) who hold executive responsibility for control of infectious disease within a community. This is a complex role which relies on teamwork and liaison between agencies including health and local authority services. (Department of Health, 1995). As a member of the Health Authority, the CCDC advises the purchasers of healthcare on contractual requirements in relation to infection control. He/she works closely with the hospital infection control teams within the district, serving on their infection control committees and collaborating with them during outbreaks of infection. The CCDC also receives notifications of infectious diseases such as food poisoning, tuberculosis or meningitis and is responsible for co-ordinating any actions necessary to protect the wider community.

The most recent addition to infection control is the community ICN. This role is being developed in many areas to respond to the demands made on the CCDC's time and the need to develop a more proactive approach to infection control in the community. Some community ICNs work alongside hospital ICNs, which has the advantages of providing mutual support and improving lines of communication. The community ICN works closely with the CCDC, covering aspects such as contact tracing in cases of meningitis or tuberculosis and providing advice to control outbreaks of infection in the wider community. In this role, he/she is also able to take a more proactive approach to the prevention of infection in establishments such as nursing homes, residential care homes, nurseries and dental and GP surgeries.

Both the CCDC and community ICN need to work closely with environmental health officers. Amongst their functions are enforcement of the Food Safety Act 1990 and investigation of outbreaks of food- or waterborne illness which obviously relate closely to the overall provision of infection control services in the community. The community infection control team has an increasingly important role in wider public health issues, including the management of environmental hazards in the locality.

The district infection control committee

It is recommended that each district should have an infection control committee that brings together representatives from hospital infection control teams within the district as well as other representatives from the wider community (Department of Health, 1995). Within this forum decisions are made regarding district-wide policies and infection control issues relevant to community establishments such as schools, nurseries and nursing homes are discussed.

Infection control nursing

An outline job description for an ICN post (ICNA, 1996), recommends that the post holder should be a 1st level Registered General Nurse with clinical experience at a senior level. The ICN should hold or be willing to undertake specialist study such as the Certificate in Professional Studies (Infection Control – ENB 329) or Diploma in Infection Control. Also advantageous is a teaching qualification such as the ENB 998 (Teaching and Assessing in Clinical Practice) or the City and Guilds 730. As in other areas of nursing, many ICNs are now studying to degree level, including Masters and PhD courses in order to practise as specialist nurses.

As one facet of the ICN's role is the promotion of evidence-based care, leadership skills and the skills necessary to manage change are essential. Under the requirements of the UKCC (1995, 1996), the professional development of an ICN can be enhanced through relevant courses and reflective practice. Continuous education, which is essential to all nurses, can also be achieved through reading professional journals, attending selected study days and Infection Control Nurse Association events such as the annual conference or area group meetings. No matter how experienced an

ICN is or how broad his/her knowledge base, as a leader of clinical practice, continual update is vital.

The personality of an ICN is an attribute that greatly influences the success of the role. As Sedgwick (1988) comments, the ICN must have the ability to deal with all grades of staff. Communication skills are essential. These include the ability to listen to the problems which staff face in their daily practice, which often compromise the standard of their infection control practices. Staff need to be confident that they can approach the ICN for advice and information without fear of reproach. In order to facilitate safe practice the ICN needs to ensure staff understand the value of their infection control practices. The ICN's response to an enquiry is not always popular, as it may involve additional or more time-consuming duties, emphasizing the need for a broad pair of shoulders!

Infection control nursing is a role full of variety and challenges and ICNs must be able to think on their feet and be prepared for all eventualities (Alderman, 1992).

Out of hours, the ICN may need to take calls to give advice, particularly if an outbreak of infection is reported – the spread of micro-organisms does not limit itself to office hours! A typical working day can involve visits to wards and departments, formal teaching sessions and meetings with colleagues or a company representative keen to demonstrate his/her latest product. In between scheduled commitments, 'on the spot' advice is often sought, and the response to any unplanned events has to be made a priority. Other background work such as consulting the literature to draft new policies or procedures, maintaining up-to-date documentation and planning new developments, teachings or research projects in infection control has to be maintained. To achieve such a variety of tasks the ability to prioritize and manage one's time is essential.

A great challenge to all ICNs is the need to instil the need for good infection control practices into others. As Bailey comments (1989), the role is advisory rather than managerial. An ICN can encourage staff to adhere to infection control practices through education and continual monitoring, and obviously every employee has a responsibility to conform to local policy. However, if, for example, an employee does not wear eye protection despite local policy, education and equipment availability, then it is that individual who holds overall accountability for his/her practice. In such circumstances it takes ingenuity on the part of the ICN to rise to the challenge and keep trying to alter practice in the face of adversity! The author's personal experience has shown the 'dripping tap' effect to be successful – when the first attempts fail, cautious persistence can eventually succeed.

One means of achieving optimum infection control influence at ward level is the development of infection control link nurses (Horton, 1988; Teare and Peacock, 1996). These nurses receive additional infection control education and act under the supervision of an ICN as a resource and role model for colleagues. This is obviously a role which requires great motivation on the part of the link nurse to attend regular meetings and to take every opportunity to update and extend his/her level of infection control knowledge. However, as emphasized by the Department of Health (1995), link nurses are not a substitute for an adequately resourced ICN service.

In summary, the above account demonstrates the qualities and experience an ICN needs to develop in order to influence the infection control practices of others. The characteristics and skills required to be a successful ICN are many and varied. It has been observed that there appears to be no limit to the knowledge required nor to the extent that the role can be extended. (Bailey, 1989). As healthcare as a whole and the roles of healthcare workers develop further, so too must the role of the ICN to ensure that practices continue to minimize the spread of infection.

References

Alderman C Never a dull moment. Nursing Standard 1992; 6 (20): 18–19.

Bailey S (1989) A day in the life of an infection control nurse. Nursing Standard 1989; 43 (3): 32–4.

Department of Health and Social Security. Hospital Infection Control – Guidance on the Control of Infection in Hospitals prepared by the joint DHSS/PHLS hospital infection working group. London: Department of Health and Social Security, 1988.

Department of Health. Hospital Infection Control – Guidance on the Control of Infection in Hospitals. London: Department of Health, 1995.

Glenister HM, Taylor LJ, Cooke EM, Bartlett CLR A Study of Surveillance Methods for Detecting Hospital Infection. London: Public Health Laboratory Service, 1992.

Hateley P Revealing answers. Nursing Times 1996; 92 (45): 65–7.

Health and Safety Executive. Health and Safety at Work Act 1974. London: HMSO, 1974.

Health and Safety Executive. The Control of Substances Hazardous to Health Regulations 1994 (COSHH) SI:3246. London: HMSO, 1994.

Horton R Linking the chain. Nursing Times 1988; 84 (26): 44–6.

Horton R Introducing high quality infection control in a hospital setting. British Journal of Nursing 1993; 2(15): 746–54.

Infection Control Nurse Association. Membership Pack. ICNA, 1996.

National Audit Office. The Management and Control of Hospital Acquired Infection in Acute NHS Trusts in England. London: The Stationery Office, 2000.

NHS Executive. Controls Assurance Standard.

NHS Executive. The Management and Control of Hospital Infection: Action for the NHS for the Management and Control of Infection in Hospitals in England HSC 2000/02.

Public Health Laboratory Service. Surgical Site Infection: Analysis of a Year's Surveillance in English Hospitals 1997–1998. London: PHLS, 1999.

Sedgwick J In control. Nursing Standard 1988; 46 Nov 5.

Shaw CD Criterion based audit. British Medical Journal 1990; 300: 649–51.

Teare EL, Peacock A The development of an infection control link-nurse programme in a district general hospital. Journal of Hospital Infection 1996; 34: 267–78.

United Kingdom Central Council for Nursing, Midwifery and Health Visitors. Code of Professional Conduct. London: UKCC, 1992.

United Kingdom Central Council for Nursing, Midwifery and Health Visitors. The Future of Professional Practice – The Council's Standards for Education and Practice Following Registration (PREP). London: UKCC, 1994.

West Midlands Infection Control Nurse Association. Infection Control Audit Pack. ICNA, 1995.

Chapter 4
Managing outbreaks of infection

LESLY FINN

> An outbreak of infection may be defined either as the occurrence of two or
> more related cases of the same infection or as the situation when the
> observed number of cases exceeds the number expected (Department of
> Health, 1994).

Outbreaks frequently occur in both hospitals and the community
and most are relatively small. What constitutes a major outbreak
involves consideration not only of the number of people involved but
also the pathogenicity of the infecting organism and the potential for
spread within hospital and community populations. For example, a
single case of diphtheria admitted from a Cub Scout camp may
require all the procedures associated with a major outbreak. The
policy document HSG(95)10, prepared in 1995 by the Hospital
Infection Working Group of the Department of Health and Public
Health Laboratory Service, includes guidance on arrangements for
the control of major outbreaks in hospitals and the community
(Department of Health/PHLS, 1995).

In England and Wales, a Consultant in Communicable Disease
Control (CCDC) is appointed by each Health Authority to its
department of public health medicine to be responsible for the
surveillance, prevention and control of all communicable disease
and infection in the district. In the majority of areas the CCDC is
also formally appointed by the Local Authority to act as the 'proper
officer' under the Public Health (Control of Diseases) Act 1984. In
Scotland and Northern Ireland this role is taken by the Chief
Administrative Medical Officer of the appropriate Health Board.

Medical staff have a statutory duty to notify certain infectious
diseases and food poisoning to the proper officer. This should be

done as quickly as possible for any infections that may have serious implications for public health, whether or not they are statutorily notifiable. These infections are often referred to as 'alert' organisms and conditions (see Table 4.1). Close collaboration between the CCDC and Infection Control Teams (ICTs) is essential if efforts to prevent spread of communicable disease in both hospitals and the community are to be successful. All those who work within the NHS have responsibilities with regard to public health and communicable disease control.

In most incidents or outbreaks of infection in hospital it is the hospital infection control doctor who takes the lead in their investigation and control. In some major outbreaks it may be more appropriate for the CCDC to take the lead. In particular, the CCDC should lead in those outbreaks with significant implications for the community; those involving many cases of a notifiable disease or food poisoning; and those involving even small numbers of cases of an infection which pose a very serious risk to public health. In the event of such an outbreak the CCDC has the responsibility to communicate and consult with the PHLS Communicable Diseases Surveillance Centre and also has a statutory duty to inform the Chief Medical Officer of the Department of Health.

Investigation of outbreaks of foodborne illness involves both Health Authorities (HAs) and Local Authorities (LAs), who hold joint responsibility. Within Local Authorities, environmental health officers (EHOs) include within their remit food safety and the prevention and investigation of foodborne illness, while necessary expertise is provided by the CCDC on behalf of the Health Authority (Department of Health, 1994). Environmental health officers also play a key role in the investigation of outbreaks, particularly those involving environmental sources of infection such as water- or airborne infections.

Surveillance of infection

Effective surveillance involves the collection, collation, analysis and dissemination of information and is essential for early identification of both outbreaks and trends in the incidence of infectious diseases. Surveillance activities are conducted at local and national levels through a variety of systems.

Table 4.1. Conditions and organisms which may give rise to hospital and/or community outbreaks

Notifiable conditions	Suggested 'alert' organisms and conditions
Acute encephalitis	Suspected infective diarrhoea/vomiting
Acute meningitis	Pyrexia of unknown origin
Acute poliomyelitis	Severe soft tissue infections
Anthrax	Legionella sp.
Cholera	Varicella-zoster
Diphtheria	Scabies
Dysentery (amoebic or bacillary)	Methicillin-resistant *Staphylococcus aureus*
Foodborne illness	Group A Streptococcal infections
Viral hepatitis	Group B Streptococcal infections (mother/infant)
Leprosy	*Pseudomonas aeruginosa*
Leptospirosis	*Stenotrophonomas (Xanth.) maltophilia*
Malaria	*Salmonella* spp.
Meningococcal septicaemia	Penicillin-resistant *Strep. pneumoniae*
Mumps	Vero-toxin producing strains of *E. coli*
Measles	Resistant Gram-negative organisms
Ophthalmia neonatorum	Other bacterial isolates with unusual antimicrobial resistance
Paratyphoid fever	Beta-lactamase producing enterococci
Plague	Rotavirus
Relapsing fever	Respiratory syncytial virus (RSV)
Scarlet fever	Influenza
Smallpox	Parvovirus B19
Tetanus	Candida species (in special units)
Tuberculosis	Aspergillus (in special units)
Typhoid fever	Cryptosporidiosis
Typhus	*Campylobacter* enteritis
Rabies	*Clostridium difficile*
Rubella	'Norwalk' virus
Viral haemorrhagic fevers	Whooping cough
Yellow fever	

The statutory notification system is the oldest established source of surveillance information. Formal notifications of foodborne and 'alert' organisms and conditions are sent on standard forms, books of which are provided to all hospitals and general practitioners by the Local Authority or Health Authority. In Scotland, notifications are forwarded to the Communicable Diseases (Scotland) Unit. Anonymized returns of data derived from these forms are sent weekly by CCDCs to the Communicable Disease Surveillance Centre and by Local Authorities to the Office of Population,

Censuses and Surveys (OPCS). Regional epidemiologists and the Communicable Disease Surveillance Centre carry out surveillance on a wider basis, using local and regional data.

The other major source of epidemiological data is the report of positive laboratory isolates which laboratories make to the Communicable Diseases Surveillance Centre. Further data on certain communicable diseases are sent by selected spotter GP practices to the Research Unit of the Royal College of General Practitioners. The CDSC collates and analyses returns and publishes regular reports in the *Communicable Disease Report*, on a weekly and monthly basis. These reports include details of the incidence of infections and particular outbreaks, as well as scientific papers, and are a valuable source of information for all those interested in infectious diseases and their control.

Outbreak recognition

A case of foodborne illness or communicable disease in the community or a health service establishment may come to the attention of any of the following agencies:

* General practitioners
* Hospital clinicians
* Environmental health officers
* Staff of the Public Health Laboratory
* CCDC or other members of the Public Health Department
* Staff of daycare or residential/nursing establishments.

These agencies should notify all such cases to the CCDC as soon as possible.

In addition, all staff need to be alert to, and report promptly, all suspected clusters of cases so that appropriate investigation and control measures can be implemented to prevent further spread. Knowledge of the usual 'background' level of infection, e.g. in a particular ward, hospital or general practice population, is an important factor in early recognition of the possibility of an outbreak. Although an outbreak situation may not be immediately apparent it should be suspected if cases appear to be linked by **time**, **place** or **person**. Documented examples are given below, but often more than one of these links may be apparent.

Time

The occurrence of cases exhibiting similar symptoms within a short space of time may denote an outbreak. Examples include two or more cases of influenza in a ward or nursing home within a 48 hour period, a sudden increase in notified cases of a particular disease, e.g. measles, shigellosis, or a cluster of postoperative wound infections caused by the same organism within one hospital or ward.

Case example 1 – viral gastroenteritis

A midwifery sister became ill within hours of the admission of a client with vomiting and diarrhoea to a maternity unit. Further cases occurred in the following 24 hours. In total, about 73 staff, 18 mothers and two babies were affected during a 17 day period.

Investigations by the ICT identified that milk and hot drinks dispensers and water coolers were not contracted for routine cleaning and staff involved with serving food had not had training in food hygiene. These may have been factors in person-to-person transmission of the illness following the initial cases (O-Dell, 1995).

Case example 2 – Hepatitis A

Environmental health officers were alerted to the possibility of an outbreak of hepatitis A infection when the number of notified cases doubled from 2 to 4 cases per month in December 1994, followed by a peak of 13 cases in January 1995. A total of 24 cases within a densely populated council estate was confirmed before the outbreak was declared over in June 1996. Investigations identified that there was a network of contact between groups, e.g. via childminding and babysitting. Control of spread would have been helped if some of the GPs had notified suspected cases more promptly, particularly where these were identified from another source (Potts and Barker, 1996).

Place

A cluster of cases of the same infection may be linked by place; for example, foodborne illness in delegates at a conference or cryptosporidiosis in a boarding school with a private water supply.

Case example 3 – Escherichia coli 0157

Twelve confirmed and 2 probable cases of *E. coli* 0157 were identified in Sunderland residents. Isolates from ten of the cases were confirmed as *E. coli* 0157 phage type 2, Vero cytotoxin 2. Nine isolates were indistinguishable on Vero cytotoxin subtyping and chromosomal DNA analysis. Epidemiological investigations found that all 14 cases were statistically associated with the consumption of several different types of pre-cooked meat from one of a chain of three shops.

Environmental health officers identified several areas of poor practice in the cooking, cooling and storage of meats which had been prepared in another of the three shops. The organism was not isolated from either food or environmental samples and it was concluded that the affected batches of meat may have been sold and eaten by the time investigations began (Stevenson and Hanson, 1996).

Case example 4 – MRSA

Over a two-month period a multi-resistant MRSA of a similar antibiogram was isolated from more than 20 patient specimens from a district general hospital, community hospitals, GP practices and a urology outpatient clinic. The majority of specimens were from surgical wounds, drain sites, supra-pubic catheter sites, midstream and catheter specimens of urine and penile swabs. Investigations identified that those affected had either recently been inpatients on the urology ward, or had attended the ward as outpatients for urological investigation or intervention.

The urodynamics and treatment rooms were found to be very dusty. Environmental screening isolated MRSA from the ultrasound machine and storage shelves housing sterile water supplies. The environmental isolates and the majority of patient isolates reacted strongly with phage type 85. Following thorough cleaning of all equipment and surfaces no further cases of colonization or infection were found on repeated screening of inpatient skin sites. Cross-infection had probably occurred through indirect transfer from contaminated equipment to the patients via staff hands (Finn, 1995).

Person

Cases may be linked by personal characteristics, e.g. age, race, sex, membership of a club, undergoing a specific treatment. For example, the first intimation of the AIDS epidemic was the appearance of opportunistic infections and rare cancers in young homosexual males in California. In a massive 'call-back' exercise in Ireland, involving 60,000 women given intravenous anti-D following child-birth, over 1,000 were found to have evidence of infection with the hepatitis C virus (Kenny, 1996).

Case example 5 – Acute hepatitis B

In 1992 and 1993, two clusters of acute hepatitis B in cardiothoracic surgery patients from two UK hospitals were investigated. The source, was identified as a carrier of hepatitis B virus who was hepatitis B e antigen (HBeAg) positive. He had not been identified during investigations of the first cluster of 4 patients when he and other members of staff, who had performed or assisted in exposure-prone procedures on these cases, were investigated and found to be HBV or HBsAg negative. Investigation of the second cluster of 2 cases revealed that the blood sample provided by the surgeon on the first occasion had been obtained from someone he believed to be unlikely to be HBsAg positive.

Further investigation of patients on whom the surgeon had performed exposure-prone procedures in the 15 months before his infectivity was recognized was undertaken. 310/323 (95%) patients were available for testing and 20 were classified as patients having acquired hepatitis B virus in association with cardiothoracic surgery involving this surgeon (Communicable Disease Report, 1996).

Case example 6 – Multi-drug resistant tuberculosis

The first outbreak of hospital-acquired multi-drug resistant tuberculosis in the UK occurred in the summer of 1995. The index case, a Portuguese male, had been admitted to an HIV unit in April 1995 and died in June that year. Seven secondary cases were subsequently confirmed – five of these had occupied beds in the same six-bedded bay with the index case, while the other two patients had only had casual contact with him. The organism was found to be resistant to isoniazid, rifampicin, pyrazinamide, rifabutin, clofazimine and ethion-amide. No other contacts developed the disease in the London cohort but a total of 50 cases of multi-drug resistant tuberculosis were isolated over the same period from a Lisbon cohort (Hannan et al., 1996).

Several outbreaks of multi-drug resistant tuberculosis have occurred in the USA amongst HIV antibody positive people and many factors have been reported to have contributed to spread. These factors include: delayed diagnosis; delayed isolation of cases; delayed recognition of drug resistance; poor response to treatment (patients remain infectious for long periods); and procedures likely to cause aerosols of sputum, particularly if performed in an inadequately ventilated environment (Communicable Disease Report, 1995).

Outbreak control

As soon as there is a suspicion that a major outbreak is occurring a Major Outbreak Control Group should be convened by the Consultant for Communicable Disease Control or hospital infection control doctor. They are responsible for deciding on the structure of the group and for convening the initial meeting by contacting members of the team. The Major Outbreak Control Group will normally be chaired by the CCDC or HICD. Core membership for both community-based and hospital-based outbreaks, together with a list of other individuals who may be required to attend, are set out in Table 4.2. In minor outbreaks it may be advisable to convene a Minor Outbreak Control Group comprising some or all of the core membership as outlined in the table.

Table 4.2 Membership of outbreak control teams

Core membership – Community-based outbreaks	Core membership – Hospital-based outbreaks	Others who may be required to attend
CCDC or named deputy	ICD or named deputy	Consultant microbiologist
Director Public Health Lab	CCDC or named deputy	EHOs from other LAs
Community ICN	ICNs	General Practitioner
Chief EHO or named deputy	Clinical consultant of	Consultant Community
from local authority	appropriate speciality	Paediatrician
Named management	Chief Executive or named	Director of Nursing
representative of any	deputy of relevant Trust	Services or deputy
establishment involved		Occupational Health
		Ambulance Service
		Head of Communications
		Water Company
		Health and Safety
		Executive

The terms of reference for an Outbreak Control Group are to:

1) Review evidence and decide whether there really is an outbreak.
2) Take all necessary steps for the clinical care of those affected.
3) Coordinate all arrangements for necessary interviews and other investigations, with the use of laboratory and epidemiological expertise, to identify the nature and source of the outbreak.
4) Agree and coordinate policy decisions on the investigation and control of the outbreak, and to allocate responsibility to specific individuals who will then be accountable for taking action.
5) Prevent further cases by taking all necessary steps to ensure that the source of the outbreak is controlled or the cause is dealt with.
6) Prevent secondary spread of the infection by controlling or isolating cases, by monitoring contacts of cases, identifying and monitoring other persons 'at risk'.
7) Provide an accurate and responsible source of information for other professionals, agencies, the media and the public.
8) Assess the need for additional supplies, staff, clerical and information technology support and clarify how these will be provided.
9) Ensure communication with the Department of Health, NHS Management Executive Regional Office, PHLS, Communicable Disease Surveillance Centre and the CCDCs of other Health Authorities as appropriate.
10) Agree arrangements for notifying and informing patients' relatives, visitors and other persons or agencies who may be directly involved.
11) Define the end of the outbreak and evaluate the lessons learned.
12) Prepare a preliminary report, ideally within the first 48 hours, interim reports if necessary and a final report.
13) Disseminate information related to the lessons learned from the outbreak.
14) Develop systems and procedures to minimize the risk of future similar episodes.

Investigating the outbreak

The role of the laboratory

Outbreaks may be recognized clinically, through signs and symptoms, or microbiologically through examination of clinical, environmental or food samples. In the latter case the role of the laboratory in the early detection and identification of the responsible organism is crucial. Additional advice regarding both microbiological sampling and specific diseases can be obtained from specialist Reference Laboratories and other centres.

Laboratory samples should be collected immediately and before control measures are introduced. Nothing should be done which interferes with the investigation of the outbreak, unless it is essential for its control or for patient care.

Liaison with the laboratory at the outset is vital so that:

a) the laboratory can make arrangements to accommodate the increased workload and to provide the facilities required to assist in the investigation and control of the outbreak, and

b) their advice can be sought regarding the appropriate specimens which need to be obtained and the correct methods of obtaining and transporting them.

The typing of isolates often plays a key role in determining whether or not a cluster of cases is in fact an outbreak, e.g. whether several cases of meningococcal disease are of the same strain or whether an isolate of *Salmonella* spp. from a suspect food is similar to that isolated from affected cases. Traditional methods comprise antigenic, bacteriophage and bacteriocine typing. Modern typing methods continue to be developed at genetic and molecular level and include protein profiling, ribotyping, restriction endonuclease analysis and DNA probes (Pitt, 1992).

Epidemiological investigations

There are two main types of epidemiological investigation: a) descriptive epidemiology and b) analytical epidemiology.

Descriptive epidemiology

The objective of a descriptive study is to provide a detailed description of the outbreak, its onset, size and progress demonstrated in an epidemic curve (Figure 4.1). Cases are identified and analysed by time, place and person. A more detailed hypothesis as to the source and method of spread may be developed and the need for further microbiological sampling or further epidemiological studies may become apparent.

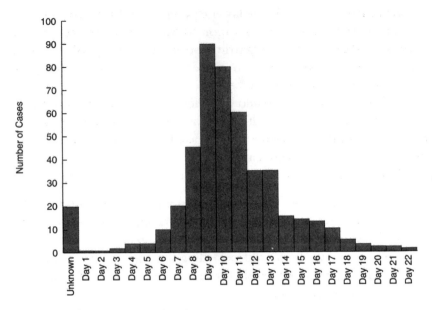

Figure 4.1 Example of an epidemic curve

Analytical epidemiology

The two designs of study used in analytical epidemiology are case control and cohort studies. The choice of design will depend on the nature of the outbreak. The decision regarding whether such a study is required will generally be made by the CCDC who has the necessary expertise and training to ensure appropriate data collection and interpretation of results (Department of Health, 1994).

The first step in any investigation will be to assess all the available information and decide whether or not the reports indicate that those affected are all suffering from the same illness and whether there is any evidence of an association between them.

A case definition should be agreed by all members of the Outbreak Control Group and the population at risk will be defined. A register of those affected, their contacts and others at risk will be drawn up and kept up-to-date.

A data collection form should be designed to ensure all necessary and relevant information is gathered in a uniform way. The data needs to be sufficient to classify all respondents as cases or not using the agreed case definition and should include the following as appropriate:

Clinical data

- Date and time of onset of symptoms
- The nature of the symptoms experienced, their severity and duration
- Hospital admission
- Antibiotic or other treatment
- Outcome of the illness.

Demographic data

- Name and address (permanent and temporary if applicable)
- Date of birth and sex
- Person giving the information, e.g. case, contact
- Occupation, work or school address
- Recreational activities, recent foreign travel
- Sources of domestic food, milk and water supplies
- History of food and drink consumed, including times and places
- Contact with domestic, farm or wild animals
- Household or other close contacts, plus whether or not these have recently been ill with similar symptoms
- Types of samples provided
- Vaccination history.

In addition to confirmed and suspected cases, others at risk may need to be interviewed depending on the infection involved.

Control measures

The control measures necessary may take a variety of forms and are dependent upon the nature and source of the infection and its mode of spread. They may include antibiotic treatment or prophylaxis, water treatments, immunization, case isolation, restriction of admissions, discharges or transfers. Education for staff or others closely involved in infection prevention is also an important element of control. Monitoring should continue once control measures are instituted in order to both assess their effectiveness and identify any further cases.

At the end of the outbreak

At the end of the outbreak the chairman of the Outbreak Control Group will prepare a final report; a copy of this will be sent to the

Communicable Diseases Surveillance Centre. A final meeting of the group will also be held to:

- review the experiences of all participants involved in the management of the outbreak
- identify shortfalls and particular difficulties encountered
- revise the Major Outbreak Plan in accordance with the above
- make recommendations, if necessary, regarding structural or procedural improvements which would reduce the chance of recurrence of the outbreak.

Dissemination of information regarding the outcome and the lessons learned should always be cascaded so that the incident becomes a positive learning experience for those involved in the implementation of the control measures.

References

Communicable Disease Report. Outbreak of hospital acquired multidrug resistant tuberculosis.CDR 1995; 5 (34): 161.

Communicable Disease Report. Lessons from two linked clusters of acute hepatitis B in cardiothoracic surgery patients. CDR 1996; 6 (9): 119–25.

Department of Health. Management of Outbreaks of Foodborne Illness. London: DoH, 1994.

Finn LF An outbreak of Methicillin Resistant Staphylococcus aureus on a Urology ward – the role of the environment. Free Paper. Infection Control Nurses Association National Conference (York). ICNA, 1995.

Hannan M, Oladele V, Fry C, Mridha L, Umasankar S, Azadian B Control of the Transmission of Tuberculosis in Hospital HIV Units, Experience from a London Teaching Hospital. Free Paper. The Fourth International Conference and Exhibition on Infection Control (Dublin). ICNA, 1996.

Hospital Infection Working Group of the Department of Health and Public Health Laboratory Service. Hospital Infection Control – Guidance on the Control of Infection in Hospitals. HSG(95)10. London: DoH/PHLS, 1995.

Kenny E Hepatitis C. Paper. The Fourth International Conference and Exhibition on Infection Control (Dublin). ICNA, 1996.

O-Dell K Personal contacts. Journal of Infection Control Nursing (NT suppl.) 1995; 91 (46): 4–6.

Pitt TL Recent developments in typing methods. PHLS Microbiology Digest 1992; 9 (4): 160–5.

Potts H, Barker A An outbreak of hepatitis A in St Helens. Environmental Health July 1996; 195–6.

Stevenson J, Hanson S Outbreak of Escherichia coli 0157 phage type 2 infection associated with eating pre-cooked meats. Communicable Disease Report 1996; 6 (8): 116–18.

Chapter 5
Design of new and refurbished buildings

JULIE BUSHELL

Introduction

The impact of the design of healthcare facilities on the quality of care provided within them should not be underestimated. Improvements in public health have frequently resulted not from medical intervention, but from improvements in sanitation, drainage and water quality; reduction in overcrowding and pollution; and the provision of shelter of an acceptable quality in short, from the consideration and application of improved environmental design (Bond et al., 1973).

Although many nineteenth century public health recommendations were devised to improve residential dwellings, the principles are equally applicable to institutions and particularly to healthcare facilities.

Hospital reformers such as Howard, Tenon and Florence Nightingale recognized the deplorable environmental conditions in these institutions during the 1800s and highlighted the need for effective ventilation, warmth, light and cleanliness, and for the reduction of overcrowding in wards (Bond et al., 1973).

Indeed, Florence Nightingale (1859) identified faults in the construction of wards which she blamed for the unhealthy conditions observed. These included defective ventilation; defective drains, sinks and sanitary facilities; poor kitchen and sanitary design; absorbent materials used for walls, which prevented cleaning; and defective ward furniture (in Maurer, 1985).

Nightingale's attempts to design the 'ideal' hospital were not entirely successful, particularly in controlling the transmission of communicable disease; however, attention to the continuing problem of hospital-acquired infection still requires greater consideration of sanitary and safety problems in hospital. Many of Nightingale's observations are still pertinent to the design of healthcare facilities today.

The general public expect high quality care to be provided in a high quality, hazard-free environment – this will only be achieved if strict environmental standards are applied to all healthcare facilities (Bond et al., 1973).

Control of infection must remain a primary consideration in the design of any health building. Involvement in the design and planning of healthcare building offers the infection control team the opportunity to positively influence the building to the potential benefit of its future occupants. It is now recommended that infection control teams are consulted with regard to all service developments (NHS Executive, 1999).

Risk assessment

Risk management and quality assurance are two complementary considerations. Risk management aims to minimize the probability of risks occurring, and to reduce its cost. This in turn results in safer practices, and premises and increases staff awareness of dangers and liabilities (Department of Health NHS Estates, 1994c). Potential hazards in the workplace must be identified before risks can be calculated.

The role of the infection control nurse (ICN) involves assessing and reacting to risk, and in particular assessing the risks involved in activities, environments or practices, which may prove hazardous to staff, patients or both. ICNs are therefore in an ideal position to identify and advise on potential infection risks which may arise; and on the main infection control issues to be considered when planning a new building, or refurbishment; in order to reduce sources and methods of spread of infection.

Department of Health NHS Estates (1994c) indicates that the identification of potential major hazards is a basic requirement that should be undertaken at the concept stage of any project. Fundamental decisions should be made after considering all aspects of the design that may require special attention to contain or eliminate hazards.

In operating theatre design, for example, special considerations include not only the type of ventilation, but also layout, disposal facilities and access. These will fundamentally affect the design of the facility.

The success or failure of the initial hazard assessment will depend upon:

- The accuracy of drawings/data used
- The technical expertise and experience of those making the assessment
- The ability of this team to visualize potential problems and identify causes and effects
- The ability of the team to determine the probability and seriousness of a particular hazard occurring (Department of Health NHS Estates, 1994c).

It is therefore essential that the ICT is involved at this stage and throughout all subsequent stages of any project to offer their broad-based technical expertise and risk management experience.

> Decisions on measures required in a particular situation ... (e.g. design of buildings) ... must be made in terms of possible benefits to patients, the hospital community and the cost of the measures. Cost–benefit is not a term to be used lightly, but a necessity. (Ayliffe et al., 1993)

This is particularly relevant to the upgrading of existing buildings which may have been modified over several years. A weak link can sometimes occur when modifications are introduced, or the building's application is changed.

The introduction of ultraclean ventilation, for example, may be both desirable and cost-effective when commissioning a new theatre complex, but it may be excessively expensive and impractical to introduce when refurbishing existing theatres suites because of the loss of headroom and technical requirements involved.

Likewise changes introduced to meet one need may result in an unrecognized hazard. Partitions introduced into 'Nightingale' wards to improve patient privacy, for example, have very little effect in reducing the transmission of communicable diseases. However, if these changes are not accompanied by increased provision of handwashing facilities, the partitions may result in reduced access to sinks, a significant factor in compliance with handwashing in practice (Caddow, 1989) which could result in an increased risk of hospital-acquired infection.

Once all the necessary information has been gathered, risks should be prioritized to allow for appropriate allocation of resources. It may be necessary for compromises to be reached on design criteria; however these are only acceptable if the requirements of legislation, such as the Health and Safety at Work Act (1974), and Control of Substances Hazardous to Health Regulations (1988) are fully met. The decision-making process must be fully documented in order that actions may be supported and justified at a later date.

Sources of information

Accurate assessment of the appropriateness of design drawings and data to the intended requirements of healthcare facilities entails not only considerable technical expertise but also experience of practical operational considerations which may result in infection control hazards in-use. In this chapter the broad issues will be discussed. There are, however, several sources of technical information to provide further specific guidance for personnel involved in the design of new buildings or in major refurbishment programmes.

These include:

- Health Building Notes (HBN)
- Health Technical Memoranda (HTM)
- Health Guidance Notes (HGN)
- Health Facility Notes (HFN).

The above publications are produced by the Department of Health, NHS Estates, to ensure the inclusion of fundamental design principles in all NHS health buildings. These provide useful information and guidance relevant to the control of infection.

Planning a new or refurbished facility: general considerations

Issues of particular relevance in reducing the sources and methods of spread of infection in healthcare environments include:

- Availability of handwashing and sanitary facilities
- Effective waste disposal
- Laundry facilities
- Food hygiene
- Isolation facilities
- Water supply.

These issues will be broadly discussed in terms of design considerations; however, references should be made to other chapters relating to catering, waste disposal and laundry provision for detail.

Handwashing and sanitary facilities

Handwashing is the single most important factor in the prevention of hospital-acquired infection (Ayliffe et al., 1993). Research indicates that compliance with handwashing by hospital personnel is often poor, and that a contributory factor is the absence of conveniently placed sinks. If nursing and medical staff have to walk to the other end of a ward or to another room to wash their hands, they are unlikely to do so (Garner and Favero, 1986). As hands are the most important vehicle of cross-infection, it is essential that effective methods are used to minimize this hazard (Ayliffe et al., 1999).

Essential requirements for effective clinical handwashing

Handwashing facilities must be readily available in all clinical areas incorporating the following requirements:

* A minimum of one sink per room (single rooms, small ward areas)
* One sink per every six beds if large multi-occupied rooms
* Hospital pattern basin – no overflow
* Handwashing under running water – no plug
* Lever action (elbow operated) taps, to avoid contamination
* Single spout (mixer tap) to achieve correct temperature
* Water temperature thermostatically or manually controlled
* Connection to concealed services.

(Department of Health NHS Estates, 1990; 1995b).

Rationale

Equipment provided should be suitable for the purpose. In ward areas where invasive/clinical procedures are undertaken, a sink with elbow-operated mixer taps, no plug and no overflow is necessary (Department of Health NHS Estates, 1995d).

Hand-operated taps must not be turned on by dirty hands because when the taps are turned off clean hands immediately become re-contaminated. Hand contact with taps should be avoided in clinical areas (Ayliffe et al., 1990). Maurer (1985) suggests that foot-operated systems provide a foolproof option, since staff frequently misuse the elbow-operated taps, defeating their purpose. Electronically operated systems are also available and may be an acceptable option particularly in new or specialist buildings, such as theatres. These options are at present more expensive than existing facilities and it is essential that all considerations including effective maintenance and replacement programmes are included and properly costed when attempting to introduce new designs.

Gram-negative bacteria colonize 'U-bends', taps and sink outlets. Taps discharging into a shallow sink or directly into the drain-hole can cause splashing which disperses contaminated aerosols. The tap outflow should not point directly into the sink outlet (Ayliffe et al., 1993).

Overflows are difficult to clean and are rapidly contaminated, becoming reservoirs of bacteria and should be avoided (Caddow, 1989).

If plugs are fitted, trapped bacteria present around the sink outlet contaminate the water. Handwashing should therefore be performed in running water and sinks should not have a plug (Ayliffe et al., 1993).

Sinks/washbasins should be sealed to the wall or placed sufficiently far from the wall to allow effective cleaning of all surfaces. Splash-backs should be included to prevent wall damage (Ayliffe, et al., 1999).

Concealed services result in smooth surfaces which are easier to clean.

The method of hand drying available is important in the maintenance of hand hygiene. Fabric towels are recognized as a source of cross-contamination and are not recommended in clinical practice (Blackmore, 1987).

Hot air dyers are waste-free and always usable provided the current is continuous. However they are generally noisy; warm air currents dry hands slowly and can only be used by one individual at any one time. This results in queues and the temptation to dry hands on clothing.

Paper hand towels dry hands rapidly, and dispensers can be used by several people at once, but they represent ongoing cost both in consumables and disposal of resulting wastes (Matthews and Newsom, 1987). They are, however, considered to result in lowest risk of cross-infection and are the preferred option in clinical practice areas.

Wall-mounted dispensers should be available adjacent to hand-wash basins, to ensure a supply of clean, uncontaminated soap and hand towels. The dispensers should be smooth surfaced and fixed flush to the wall to enable effective cleaning and prevent the accumulation of dust. Reference should also be made to HTM 64 (Department of Health NHS Estates, 1995d) for specifications for patient handwashing facilities and handwashing requirements in other departments; e.g. kitchens.

WCs, bathrooms and shower rooms

Many of the requirements for handwashing facilities are also applicable to other sanitary assemblies; for example, splash-backs, concealed services and wall-mounted taps are also advised for baths and bidets to enhance cleanliness and prevent water damage.

Bidets should be rimless and should not have plugs. This prevents the patient from filling the bidet and contaminating themselves with bacteria or bloodborne viruses which may be present in the outlet and other surfaces such as the rim (Department of Health NHS Estates, 1995d).

All WCs must have provision for handwashing, and since patients may wish to use the WC before or after bathing or showering, a WC and handbasin should be provided in each bathroom/shower room (Department of Health NHS Estates, 1990).

HBN 4 (Department of Health NHS Estates, 1990) also recommends that toilet facilities should be no more than 12 metres from dayrooms or bed areas; and that toilet paper should be readily available in wall-mounted dispensers to minimize potential cross-contamination.

Disposal of waste

Essential requirements

- Secure (lockable) storage areas for clinical waste and sharps
- Effective segregation of domestic and clinical wastes

- Waste bins
  - foot-operated
  - spillage and puncture proof
  - easily cleaned
  - clearly labelled
  - accessible
- Sharps boxes – manufactured to BS 7320 (British Standards Institute, 1990) and UN 3921.

Rationale

Current legislation relevant to clinical waste and its disposal includes:

- Health and Safety at Work Act 1974
- Control of Substances Hazardous to Health Regulations 1998
- Environmental Protection Act 1990 (and associated Duty of Care orders)
- Controlled Waste Regulations 1993
- Special Waste Regulations 1980.

> Plus any future regulations resulting from EU directives (Department of Health NHS Estates 1995b).

Some of the statutory requirements place criminal liability upon individuals responsible for the management of waste. Department of Health NHS Estates (1995b) states: 'It is the responsibility of Chief Executives, general managers and managers to ensure that the premises for which they are responsible meet the requirements of all statutes'.

Correct specifications for disposal areas and containers are therefore essential considerations for any building's design and should form the basis of an effective policy for the disposal of clinical waste and sharps.

Waste storage areas

These must conform to all standards necessary to satisfy 1991 Building Regulations. They must, for example, be easily accessible for people to transport waste within the building, and in addition there must be easy access from the place of storage to the final collection area (Health and Safety Commission, 1992). Any waste storage area must be easy to clean, in case of spillage. It should be roofed, properly drained and pest proof (particularly rat proof) (Ayliffe et al., 1993).

Dirty utility areas are generally considered secure in most healthcare facilities; however, the quantities of waste produced frequently result in storage difficulties and reduced access to other equipment or services located within them. Segregation of wastes is also difficult where space is limited. These problems can be alleviated by improving collection times or preferably by providing dedicated 'disposal rooms' in new or refurbished facilities.

Clinical waste and sharps must be stored in a room or area of adequate size and dedicated for that sole purpose. It is essential that the area is secure (preferably locked) (Department of the Environment, 1991).

Waste bins

Separate containers/bins must be available for clinical and domestic waste, and should be clearly labelled. It is essential that bins appropriate to the needs of the specific area are readily available if effective waste segregation is to be achieved. Since items contaminated with blood and body fluids are considered 'clinical waste' there is no value in placing clinical waste bins in clean utility rooms where the majority of waste consists of clean paper wrappings produced during the preparation of items for clinical procedures. Only a domestic waste container is required in this situation. If clinical waste bins are available, staff may return contaminated items to the clean utility area rather than to the dirty utility or disposal areas.

Many clinical areas produce only small amounts of clinical waste, when, for example specific procedures such as wound dressings are undertaken. In these cases a clinical waste bin placed in the dirty utility area and domestic waste bins in wards areas would be most appropriate. However, if large amounts of clinical waste are generated, as in nursing home or elderly care wards, consideration should be given to providing two clearly labelled bins for clinical and domestic waste in each bed or ward area in addition to the dirty utility room. However this may lead to unpleasant odour problems and the bins need to be emptied frequently to avoid this.

Waste containers should be foot-operated, to prevent hand cont-amination (Ayliffe et al., 1993) and should be capable of being suit-ably cleaned and disinfected.

Sharps boxes

These must conform to UN standards and BS7320 (British Stan-dards Institute, 1990) and UN 3921. Sharps boxes are brightly coloured and can be easily mistaken for toy containers by children. Care should therefore be taken when positioning them. Various devices are available for fixing sharps boxes to walls or permanent fittings to reduce the incidence of deliberate or accidental tampering. These may be particularly appropriate in paediatric or antenatal departments and general practice surgeries.

Disposal of body fluids (urine and faeces)

Essential requirements

A minimum of one maceration or bedpan washer/disinfector is required per ward or care area. (If only low level, intermittent use is likely, this may not be cost effective, and the use of disposable bedpans and urinals with ultimate disposal as clinical waste may be more appropriate.)

Rationale

The risk of cross-infection for patients and staff from washing commodes and bedpans by hand is not acceptable under the COSHH Regulations – The Health and Safety at Work Act (1988).

Two options exist: *washer/disinfectors* or *macerators*.

The Central Sterilising Club (in Collins and Phelps, 1985) indi-cated the potential for serious deficiencies in many bedpan washing machines, including failure to maintain correct temperature for sufficient duration to achieve thermo-disinfection, and failure to remove soiling on all surfaces. Bedpans are extremely difficult to clean effectively and faeces can bake on, resulting in the need to either re-process, or to soak and scrub the pan by hand risking unnecessary exposure of staff to microbiological hazard (COSHH Regs., 1988).

Bedpan washer/disinfectors can often only process one item at a time and the cycle is slower; macerators can process several items rapidly. Several washes may be required to equal the output of one macerator (Collins and Phelps, 1985). Washers are therefore frequently inadequate for high-use areas.

Disposable bedpans reduce the need for handling and risk of contamination with body fluids. There is no physically contaminated item passing between patients and the infection risk is removed. Only the bedpan support requires cleaning regularly and this can be undertaken safely by hand using detergent and hot water because gross contamination is rare (Johnson, 1989).

The machinery involved in macerators is less complex than in bedpan washer/disinfectors. This results in cheaper capital costs. The revenue costs involved are usually equivalent; washer/disinfectors involve high energy and water costs, whilst the cost of disposables represents the ongoing revenue costs of macerators. Maintenance time, however, is far shorter for macerators and maintenance is offered as a service by many suppliers (Fairbrother, 1988). Macerators are the preferred option of many ICTs; however the subject continues to arouse much discussion and careful consideration of all relevant data is essential when purchasing these items.

Linen and laundry services

Essential requirements

Provision of linen and laundry services in healthcare facilities must meet the requirements of HSG (95) 18 (Department of Health NHS Estates, 1995f):

- Secure (lockable) storage areas for fouled and infected linen
- On-site laundry services should include:
  - industrial washing machines with sluice facilities
  - industrial tumble dryers
  - monitoring systems to ensure thermo-disinfection temperatures are achieved
  - areas for flat-drying of items
  - facilities for processing heat-labile items
  (e.g. dosing low-temperature washes with a chlorine-based disinfectant).
- Domestic washing machines in smaller units should achieve similar microbiological standards to industrial/commercial washers.

Rationale

In large establishments the quantity of linen processed requires specialized machinery, which may include tunnel washers, industrial tumble dryers, etc. (Barrie, 1994). Alternatively, linen services may be contracted out to commercial companies. If laundry services are to be provided on-site there must be sufficient industrial machines with sluicing facilities and industrial tumble dryers available to process loads (particularly contaminated items) promptly. If 'infected' linen is to be processed on-site, the laundry facility should include a monitoring system to ensure thermo-disinfection temperatures are achieved (HSG (95)18).

Domestic-style washing machines are frequently the preferred option for small community units, for example, for the laundering of personal clothing in mental health and learning disabilities community homes. These machines are acceptable where clients live in small permanent 'family groups' and are physically healthy. However, alternative arrangements may still need to be considered for 'infected' items.

Ayliffe (1993) states that microbiological standards lower than those obtainable in commercial machines used in hospitals should not be accepted without full consideration of the infection risks present in the proposed area of use.

If a small unit is expected to process predominantly fouled linen, industrial machines with sluicing facilities should be provided. Sluicing of fouled items by hand is not acceptable since this may expose staff to unnecessary microbiological hazards (COSHH Regs. 1988).

A secure (lockable) area must be available for the storage of fouled and infected linen to prevent pilfering and to ensure protection from pests. A separate area is required for the storage of clean linen.

Fixtures and fittings: wall, floors and ceilings

Essential requirements

- Low dirt retention – easily cleanable and washable
- Materials should be jointless, or where unavoidable joints should be sealed or welded
- Maintenance and cleaning programmes must be fully considered when choosing the finish.

Rationale

The majority of organisms present on hospital floors are non-pathogenic (Caddow, 1989). Although soiling can accumulate in cracks, joints and corners it rarely results in infection (Ayliffe et al., 1999). It does, however, appear unpleasant and inhibits cleaning. Any joints should therefore be welded or sealed where they are unavoidable. HTM 61 provides detailed information on the following aspects (Department of Health NHS Estates, 1995c). Sealing of joints also prevents damage due to water ingress under the flooring. Skirtings should be made from the same material as the floor and fully sealed both to the wall and floor, to give an impervious finish.

Wide-ranging considerations are necessary when selecting, specifying and installing new flooring – whether in a new or existing facility. The major choice exists between hard or soft finishes, i.e. thermoplastics (vinyl), natural stone, cement, resin or textile (carpet).

Carpets are often the popular choice in new facilities, health centres and general practice surgeries, because of the non-clinical, comfortable associations. Carpets with water-impervious backing are available, and providing they are cleaned and maintained correctly there is little evidence to indicate that they present a greater infection risk than flooring made of hard finishes (Ayliffe et al., 1999; Caddow, 1989).

Modern steam cleaning machines provide an effective means of cleaning carpets; however, it would be impractical to advise steam cleaning on a daily basis. Carpets are also associated with retention of odour, particularly in facilities which experience frequent body fluid spillage. They are also readily damaged (bleached) by chlorine-releasing disinfectants used for decontamination of blood and blood-stained body fluid spillage (UK Health Department, 1990). Carpets are therefore considered less suitable for clinical areas where body fluid spillage frequently occurs and also where food and drink frequently cause soiling; ultimately resulting in odour problems. Correct and effective cleaning and maintenance of any flooring is essential. Certain cleaning agents can, for example, cause shrinkage in PVC flooring, resulting in joints opening or the rupture of welded seams. Permanent records must be available containing all details of the flooring used. This should include manufacturer, finishes, any adhesives, screed and damp proof membranes used; the structure of the floor base and finally manufacturers' instructions for cleaning and maintenance.

If the manufacturer-recommended programmes have been properly maintained the facility may have recourse to them if damage occurs or if the material fails to meet the required specifications.

Walls and ceilings present very little risk of infection (Ayliffe et al., 1999; Caddow, 1989). Smooth, hard impervious surfaces are recommended in patient treatment areas because these are easier to clean and bacteria cannot readily adhere to them.

False ceilings, however, may be associated with accumulation of dust and fungi, and can harbour pests. It is therefore essential that buildings are checked on completion to ensure that no unwanted materials from the building works remain and that there is no access for pests (Ayliffe et al., 1999).

Ceilings with removable tiles or perforated ceilings can allow dust to fall onto the area below, especially if they are disturbed during maintenance work. It is therefore advisable to avoid this type of ceiling in operating theatres and treatment rooms (Ayliffe et al., 1999). Careful risk assessment should also be undertaken whenever this type of maintenance is proposed on occupied ward areas.

Food hygiene: kitchen area

It is not possible to cover all the requirements necessary in catering facilities in this chapter. A limited number of issues will be considered as follows:

- General requirements to reduce infestation with pests
- Facilities for dishwashing
- Handwashing facilities.

Close cooperation is essential between the ICT, hotel services/catering department and Local Authority environmental health officers when planning a new or refurbished kitchen, to ensure safe food production for the client group served. Crown immunity against prosecution was removed from hospitals following a major outbreak of food poisoning at Stanley Royd Hospital in 1986. Hospitals and healthcare facilities must therefore meet all the requirements of Local Authority environmental health inspections (Department of Health NHS Executive, 1996).

Any building used for food preparation and production should be of sound structure and well maintained. This includes covering of any drains and prompt repair of leaking pipe work, damaged surfaces, etc. (Ayliffe et al., 1993).

Cracks in walls, unsealed pipe work, damaged tiles and poorly fitted equipment or kitchen units can all provide access for pests. Some protection can be achieved by ensuring that doors and windows fit tightly, and through the provision of fly-screens and bird netting. Surfaces should be smooth, water impervious and readily cleanable (Department of Health NHS Estates, 1995c). Pest control systems, e.g. rodent and cockroach traps should also be employed.

The purpose of dishwashing machines in hospitals is to provide hygienically safe crockery and cutlery. Kitchen and service utensils and tableware should be washed at temperatures and for lengths of time which will destroy bacteria and allow drying without danger of recontamination. Domestic Service Advice Note 2 (Department of Health and Social Security, 1976) recommended heat treatment as the most effective method. Two cycles are necessary:

a) A detergent wash to remove food and grease (60 °C)

b) A rinse cycle to thermo-disinfect, i.e. kill all vegetative bacteria including those which cause communicable disease.

Effectiveness depends on the temperature achieved and the duration for which the organisms are exposed to the heat. The Central Sterilising Club Working Party (in Collins and Phelps, 1985) recommended a scale ranging from 71 °C for 3 minutes to 90 °C for one second to achieve effective thermo-disinfection. Since handwashing cannot achieve these temperatures safely, machine washing is preferable. Monitoring systems must be available to ensure thermo-disinfection temperatures are achieved in use (Department of Health NHS Executive, 1996).

Washing up at ward level is difficult to supervise. Central washing up facilities should be introduced wherever possible, particularly in large healthcare establishments. In small units, daycare facilities and wherever washing up is undertaken locally, sufficient dishwashers should be available to ensure prompt processing of all used items after each meal (Maurer, 1985).

Dedicated handwashing facilities must be available to prevent cross-contamination of foods and items used for food preparation, and to ensure that staff can effectively decontaminate their hands as necessary before and after food handling.

Isolation facilities

Essential requirements

- A minimum of four single rooms (two with en-suite WC and shower) must be provided per adult ward.
- These rooms must have a door which can be closed.
- (Reference should be made to relevant NHS Estates documents for requirements for isolation facilities in specialist units such as paediatrics).

Rationale

Several factors influence the practicality of carrying out isolation precautions. These include the availability of single rooms; the mix of patients in a ward or unit; staffing levels; general facilities, e.g. hand-wash basins, bedpans, macerator/washer, etc.; availability of staff trained in isolation techniques and the overall condition of the patient.

Standard isolation precautions are the minimum requirements necessary to prevent the spread of communicable infection. The safety of all concerned depends on compliance with these minimal requirements:

- Effective handwashing
- Use of protective clothing
- Correct decontamination of equipment
- Single-room accommodation where necessary.

The absence of single-room isolation facilities results in a risk to other patients within multi-bedded rooms, particularly if existing handwashing facilities are inadequate. Even where illnesses are potentially airborne, e.g. viral gastroenteritis, isolating the patient in a side room can limit the risk to others (Ayliffe et al., 1993).

An admission policy can divert potentially infectious patients to more appropriately equipped or specialist isolation units. It does not reduce the potential for infections to arise within the unit, or for delayed or inaccurate initial diagnosis to result in infection hazards. Isolation accommodation can vary from a ward side room to a fully equipped suite with an airlock. The minimal requirement is a side room of a main ward with a handbasin and preferably en-suite WC and shower. All surfaces must be washable and furniture, fixtures and fittings should be kept to a minimum (Ayliffe et al., 1999).

Health Building Note 4 (Department of Health NHS Estates, 1990) indicates that for each new or upgraded ward accommodation at least two single bedrooms should be provided with en-suite WC and shower. At least 4 single rooms should be available in total. These rooms may be used for patients whose condition cannot be treated within a multi-bedded room but who do not require *strict* isolation (Ayliffe, 1993). Present trends indicate a continued increase in the number of patients colonized or infected with antibiotic resistant organisms such as methicillin-resistant *Staphylococcus aureus* (MRSA) and vancomycin-resistant enterococcus (VRE), and also an increasing incidence of communicable diarrhoeal illnesses such as *Clostridium difficile*, salmonella, *Escherichia coli* 0157, etc. (Department of Health, 1994a). Recommendations for the care of these patients include the need for isolation. The demand for single-room accommodation is therefore very high and likely to increase. The required numbers of single rooms should therefore be carefully reviewed and probably revised upward if the Department of Health's recommendations are to be achieved.

Patients with a communicable respiratory or airborne disease, e.g. chicken pox or untreated pulmonary tuberculosis (especially multi-drug resistant TB) require isolation involving a ventilation system which may be provided within a dedicated 'infectious disease unit'. These units frequently consist of fully equipped suites with gowning lobby, negative pressure ventilation, en-suite facilities and airlock (Ayliffe et al., 1999). Design specifications for this type of unit can be found in HTM 2025 (Department of Health NHS Estates, 1994b). This level of isolation may also be desirable for other patients, for example those who are heavy dispersers of staphylococci, and particularly patients who are colonized or infected with MRSA, or who have exfoliating skin conditions, chest infections, etc.

Patients with severely reduced immunity may require protective isolation, which can include positive pressure ventilation systems producing 8–10 air changes per hour and effective filters. In all other respects the requirements for isolation rooms for these patients are identical to those described for infectious patients.

A safe water supply: control of Legionellae

Source water obtained from the mains supply is usually of a good bacteriological quality (Ayliffe et al., 1993). Chemicals such as hypochlorite are frequently added by water companies to prevent the multiplication of bacteria, and the water is considered safe to drink without further treatment (Department of Health NHS Estates, 1993). However, where water is stored in tanks, contamination by algae, bird droppings, insects and dead birds may neutralize the hypochlorite, resulting in increased bacterial counts. Contamination can also occur during construction or refurbishment, and during routine inspections.

Hospital sites are generally large, have complex water storage and air-conditioning systems and contain particularly susceptible individuals. Therefore control of legionella, by means of effective design and maintenance of these systems, must be a serious consideration for the planning team.

Design and installation of cold and hot water services in NHS premises must comply with the following:

- Current water bylaws
- BS 6700: British Standard Specification for design, installation, testing and maintenance of services supplying water for domestic use within buildings and their curtilages (1987)
- HT27: Cold water supply storage and mains distribution (Department of Health, 1978)
- HTM 2040 Control of Legionellae in Healthcare Premises (Department of Health NHS Estates, 1993).

Legionella pneumophilia is an organism often associated with the growth of algae and protozoa in water systems. It is therefore vitally important that correct storage and distribution temperatures are maintained and measures taken to prevent water stagnation.

Legionellae multiply actively at temperatures between 20 and 45°C (and most rapidly at 36°C). The survival of the organism at higher temperatures is dependent on the time of exposure to a given temperature. At 60°C, for example, 90% of Legionellae will die after 2 minutes (Department of Health NHS Estates, 1993).

In hot water systems the temperature at the outflow point from the calorifier should achieve 60°C (with a control tolerance of +/- 2.5°C). At this temperature Legionellae survive for only short periods of time, and the organism is unlikely to be distributed in sufficient numbers to be of harm to the patients (Department of Health NHS Estates, 1995e).

Temperatures above 60°C are undesirable for the following reasons:

- risk of scalding increases dramatically
- increased deposits of scale occurs
- increased corrosion and production of corrosion products (HTM 2027).

Mental health, learning disability, elderly care and paediatric wards require thermostatic mixing valves to control the temperatures at the outlets to reduce the risk of accidental scalding, without having to reduce the temperatures at the outflow from the calorifier. Hot water circulating pumps must be of adequate performance to ensure that a minimum circulation temperature of 50°C is achieved (Department of Health NHS Estates, 1993).

Cold water should be kept below 20°C; therefore supply should be kept away from areas where it is prone to thermal gains (see Figure 5.1 for optimal 'hot and cold water services distribution').

Stagnation can be avoided by limiting taps, or other outlets, to areas that will be used regularly (more than once a week) and by avoiding installation of outlets on the ends of lines, called 'dead legs' (Department of Health NHS Estates, 1993).

Where taps are unavoidably sited in remote areas they should be flushed through for several minutes on a weekly basis. WCs should also be flushed. This also applies where wards or departments are temporarily closed. If this is impractical., the system should be disinfected throughout before being returned to service (Department of Health NHS Estates, 1993).

Legionellae may colonize other areas where droplets of contaminated water of a size suitable for deep inhalation are generated. Aerosol-generating plant and equipment should not be installed next to patient accommodation. Showers and shower-heads are not considered to pose a great hazard. It is now no longer necessary to disinfect shower-heads (Department of Health NHS Estates, 1995e).

Routine testing for legionella is not recommended, unless the system is suspected as a source of hospital-acquired infection. A study by the Public Health Laboratory Service in 1991 concluded that Legionellae can be found in most water systems without resulting in disease (in Health and Safety Executive, 1993).

Reference should also be made to Health Technical Memoran-

Note: All pipes to be insulated

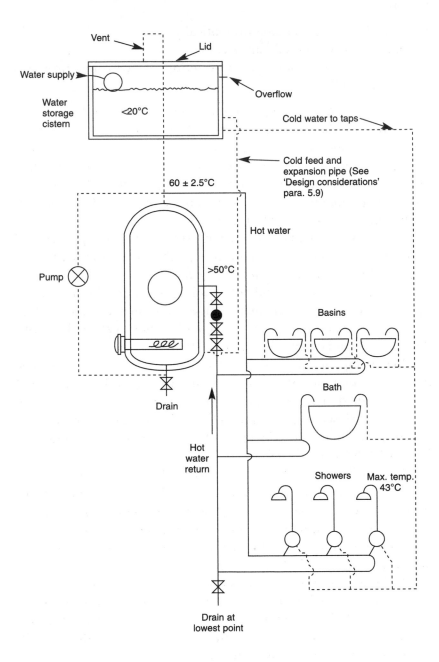

Figure 5.1 Hot and cold water distribution services

dum 2040 (Department of Health NHS Estates, 1993), for specific information concerning:

- hydrotherapy pools/whirlpool baths/spa baths
- portable room humidifiers
- non-portable water storage
- deluge showers
- trolley wash procedures
- lawn sprinklers/hoses
- vehicle washing plant
- ornamental fountains
- ice-making machines

Health Technical Memorandum 17 Commissioning of Hospital Engineering Services, 1978 (Department of Health, 1978) should be referred to regarding the commissioning and testing of any new or refurbished water services.

Additional requirements in specialist facilities

Operating theatres

Major historical developments in surgery, such as improvement in surgical technique, anaesthesia and antisepsis which occurred in the nineteenth century are well documented. These milestones were, however, achieved without recognition of the potential role of the environment in limiting postoperative infection. The development of specialist operating theatres with controlled environments is relatively new. Positive pressure (plenum) ventilation, for example, was first introduced in the 1940s (Holton and Ridgway, 1993) and it was not until 1962 that the Medical Research Council published six design requirements to control infection in operating suites, as follows:

- separation from the general traffic/airflow of the hospital
- provision of increasingly 'clean zones' between the entrance to the suite and the operating theatre
- control of airflow out from 'clean' to less clean areas
- easy movement of staff between 'clean' areas without passing through 'dirty' areas
- removal of dirty materials/waste without passing through 'clean' areas

- heating and ventilation to ensure comfortable conditions for patients and staff.

Many of these recommendations have not been scientifically validated because of the wide range of variables encountered when attempting to prove causation in reduction of postoperative wound infection rates. Some recommendations are no longer considered to be valid; for example, specific disposal zones are not required if the waste is removed from the theatre in sealed bags, and single corridor layouts can be accepted without any decrease in microbiological standards (Department of Health NHS Estates, 1991a).

Points to consider at the initial planning stage of any new theatre development include:

The type of theatre required

The type of surgery to be performed, general or specialized, will dictate the type of equipment used and size of the scrub team and therefore the size and configuration of the theatre.

The site of the department

Location should be based on convenience and easy access to complementary departments such as ITU, A and E, X Ray, sterile supplies, etc. (Department of Health NHS Estates, 1991a). Ventilation systems are more easily installed if the department is situated on the top floor, therefore this is the preferred site, but is not essential (Humphrey, 1993).

The number of theatres required

This relates to the department's projected workload and can be predicted by considering:

- the total number of surgical beds
- bed occupancy
- departmental throughput
- anticipated caseload per session
- plus an allowance for regular maintenance and servicing (Humphrey, 1993; Ayliffe et al., 1993).

Theatres are expensive to run and equip and in order to be economical they must be extensively used. It is a false economy to underestimate requirements because extending existing premises in the future can prove to be expensive, logistically demanding and disruptive (Department of Health NHS Estates, 1991a; Johnson and Hunter, 1984).

Zoning and access

The layout of the theatre must allow for efficient movement of staff, patients, supplies and equipment. Possible segregation arrangements are shown in Figure 5.2.

Single-corridor arrangements provide the simplest and most economical layout without compromising microbiological standards. However, corridors must be wide enough to permit movement of beds and trolleys. Fire safety must also be built into the design. The latter in particular may necessitate a two-corridor arrangement (Ayliffe et al., 1993).

Most theatres are now designed in 'zones':

- Aseptic (operative zone): theatre and lay-up rooms
- Clean (restricted access zone): anaesthetic/scrub rooms
- Protective (limited access zone): entrance, recovery, changing rooms
- Disposal (general access zone).

(Medical Research Council, 1962; Department of Health NHS Estates, 1991a).

Ayliffe et al. (1993) suggests that this type of zonal layout can be used to enhance theatre discipline and focus attention on good practice. Acceptance of the zoning arrangements means that parents can accompany their children into the anaesthetic room without changing into theatre clothing and without compromising microbiological standards in the operating room itself.

When ventilation pressures are arranged to ensure that air flows out from the aseptic zone to the disposal or general access zone, the pressure gradient achieved prevents the entry of bacteria into the operating room from these outer areas (Holton and Ridgway, 1993). Benefits may also exist in terms of security. The effectiveness of this

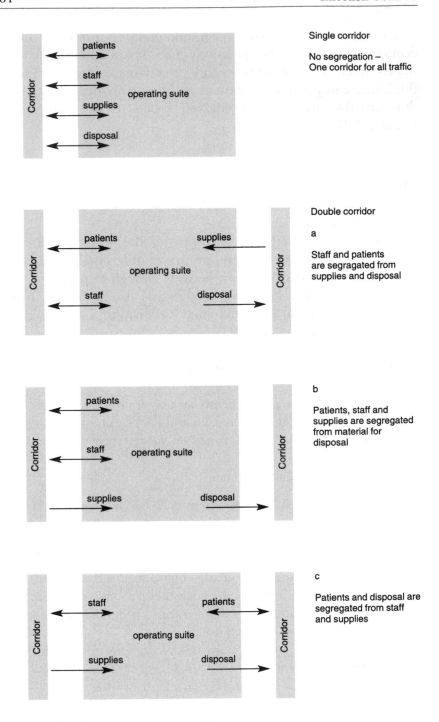

Figure 5.2 Possible theatre segregation policies

arrangement in reducing surgical wound infection rates has not, however, been scientifically validated (Ayliffe et al., 1993).

Ventilation requirements

The purpose of ventilation in operating suites is to provide a supply of filtered air to the operating room, at a controlled temperature and humidity resulting in:

- removal of airborne bacteria released within theatre (e.g. by staff)
- prevention of entry of bacteria from external areas (e.g. from outside the hospital)
- removal of anaesthetic gases
- reduction of electrostatic spark.

Therefore the dual benefits of increased safety and comfort for the staff and patients and reduced incidence of wound infection may be achieved (Ayliffe et al., 1993).

Most standard (non-orthopaedic) theatres are plenum ventilated at 20 air changes per hour in the aseptic zone without re-circulating the air. Lower input is maintained in the clean zone with low, or no, input into the protective and general access zones. This maintains the pressure gradient mentioned above (Lidwell, 1972; Ayliffe et al., 1993; Humphrey, 1993).

The ventilation plant should consist of filtration, heating, cooling and humidification systems and should be organized so that the ventilation of a particular theatre can be inactivated, for maintenance for example, without affecting the other theatres (Department of Health NHS Estates, 1991a). Time clocks should also be included to allow the system to be switched on in advance of the operating sessions whenever the system has been temporarily shut down. It is important to locate the plant's air intake as far away as possible from bacterial contamination, preferably on the roof of the building, and to take care to protect the intake from adverse weather conditions (Humphrey, 1993). The efficiency of the ventilation system should be monitored daily using engineering parameters, such as air switches which indicate on theatre panes whether the correct volume of air is being supplied by the plant. Alternatively, manual measurements of airflow at ventilation grilles and room pressure measurements may be undertaken. Results should be recorded in a daily log book and ventilation rates checked periodically by an engineer. Reduced pressure and air turnover can indicate a blockage in the filters which requires immediate replacement (Ayliffe et al., 1993).

In conventional theatres filtration is generally carried out in stages:

- Pre (or primary) filters prevent dirt or large bacteria carrying particles (>5 microns) from entering the plant. They are positioned on the negative pressure side of the fans
- Secondary filters reduce the particle count and remove pathogens. They are placed on the positive pressure section of the system. They are protected by primary filters.

High Efficiency Particulate Air (HEPA) filters allow for re-circulation of air, but are not considered to be necessary for conventional theatres (Department of Health NHS Estates, 1991a; Humphrey, 1993).

Ultraclean ventilation

Cost–benefit analysis supports the use of ultraclean air on economic as well as clinical grounds for orthopaedic theatres because pathogens are more likely to result in infection in the presence of a prosthesis than in general surgery (Lidwell, 1984).

In conventional theatres the effect of the ventilation system is reduced in practice by convection movements caused by the turbulence created by the movement of staff and the opening and closing of operating room doors (Ayliffe et al., 1993). The ultraclean system renders the zone immediately adjacent to the operator totally free from micro-organisms (Department of Health NHS Estates, 1991a). This is achieved by the development of 'laminar' or uni-directional airflow from a diffuser or filter bank directly downward over the operating site. A larger area of diffusion and a greater volume of air (300 air changes per hour) are required in comparison with conventional theatre ventilation, and re-circulation using HEPA filters is essential to reduce costs (Humphrey, 1993; Ayliffe et al., 1993; Department of Health NHS Estates, 1991a). Vertical airflow reduces the possibility of operators introducing bacteria into the airstream, however care must be taken in siting the lighting configurations so that there is minimal disruption to the airflow.

Typical ventilation airflow patterns are shown in Figure 5.3. Horizontal airflow ultraclean systems are available but are not widely used because many of the benefits are reduced if personnel shed bacteria 'upstream' of the wound.

The cost of installing ultraclean ventilation, fully integrated with a conventional system, and including lighting and service outlets in a new building may not be significantly greater than for a conventional system alone, and can result in greater flexibility in the ultimate use of the operating theatre. However, care should be taken regarding the introduction of this system into existing or refurbished buildings, not only on grounds of cost, but also because the canopy (partial wall) can reduce headroom and may necessitate re-configuration of the lighting, resulting in unsatisfactory working conditions. It is therefore essential that a full cost–benefit analysis is undertaken at the planning stage prior to committing resources to the project.

Bacteriological requirements

Blowers and Crew (1960) recommended that the air delivered to the operating suite by conventional ventilation should contain no more than 1 colony of *Clostridium welchii* or *Staphylococcus aureus* in a sample of 30m^3 of air, and that aerobic cultures on non-selective media should not contain more than 35 bacteria particles in 1 m^3 of ventilating air.

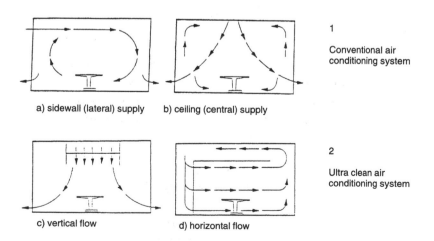

a) sidewall (lateral) supply   b) ceiling (central) supply

1

Conventional air conditioning system

c) vertical flow   d) horizontal flow

2

Ultra clean air conditioning system

Figure 5.3 Typical airflow patterns

Routine air testing in conventional theatres is no longer considered to be of value. However, measurement of bacterial counts is still widely recommended when filters are changed or ventilation circuits disrupted, and particularly during the commissioning of new or refurbished theatres (Humphrey, 1993; Ayliffe et al., 1993, Department of Health NHS Estates, 1991a) (see Figure 5.4).

By contrast, ultraclean theatres require regular routine testing (3-monthly), because of the need to identify and repair promptly any faults. This is because infections post joint surgery may take several weeks or months to incubate (Holton and Ridgway, 1993).

The validity of accepting air counts as a measurement of theatre air quality has recently been questioned, particularly where ventilation systems are checked daily or during commissioning by hospital engineers, and where the systems are appropriately cleaned, serviced and maintained, since it is considered that these measures are more reliable indicators of the effectiveness of the ventilation plant (Mennie, 1997).

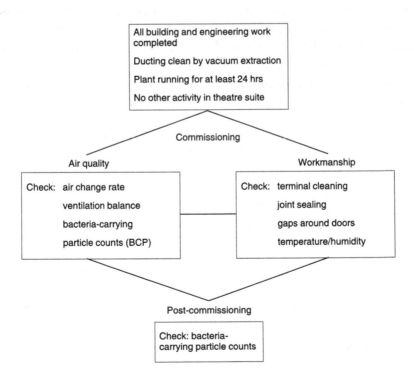

Figure 5.4 Plan for commissioning of operating theatres

Additional requirements

- Anaesthetic room: this should be adjacent to the theatre and equipped with a clinical handwashing basin and facilities for the disposal of waste and sharps.
- Scrub-up and gowning areas: these must be accessible from the limited access zone and lead directly into the operating room.
- Storage space (shelves): must be provided for sterile gloves and gowns. They must be positioned or placed on a trolley so that accidental splashing is prevented.
- Scrub facilities: described in Health Technical Memorandum 64 'Sanitary Assemblies' (Department of Health NHS Estates, 1995d).
- Lay-up room: separate lay-up areas or rooms should be provided within the aseptic zone, adjacent to the operating room. Trolleys should not be laid up in advance within the operating room, because of the risk of contamination during the opening and closing of the doors.
- Domestic waste bins: must be available for the disposal of used hand towels and wrappers.
- 'Tacky mats': mats with disinfectant-coated surfaces placed at the entrance to the theatre suite are not recommended. They offer little protection against bacterial contamination of the operating room floor. If they are not cleaned regularly they may increase the number of organisms transferred into the theatre (Department of Health NHS Estates, 1991a; Medical Research Council, 1962).

Intensive care units

Detailed specifications for the design of general intensive care units (ITUs) are provided in Health Building Note 27 (Department of Health NHS Estates, 1992b). This document recommends that specific advice should be sought when considering design features necessary for specialist ITUs, e.g. neurosurgery, burns, cardiothoracic, neonatal units, since there may be additional requirements for isolation of patients, bed space for equipment, etc.

In addition to the general requirements for healthcare premises, the following recommendations are particularly relevant for the control of cross-infection in ITUs.

Space

The functional unit for an ITU is the 'bed'. The recommendations
contained in Health Building Note 27 (Department of Health NHS
Estates, 1992a), refer to ITUs of 6–10 beds, but can be adapted for
larger units.

The design layout must allow sufficient space around each bed
for all-round access to the patient, to equipment and to handwashing facilities without encroaching upon other bed spaces. Allowance
should also be made for staff working in protective clothing and for
the storage of these items. 'Island' bed spaces are generally considered to achieve these requirements in the most effective, ergonomic,
manner (Kitchen and Ware, 1994).

The design must facilitate observation of the patients and effective deployment of staff. Prevention of cross-infection is fundamental
to patient care in ITUs and a high standard of hygiene must be
promoted in all areas. Facilities for handwashing and drying, and for
the disposal of waste and sharps, must be provided at every bed
space.

Single-room accommodation

At least two single rooms should be provided within each unit of
6–10 beds. Each must be equipped with a ventilation system to
provide positive and negative pressure as required for source or
protective isolation.

Ideally, entry should be via a gowning lobby which acts as an
airlock preventing the escape of significant microbial contamination
into the open unit, or in cases of protective isolation, into the single
room itself. The gowning lobby should include a clinical handwash
basin, plastic apron dispenser, storage for white coats and disposal
facilities for waste and sharps. The single room should also be
equipped with a clinical handwash basin. Ceilings, walls and doors
should be tight-fitting with seals to prevent air transfers.

Ventilation

In addition to the requirements for specific systems for ventilation of
single rooms, the ITU should be mechanically ventilated, providing
fresh air moving from clean towards dirty areas. The ventilation
plant should include filters which are readily accessible for replace-

ment and maintenance and should also control temperature and humidity (Department of Health NHS Estates, 1992a).

Laboratory

A status laboratory is often required for blood-gas analysis, etc., within the unit. The main requirements usually include a sink; laboratory benching made from water-impermeable material; space to perform tests and for equipment; a specimen fridge; disposal facilities for waste and sharps; and access to a computer. In addition, a separate handwash basin should be available. These requirements should be applied 'as far as reasonably practicable', when upgrading existing facilities (Department of Health NHS Estates, 1992a).

General practice surgeries and health centres

The relevance of infection control within the primary sector has increased in the last decade. Relevant factors include:

- safety of patients, staff and visitors
- legal requirements and professional guidance, such as Health and Safety legislation
- increased likelihood of litigation in cases of alleged negligent practice (including acquisition of infection)
- ethical and professional issues such as accountability
- changing patient profile as a result of early hospital discharge
- increase in invasive procedures within primary care such as minor surgery.

Although it may not be appropriate to attempt to apply identical standards to both primary and secondary sector facilities, general practitioners should be aware that poor design of their premises can not only reduce the effectiveness of measures to control infection but can also hinder the work of the team.

When considering the design of surgeries and health centres, practitioners should make a careful assessment of the activities of the centre, including any past changes in practice and any anticipated future changes (Department of Health NHS Estates, 1991b).

Schemes which provide financial incentives to general practitioners to encourage high standards in the accommodation are often dependent upon Health Authority involvement in the project.

General design

Effective layouts must allow for the following requirements:

Patient treatment areas

This includes examination rooms, nurse treatment rooms, minor surgery, podiatry, etc. Adequate space must be available for patient treatment. All treatment areas must have the following facilities:

- clinical handwashing and drying
- clinical waste and sharps disposal (sharps containers must be placed in a secure area away from access to children and other vulnerable people)
- treatment trolley/tray preparation area
- cleaning and decontamination areas, including a separate utility sink and space for an autoclave
- drug storage cupboard and fridge
- specimen fridge.

(Department of Health NHS Estates, 1991b; British Medical Association, 1990).

A separate utility room may avoid the need for many of the above features elsewhere and has the advantage that the utility room may be used by all staff without disrupting treatment sessions.

Collection and testing of samples

This an increasingly important aspect of primary care. Some specimens may be brought in by patients from home, whilst others are collected on site. In larger practices it may be possible to include a dedicated toilet for collecting urine samples, connected by a hatch to the treatment or utility room. The hatch should have acoustically sealed double doors with a shelf in between which can be cleaned easily. A specimen fridge should be available for storage of samples awaiting transportation to the laboratory. This must not contain items other than specimens (Worsley et al., 1994).

Working practices within primary care differ from those in acute care settings in that the practice nurse may be able to arrange the schedule to avoid mixing 'clean tasks' such as minor surgery with 'dirty tasks' such as specimen collection and instrument cleaning.

Therefore clean and dirty zones are not necessarily required. However all surfaces within treatment and utility rooms must be easily cleaned and have adequate storage space to avoid cross-contamination.

In larger premises, where there is a greater workload and many staff sharing the facilities, it may be necessary to separate clean and dirty activities to limit the risks of cross-infection (Department of Health, 1991b).

Commissioning a new or refurbished building

Building projects can be considered in phases:

- Design: service requirements are reviewed and alternative concepts explored.
- Planning: detailed specifications, room layouts and configurations are presented. Architectural plans and room activity data sheets are developed and carefully evaluated by the users and other relevant personnel such as housekeepers and the infection control nurse. Changes can be debated and implemented at this stage with little disruption or cost.
- Construction: building work begins. Site visits are advisable and can assist in identifying problems at the earliest opportunity. The contractor must be involved in the visits and discussions. The building does not become the property of the Authority until final transfer.
- Commissioning: is generally considered to be the period when the building is transferred from the contractor to the user, it is furnished and opened.

(Department of Health NHS Estates, 1995a; Millard, 1981).

Activities undertaken during the commissioning period before the service is opened include:

- equipping the facility
- completion of final risk assessment
- technical commissioning, including checks of the standard of workmanship, services and equipment
- post-project evaluation.

Decommissioning of any vacated premises will be carried out at this time (Department of Health NHS Estates, 1994e).

Effective commissioning should actually begin at the point of awarding the tender. It requires careful leadership and planning throughout to prevent costly errors occurring. Most problems can be avoided by ensuring that there is good communication between all parties (architects, engineers, users, management, accountant, infection control, support services) throughout the planning, construction and commissioning stages of any project.

As with many aspects of infection control, people are the key to reducing potential environmental infection risks. Communication and attention to detail are vital in producing a building that is not only fit for its purpose, but is better by design.

References

Ayliffe GAJ, Collins BJ, Taylor LJ. Hospital Acquired Infection: Principles and Prevention. London: Butterworth-Heinemann, 1999.

Ayliffe GAJ, Lowbury EJL, Geddes AM, Williams JD. Control of Infection: A Practical Handbook, 3rd Edition. London: Chapman and Hall Medical, 1993.

Barrie D. How hospital linen and laundry services are provided. Journal of Hospital Infection 1994; 27 (3): 219–35.

Blackmore M. Hand drying methods. Nursing Times 1987; 83 (37): 71–4.

Blowers R, Crew B. Ventilation of operating theatres. Journal of Hygiene, Cambridge 1960; (58): 427.

Bond RG, Michaelsen GS, De Roos RL (eds). Environmental Health and Safety in Healthcare Facilities. New York: Macmillan Press, 1973.

British Medical Association. A Code of Practice for the Safe Use and Disposal of Sharps. London: BMA, 1990.

British Standards Institute. Specification for Sharps Containers (BS7320). London: BSI, 1990.

Caddow P. Applied Microbiology. Oxford: The Alden Press, 1989.

Collins BJ, Phelps M. The Evaluation of Bedpan Washer/disinfectors. (In association with the Central Sterilising Club Working Party on washer/disinfectors). Birmingham: Hospital Infection Research Laboratory, 1985.

Control of Substances Hazardous to Health (COSHH) Regulations, 1994.

Department of the Environment. Special Wastes: A Technical Memorandum Providing Guidance on Their Definitions (Waste Management Paper 23). London: HMSO, 1981.

Department of the Environment. Environmental Protection Act 1990, Section 34: Waste Management, The Duty of Care Code of Practice. London: HMSO, 1991.

Department of Health. Health Technical Memorandum 17: Commissioning of Hospital Engineering Services. London: HMSO, 1978.

Department of Health NHS Estates. Health Building Note 4: Adult Acute Wards. London: HMSO, 1990.

Department of Health NHS Estates. Health Building Note 26: Operating Department. London: HMSO, 1991a.

Department of Health NHS Estates. Health Building Note 46: General Medical Practices Premises. London: HMSO, 1991b.

Department of Health NHS Estates. Design Guide: The Design of Community Hospitals. London: HMSO, 1991c.

Department of Health NHS Estates. Health Building Note 27: Intensive Therapy Unit. London: HMSO, 1992a.

Department of Health NHS Estates. Health Guidance Note: Safe Hot Water and Surface Temperature. London: HMSO, 1992b.

Department of Health NHS Estates. Health Technical Memorandum 2040: Control of Legionellae in Healthcare Premises – Design Considerations. London: HMSO, 1993.

Department of Health. Management of Outbreaks of Foodborne Illness. London: Department of Health Central Print Unit, 1994a.

Department of Health NHS Estates. Health Technical Memorandum 2025: Ventilation in Healthcare Premises – Design Considerations. London: HMSO, 1994b.

Department of Health NHS Estates. Health Technical Memorandum 2050: Risk Management in NHS Estate – Design Considerations. London: HMSO, 1994c.

Department of Health NHS Estates. Pursuit of Excellence in Healthcare Buildings: Better by Design. London: HMSO, 1994d.

Department of Health NHS Estates. Capital Investment Manual: Commissioning a Healthcare Facility. London: HMSO, 1994e.

Department of Health NHS Estates. Health Facilities Note 06: Operational Commissioning Strategy – A Manager's Guide. London: HMSO, 1995a.

Department of Health NHS Estates. Health Guidance Note: Safe Disposal of Clinical Waste: whole hospital policy guidance. London: HMSO, 1995b.

Department of Health NHS Estates. Health Technical Memorandum 61: Building Components – Flooring, 2nd Edition. London: HMSO, 1995c.

Department of Health NHS Estates. Health Technical Memorandum 64: Building Components – Sanitary Assemblies. London: HMSO, 1995d.

Department of Health NHS Estates. Health Technical Memorandum 2027: Hot and Cold Water Supply – Design Considerations. London: HMSO, 1995e.

Department of Health NHS Executive. Health Service Guidelines: Hospital Laundry Arrangements for Used and Infected Linen (HSG(95)18). London: HMSO, 1995f.

Department of Health NHS Executive. Health Service Guidelines: Management of Food Hygiene and Food Services in the NHS (HSG(96)20). London: HMSO, 1996.

Department of Health and Social Security. Capricode: Health Building Procedures. London: HMSO, 1986.

Fairbrother C Good riddance. Hospital Equipment and Supplies 1988: 19–20 August.

Garner JS, Favero MS CDC. Guideline for handwashing and hospital environmental control 1985. Infection Control 1986; 7 (4): 231–5.

Hambraeus A. Aerobiology in the operating room: a review. Journal of Hospital Infection 1988; 11 (suppl. A): 68–76.

Health and Safety Commission. Safe Disposal of Clinical Waste. London: HMSO, 1992.

Health and Safety Executive. The Control of Legionellosis including Legionnaires Disease HS (G) 70. London: HMSO, 1993.

Holton J, Ridgway GL Commissioning operating theatres. Journal of Hospital Infection 1993; 23: 161–7.

Humphrey H Infection control and the design of a new operating suite. Journal of Hospital Infection 1993; 23: 61–70.

Johnson A Bedpans: Disposable or reusable? Nursing Times 1989; 85 (41): 72–4.

Johnson IDA, Hunter AR The Design and Utilisation of Operating Theatres. London: Edward Arnold, 1984.

Kitchen J, Ware R Intensive planning. Healthcare Design September 1994: 42–3.

Larson E A causal link between handwashing and risk of infection? Examination of the evidence. Infection Control and Hospital Epidemiology 1988; 9 (1): 28–36.

Lidwell OM (Chair) The Report of a Joint Working Party, Department of Health and Social Security Ventilation in Operating Suites. London: HMSO, 1972.

Lidwell OM The cost implication of clean air systems and antibiotic prophylaxis in operations for total joint replacement. Infection Control 1984; 5 (36): 36–7.

Matthews JA, Newsom SWB Hot air electric hand driers compared with paper hand towels for potential spread of airborne bacteria. Journal of Hospital Infection 1987; 9 (1): 85–8.

Maurer IM Hospital Hygiene, 3rd Edition. London: Edward Arnold, 1985.

Medical Research Council. Design and ventilation of operating suites. Lancet 1962; (ii): 943.

Meers PD, Leong KY Hot-air hand driers. Journal of Hospital Infection 1989; 14: 169–81.

Mennie K Air today, gone tomorrow. Nursing Times Infection Control Supplement 1997; 93 (11).

Millard G Commissioning Hospital Buildings: A King's Fund Guide. London: King Edward's Hospital Fund for London, 1981.

Mims CA, Playfair JHL, Roitt IM, Wakelin D, Williams R, Anderson RM Medical Microbiology. London: Mosby, 1993.

NHS Executive. Guidelines for Implementing Controls Assurance in the NHS (Guidelines for Directors) Leeds: NHSE, 1999.

Public Health Medicine Environmental Group (PHMEG). Guidelines on the Control of Infection in Residential and Nursing Homes. London: PHMEG, 1995.

Stevens J, Miller J Opening a Hospital is Easy ... Isn't It? South East Thames Regional Health Authority, 1982.

Wilson J Infection Control in Clinical Practice. London: Bailliere Tindall, 1995.

Worsley MA, Ward KA, Privett S, Parker L, Roberts JM Infection Control: A Community Perspective. Cambridge: Infection Control Nurses' Association, 1994.

UK Health Department. Guidance for Healthcare Workers: Protection Against HIV and Hepatitis Viruses. Recommendations of the Expert Advisory Group on AIDS. London: HMSO, 1990.

Chapter 6
Waste management

JANET MCCULLOCH

Introduction

A fully functioning waste disposal system does not cause a second thought, but when the system breaks down the relentless daily generation of waste quickly becomes visible and unacceptable, as noxious odours are emitted and vermin attracted. Happily such events are rare, and waste is generally collected regularly and carted off for final disposal either to a landfill site or an incinerator. However, in recent years it has become clear that the disposal of waste is placing increasing pressure on the environment, whatever its final destination.

Until recently incinerators for the burning of clinical waste could be found in many hospitals, large and small, and in nursing homes bonfires would be lit for this purpose. There was little control over the maintenance or operating standards of these incineration methods. The disposal of sharps in the past was also very different to today. Used needles might be bent or inserted into the rubber plunger of the syringe before being discarded into cardboard boxes which were sealed with tape and labelled 'sharps' with a felt tip pen. Concerns over health and safety and the environment resulted in the introduction of legislation which now affects us all, but particularly those of us engaged in healthcare in hospitals, the community or even in the patient's own home. This legislation is becoming increasingly complex and rigorous, requiring careful consideration and implementation.

Legislation

In 1991 the government published the Environmental Protection Act (EPA), 1990 (Department of Environment, 1991) which removed

Crown Immunity from the health service and introduced the concept of a Duty of Care in the disposal of waste. This Duty of Care requires managers to prevent others from committing offences, prevent the escape of waste, transfer waste to authorized individuals only and complete required documentation. Failure to comply with these requirements is a criminal offence and managers have legal and personal liability (NHS Executive, 1994). Ordinary householders are exempt from the Duty of Care, even if they generate waste which may be classified as controlled waste in clinical settings. The EPA also specified standards for operational incinerators to ensure that the by-products of incineration (both solid waste and smoke emissions) are controlled. The costs of attempting to meet the new standards will be very high for individual hospitals so the use of private sector incinerators will inevitably become more commonplace (NHS Executive, 1994a). Legislation also requires that waste is accompanied by documentation and that those involved in the process, including transport and disposal, are licensed (NHS Estates, 1997). Alternatives to incineration, such as microwaving, are being developed.

In response to the legislation the NHS Executive produced guidelines to help NHS managers develop their waste policies so that they comply not only with the EPA, but also the Health and Safety at Work Act 1974 (HASAW) and the Control of Substances Hazardous to Health Regulations 1988 (COSHH). These Acts aim to protect the employee and any others who may come into contact with hazards such as waste either directly or indirectly. The key themes of the guidance produced by the NHSE were: risk assessment; categories of waste; segregation of waste; storage; specification of containers; transport; handling; training; protective clothing; accident and incident reporting and investigation; spillage procedures and final disposal. All of these elements will be considered later in this chapter. The Audit Commission (1997) found that the NHS was wasting a great deal of money by inappropriately managing waste, therefore managers should review existing procedures and examine methods of minimizing the volume of waste generated by their organization.

Waste minimization

Minimization of the volume of waste generated can help to ease pressure on the environment and produce a more sustainable society as well as reduce the costs of disposal. The concept of 'the polluter pays' is increasingly being incorporated into public policy, for example the disposal of waste by landfill is subject to a 'landfill tax' which will increase the costs of the disposal of waste by this method; some waste is categorized as 'special waste' requiring additional documentation and fees.

Waste minimization can be achieved in a number of ways, as outlined below.

Minimize volume of waste

Reduce the volume of waste coming into the organization, for example by replacing disposable boxes used to transport supplies with re-usable baskets.

Re-use items

Purchase returnable items where possible. For example some suppliers may be able to re-use the cardboard containers they use for delivery. Repair items rather than discard them, to prolong their lifespan and reduce waste. Re-allocate items; for example an obsolete cardiac monitor in one intensive care unit could be high technology elsewhere; unwanted or obsolete beds and mattresses might be of use to others. Items can be sold or given away if they are serviceable.

Recover materials

Some waste may be recovered for further use. For example, waste water in certain dishwashers is used as the pre-wash in the next cycle. Energy and heat may also be recovered. Recycling of materials such as paper, glass, plastics, oils and fabrics is also possible, although sometimes this can be an expensive option depending upon market forces.

Risk assessment

Risk is related to the probability of loss, injury or infection as a result of exposure to a hazard. The main aim of risk control is to reduce the risk to the lowest possible level by either eliminating or avoiding the hazard (NHS Estates, 1994b). The EPA states that 'any waste can be hazardous if it is wrongly managed'. The hazards associated with the disposal of waste include manual handling problems, the presence of sharp objects and the containment of waste and microbiological hazards. In addition to the known hazards of waste, there is also an issue of aesthetics. It is not pleasant to be in contact with, or even to see, items such as used nappies, incontinence pads, stoma bags, etc. and in particular human tissue such as placentae or amputated limbs.

According to Ayliffe et al. (1992), the risks of infection associated with waste from clinical settings, which is generally termed 'clinical waste', are no greater than waste which arises from the home. The micro-organisms that cause most concern require specific conditions for life and die easily. Keene (1991) describes them as truly 'bio-degradable'. Therefore it would seem paradoxical to separate out clinical waste for special treatment in that the nature of the waste, and the micro-organisms contained in the waste, are usually indistinguishable from waste disposed of in the home. For example, in gynaecological wards sanitary towels are treated as clinical waste yet they are put into the dustbin once the same patients are at home. There is little difference between incontinence pads from patients on an elderly care ward and babies' nappies, yet the pads are carefully put into a yellow bag and incinerated whilst the nappies are destined for landfill. A person who is admitted to hospital, having contracted gastroenteritis from a contaminated chicken, will find that their waste will be classified as clinical waste but the offending chicken will have been put out with the rest of the rubbish at home.

Collins and Kennedy (1992) argue that the fears associated with clinical waste have no scientific basis. If it is handled, packaged, transported and disposed of with care the risk to public health is insignificant. Unfortunately these steps cannot always be guaranteed and, with the added problem of public fears, healthcare managers are required to comply with legislation and national guidance on the disposal of waste. In the home there is often more room for flexibility because the waste generated at home is considered to be of low risk and produced in small volumes. In some circumstances in the home it may be possible to dispose of clinical waste in the household waste stream (Report of the Working Party of the RCN, 1994). However, higher risk waste such as sharps and contaminated waste from patients with highly communicable diseases must have special arrangements made for its disposal. Some waste may need to be categorized as 'special waste' because it has specific safety requirements.

A waste disposal policy, which includes guidance for staff on the assessment of risk, should be agreed between the local environmental agency and the Consultant for Communicable Disease Control. In hospitals an individual manager must be assigned the responsibility for ensuring that such a policy is in place and for monitoring its implementation.

Segregation of waste and methods of disposal

Segregation of waste must occur at all stages of the waste handling process. Segregation begins at the point of generation and initiates a series of actions that ensure the waste reaches its final destination with minimal hazard. Incorrect segregation may result in either clinical or special waste entering the household waste stream, for which senior managers may be prosecuted; or household waste entering the clinical waste stream to be needlessly incinerated, which is expensive.

A national colour coding system which is based on the principles of risk assessment was described by the Working Group of the Health Services Advisory Committee (1992). Five categories of waste were identified which are applicable in all settings including the home, hospitals, nursing homes, GP practices, laboratories, dentists, chiropodists, ambulances, etc. The colour coding of the waste bags acts a visual indicator denoting the nature of the waste (see Table 6.1).

The location and size of waste containers are of crucial importance to the correct segregation of waste. Health Technical Memorandum 2065 provides guidance in determining best practice in local areas (NHS Estates, 1997). It is also important to ensure the provision of adequate supplies of good quality bags, sharps containers, pedal bins and storage room. In clinical areas it may be tempting to place yellow bags in every bin, but this will discourage segregation of waste. In addition, discarding clinical waste such as dressings and incontinence pads into bins in patient areas will inevitably lead to offensive odours permeating the ward or bedroom. To avoid this, clinical waste should be bagged at the bedside and then taken to a designated area such as a dirty utility room or waste disposal point for storage. Double bagging is unnecessary, even for waste from isolation rooms, unless the first bag splits (Maki et al., 1986).

Table 6.1 Waste disposal policy: colour coding

Container colour and type	Waste type
Black plastic bags	Paper towels; flowers; all domestic, normal household waste EXCEPT broken glass, china.
Yellow plastic bags	Dressings; swabs; contaminated waste; large quantities of sanitary towels; nappies. Tied and labelled with ward name.
Yellow sharps containers	Sharps; needles; syringes; glass ampules; blades; razors, etc. - Cytotoxic waste labelled. - Low-level radioactive waste labelled.
Marked pedal bin • Clear liner • Black liner	 Glass; china; cans. Food waste.
Yellow approved lockable container	Human tissue; placentae; blood, contaminated equipment, e.g. drains. - Cytotoxic waste labelled. - Low-level radioactive waste labelled.

Laboratory clinical waste

It is usually recommended that contaminated laboratory waste such as culture plates, used swabs, etc., should be autoclaved before being incinerated. However, there may be a local agreement that the waste is secured in a locked bin before incineration as an alternative to autoclaving (Ayliffe et al., 1992). The locked bin prevents the escape of waste.

Blood and body fluid waste

At times large quantities of body fluids, including blood, will need to be disposed of. Often the best method of disposal is to use a macerator, slop hopper or bedpan washer and discharge the waste into the sewerage system (Philpott-Howard and Casewell, 1994). Health service managers must ensure that any discharge into the sewerage system complies with current regulations. Contractors, especially on hospital sites, may wish to be informed of this and the best advice to them is to remind them of universal precautions and the use of appropriate protective clothing.

It is important to continually assess the method of disposal and seek safer methods which eliminate the risk of personal contamination. For example, suction waste can be made safer by introducing disposable suction liners which contain the fluid until it is incinerated. Liquid waste can be turned into a gel by using a desiccating powder. This may be particularly useful on ambulances and for patients who often spill the contents of their urinals due to poor eyesight or shaky hands. The gel is easily removed by running water or can be macerated. Liquid waste from home births can be contained in rigid clinical waste containers which have lockable lids, are puncture-resistant and leak-proof. As they are opaque, handlers cannot see the contents which they may have found distressing or offensive. Similar containers may be used for the containment of used surgical drains, blood administration sets and bags of venesected blood.

Foetal tissue

Foetal tissue and foetuses arising from miscarriage or termination of pregnancy are particularly sensitive. The parents may feel distressed if they believe that the remains of their child are not handled with respect. Guidance on this issue has been produced by the NHS Executive and this should provide the basis for local policy (NHS Management Executive 1991 a and b). The basic principles of the guidance are that the remains must be incinerated or cremated, but must never be macerated or sluiced; the wishes of the parents must be taken into account; opaque containers must be used for storage until final disposal; support services staff must not be compelled to handle the remains against their wishes.

Other human tissue

Human tissues, such as amputated limbs, must not be mixed with the general clinical waste and must be treated with respect; therefore security is essential. In the past the incineration of such waste would be witnessed by a responsible person such as the head porter. However, today incineration often takes place off-site, perhaps many miles away from the point of origin. Consequently the waste must be secured at all stages and refrigeration may be necessary if collection is delayed (Working Group of the Health Services Advisory Committee, 1992).

Clinical waste from the home

There are various possible methods of managing clinical waste arising from the home, and it is important to refer to local policy. Low-risk waste from the patient's own home could be carefully wrapped in at least one plastic bag and stored away from scavengers awaiting transportation to the landfill site. This must be placed in either a black plastic bag, or a yellow bag with a black stripe. High-risk clinical waste should be placed in a yellow plastic bag and a special collection arranged with the waste disposal agency.

Some community health providers require their staff to carry the waste in purpose-built containers in their vehicles (Wilson, 1995). Problems with this include: the frequency of handling waste is increased; there is a risk of contaminating sterile or clean items which may also be transported; personal items such as groceries may also be contaminated; there may be problems with the volume of waste to be carried.

Sharps containers must always be incinerated and need to be taken either to the surgery or to a local hospital by the patient, a friend or the healthcare worker. Alternatively, a special collection may be arranged with the disposal agency. If the container is taken to a hospital this needs to be agreed in advance. Patients who inject themselves should be supplied with a sharps container. Needle clippers are the next best option, but the clipper usually leaves a small stump of needle which must be discarded with great care. General practitioners must not neglect their responsibility for ensuring that the by-products of treatment are disposed of safely.

Storage

Waste must be stored in safe manner, but procedures will vary depending upon the individual circumstances. As a general rule waste should not be stored in corridors or other public areas and the storage area must be secured to prevent vandals and scavengers from tampering with the waste. The area should also be protected from the weather, well lit and access restricted to authorized personnel only (HSAC, 1999). The frequency of collections will depend upon the volume of waste generated and the nature of the waste.

The waste must at all times be securely packaged in appropriate containers and systems must be in place to prevent unnecessary handling, which would increase the risk of injury. Ideally as the waste is produced it should be placed directly into the container that will transport it to its final destination, i.e. incinerator or landfill site. Unfortunately such systems are not always available and bags of waste are often decanted from one container to another (NHS Estates, 1997).

Containers

Pedal bins

Pedal-operated containers should be available for the immediate storage of waste, and they should be lined with a plastic bag of the appropriate colour. The pedal bins must be of a size appropriate for the volume of waste generated at the location and placed wherever needed. They should also be washable and cleaned regularly using detergent and water. The foot-operated mechanism must be checked and maintained. Staff must not use their hands to lift the lid of the container because this will contaminate their hands.

Other types of container

Containers such as wheelie bins are often used to store several bags of waste whilst awaiting collection. These must be of an appropriate size, lockable and kept locked at all times; all relevant staff must therefore be provided with a key. Keene (1991) identified the safe transportation of waste as a key factor in a safe system of waste disposal. This involves designating vehicles for this purpose alone and ensuring their cleanliness, security and roadworthiness. The containers should be cleaned on a regular basis and after any spillage of waste. Sometimes a steam cleaner or disinfectant (such as hypochlorite) may be recommended. In either case the operator must wear personal protective clothing. Containers do not need to be soaked in a disinfectant or deodorized if they are kept clean and dry.

Waste bags

Plastic sacks must comply with current regulations and be marked 'clinical waste for incineration'. They must never be more than two-thirds full. This allows room for tying, prevents the bag bursting because of excessive pressure, avoids the need to decant waste into a second bag, and protects handlers from lifting heavy loads. There are a number of methods for tying clinical waste bags to prevent spillage of waste from the bag in transit. These methods include using a plastic tie or clip, tying a knot or using tape. If a knot is tied, the spare material should be able to function as a handle.

It should be possible to trace the source of the waste in the event of an incident in order to help assess the risks to the injured party, or for audit purposes to identify areas of poor compliance. Ties, clips and tape can be produced pre-printed with a code number or the name of the site where the waste was produced. Sticky labels are an alternative method, or the name of the source could be printed directly on the bag in indelible ink. From 1 January 2002 clinical waste must be transported in rigid containers (Carriage of Dangerous Goods Act, 1999).

Sharps containers

Sharps containers must not only conform to British Standard BS7320 (See Table 6.2) and UN 3921. Sharps containers must be available where needed so that used sharps do not have to be carried long distances. They must be assembled correctly and checked before use to ensure that the lid is firmly attached. The aperture should be closed between uses to prevent accidental spillage and to stop children and others from putting their fingers inside. Brackets can usually be used to position the containers out of reach of children. The aperture must be locked when the container is two-thirds full to prevent needlestick injury and avoid carrying heavy loads.

The source must be identified either by completing an attached label or printing in indelible ink. Sharps containers must always be carried by their integral handle and should never be placed within a plastic bag because of the danger of unseen protruding sharps causing injury in the event of a spillage.

Hypodermic needles should not be re-sheathed before disposal. Re-sheathing is associated with needlestick injury, with the BMA claiming that 33% of such injuries result from re-sheathing (BMA,

Table 6.2 BS7320, UN 3921 Sharps containers

- Must have a handle if appropriate
- Must be ready assembled, or have assembly instructions
- Must have apertures which close securely
- Must be rigid and puncture-resistant
- Must have a line indicating the fill level
- Must have the maker's name
- Must not leak
- Must not come apart once assembled
- Must be yellow
- Must be marked 'Danger, contaminated sharps only, destroy by incineration'
- Should show the kite mark

Adapted from Legge (1996)

1990). It is the responsibility of the individual user of the needle or sharp object to dispose of it him- or herself. Practitioners should be in the habit of taking a sharps container with them whenever they use a sharp instrument so that it can be discarded directly into the sharps container immediately after use. It is unacceptable to expect another person to clear away trays and dressing trolleys, etc., especially when needles, sutures, scalpels, etc., have been used. Failure to comply with this should result in disciplinary action being taken. Unfortunately it is not always possible to identify the offender, even though the consequences for the injured party can be life-threatening. Collins and Kennedy (1987) reviewed the literature concerning the microbiological hazards of needlestick injuries and described the range of infections which could be transmitted percutaneously. These included human immunodeficiency virus, hepatitis B and C, streptococcus, herpes and diphtheria, amongst many others. They quote many studies into needlestick injuries which demonstrate that such injuries not only affect nurses and doctors – the main users of needles – but also domestics and porters. Begley (1994) describes an incident in which a nurse lost a finger through systemic infection which developed after sustaining an injury caused by a scalpel. Many of these injuries could be prevented by adopting safe systems of handling sharps, including not re-sheathing needles, using 'sharpless systems' such as the Unistik lancet which has a retractable sheath, and by safe disposal.

Staff health

In compliance with the Health and Safety at Work Act (1974) and Control of Substances Hazardous to Health Regulations (1988), staff who are engaged in the handling of waste must be provided with the necessary training, personal protective clothing, immunization against tetanus and hepatitis B and have knowledge of the agreed procedures for general handling of waste and the management of spillages and other unforeseen incidents (NHS Executive, 1994b).

Training

Training in the management of waste must be compulsory for all staff according to their degree of involvement in the process. Training programmes should involve issues such as: the hazards of waste disposal; the segregation of waste and the colour coding system; the legislation and responsibilities of employers and employees; correct procedures and protective clothing to be worn; and procedures for dealing with spillages and injuries (NHS Estates, 1995). Training should be provided on induction and at regular follow-up sessions (Branson, 1995).

Visual reminders are useful in maintaining awareness, and posters which show the local policy in an interesting way should be displayed prominently (Collins and Kennedy, 1987). Manufacturers often produce attractive posters that can be used on a rotational basis or for specific sharps awareness campaigns. Messages can also be displayed on computer screens, in newsletters and on notice boards, together with information such as the results of audits of waste disposal, or the number and causes of reported incidents, etc.

Protective clothing

Good quality gloves are the most important type of protective clothing needed for handling waste. Nurses and domestics usually wear disposable latex or vinyl gloves for this purpose. This is because they handle relatively small volumes of waste in controlled circumstances, i.e. they know what they are dealing with. Porters and others involved in the transportation of waste from place to place should have heavy-duty gloves which are able to withstand the wear and tear of carrying large volumes of waste and moving heavy cages or wheelie bins. The gloves should also provide a certain degree of protection from sharps injuries. Heavy-duty gloves are re-usable and should be checked to ensure they are in good condition and remain puncture-free. They should be kept clean by washing with detergent and water after use and dried thoroughly. Hands should always be washed after removing gloves of any kind.

Staff should also wear sturdy shoes to protect them from falling objects, etc., but this is particularly important for porters who manoeuvre vehicles and large containers (HSAC, 1999). Eye protection may also be necessary for those operating steam cleaners; and plastic aprons, or overalls, worn if splash is anticipated or when spillages are dealt with.

Management of incidents

Injuries are often sustained through the incorrect disposal of waste. Many of these injuries could be prevented through education and safer working practices. However, when they do occur it is important that the correct procedures are then followed to minimize the risk of serious infection. Every workplace where needles or other such sharp instruments are used should have a written inoculation injury procedure in place which has been agreed in collaboration with the occupational health department, trades unions and infection control team. Staff must have ready access to this either in poster form, within a policy manual or as a personal aide-memoire. Managers and safety advisers should analyse local incident statistics and trends to identify their main causes and introduce safer procedures where possible.

People who sustain an injury from a sharp object in the street, especially if contaminated with blood, should carry out the first aid measures and then discuss the incident with their GP who should offer advice regarding the risks of infection and administer any required treatment. Healthcare workers who are involved in the management of waste should all receive immunization against hepatitis B and tetanus.

The management of spillages of waste

Procedures for the management of spillages of sharps and other waste should always be included in a waste disposal policy. The main aims are to prevent immediate injury, render the waste safe and prevent further injury or contamination. Examples can be seen in Tables 6.3 and 6.4.

Table 6.3 Management of spillage from a clinical waste bag

- Wear heavy-duty gloves
- Place the damaged bag together with its remaining contents into a second yellow bag
- Collect the spilled contents and carefully place into the second bag
- Avoid contaminating the outside surface of the second bag
- Secure the second bag in the usual manner
- If appropriate clean the contaminated surface and leave dry
- Wash the gloves (or discard) followed by handwashing

Table 6.4 Management of spillage from a sharps container

- Wear-heavy duty gloves
- Secure the damaged container if possible
- If this is not possible then place it inside a second larger container
- Carefully collect the spilled contents, using a dustpan and brush or forceps
- Place the sharps into either the original or the second container
- Lock the container and dispose of it in the usual manner
- Clean the contaminated area if necessary
- Wash the gloves (or discard) followed by handwashing

Audit

As part of risk management and infection control programmes the audit of waste disposal procedures should be incorporated into an annual plan. Incidents should be reported as they happen and these reports should be reviewed and analysed on a regular basis and the findings communicated to senior managers and relevant staff groups. An audit tool should be devised and implemented either by managers, staff or audit assistants. Issues which should be audited include: segregation of waste, correct loading and tying of waste bags, wearing of protective clothing, handling of waste, locking of bins, safe storage, correct disposal of sharps.

Table 6.5 presents an example of a simple audit tool which was devised to audit the disposal of sharps on an ongoing basis. Responsibility for this may be delegated to one member of staff who regularly examines every sharps container in the locality and indicates correct procedure with a ✓, and incorrect procedure with a ✗. These are counted and the percentage score for compliance with each element of the standard is calculated.

Table 6.5 Sharps audit tool

Assessment criteria	Y/N	Comments	Score
Sharps disposal			
Containers are securely fastened	✓✓✗		66%
Containers are less than two-thirds full	✓✓✓		100%
Containers are labelled with name of ward/dept	✓✗✗		33%
No sharps are protruding from the container	✓✓✓		100%
Average score			75%

References

Audit Commission. Getting Sorted –The Safe and Economic Management of Hospital Waste. London: Audit Commission, 1997.

Ayliffe GAJ, Lowbury EJL, Geddes EM, Williams JD Control of Hospital Infection: A practical handbook, 3rd edition. London: Chapman and Hall Medical, 1992.

Begley DK Undiscarded contaminated sharps are lethal weapons. Journal of Emergency Nursing 1994; 20 (6): 444.

Branson M Hazards of sharps disposal. British Journal of Nursing 1995; 4 (4): 193–5.

British Medical Association. A Code of Practice for the Safe Disposal of Sharps. London: BMA, 1990.

Carriage of Dangerous Goods Act 1999. Classification, packaging and labelling Regs 1996 Amendment.

Collins CH, Kennedy DA Microbiological hazards of occupational needle-stick and sharps injury. Journal of Applied Bacteriology 1987; 62: 385–402.

Collins CH, Kennedy DA Microbiological hazards of municipal and clinical waste. Journal of Applied Bacteriology 1992; 73: 1–6.

Daschner F Unnecessary cost of hospital infection. Journal of Infection 1991; 18 (suppl. A): 73–8.

Dept of Environment. Environmental Protection Act (1990). London: HMSO, 1991.

Health Services Advisory Committee (HSAC). The Safe Disposal of Clinical Waste. Norwich: HMSO, 1999.

Jagger J Rates of needle-stick injuries caused by various devices in a university hospital. New England Journal of Medicine 1988; 318: 284–8.

Keene JH Medical waste: a minimal hazard. Infection Control Hospital Epidemiology 1991; 12 (11): 682–5.

Legge A Sharps disposal systems. Professional Nurse 1996; 12 (1): 57–62.

Maki DG, Alvarado C, Hessemer C Double bagging of items from isolation rooms is unnecessary as an infection control measure. Infection Control 1986; 7 (5): 35–7.

NHS Estates. Health Service Guidance Note: Safe Disposal of Clinical Waste, Whole Hospital Policy Guidance. London: HMSO, 1995.

NHS Estates. Health Technical Memorandum 2065: Healthcare Waste Management – Segregation of Waste Streams in Clinical Areas. London: Stationery Office, 1997.

NHS Executive. Health Service Guidance: Clinical Waste Management (HSG(94)50). Heywood: BAPS, 1994a.

NHS Executive. Risk Management in the NHS. Heywood: BAPS, 1994b.

NHS Management Executive. Health Service Guidelines: Disposal of Foetal Tissue HSG(91)19. Heywood: BAPS, 1991a.

NHS Management Executive. Sensitive Disposal of Dead Foetus and Foetal Tissue EL(91)144. Heywood: BAPS, 1991b.

Philpott-Howard J, Casewell M. Hospital Infection Control: Policy and Practical Procedures. London: WB Saunders Co Ltd, 1994.

Report of the Working Party of the RCN. Disposal of Healthcare Waste in the Community. London: RCN, 1994.

Wilson J Infection Control in Clinical Practice. London: Baillière-Tindall, 1995.

Chapter 7
Laundry issues

JANET McCULLOCH

Introduction

The National Health Service produces thousands of pieces of used linen every day of the week, much of this is heavily fouled with body fluids, sometimes of an infectious nature. Added to this are the many items produced within nursing and residential homes and in the home setting, where so much healthcare is carried out today.

Sometimes laundering of soiled linen will be undertaken on-site, but often laundry is transported great distances to a commercial laundry. The risks of cross-infection occur at all stages of the laundry process: handling; packaging; transporting; laundering and delivery of clean supplies. These risks need to be minimized to safeguard the health and wellbeing of staff and patients. For this reason it is important that all organizations which are responsible for the care of the ill or vulnerable consider the risks and processes involved and develop workable policy and procedures which are consistent with current national guidelines.

Risks of cross-infection

Although linen may be contaminated with body fluids which may carry disease, or with mites such as scabies, head lice, pubic lice, etc., which can be disturbing for laundry handlers, there is little risk if correct procedures are followed.

Cross-infection has occurred where contaminated linen has caused gastroenteritis in laundry workers in a nursing home (Standaert et al., 1994), and has also been identified as a possible source of *Bacillus cereus* meningitis in patients following neurosurgery (Barrie et al., 1992) (see Table 7.1). Sharps injuries may also occur if items such as used needles and instruments are carelessly discarded into laundry bags. These, and more innocuous objects such as bedpans and pot-plants, may damage the washing machines or cause injuries if not found and removed.

However the risks to health and equipment may be negligible if sensible precautions are taken in the safe handling and thermal disinfection of used linen and the prevention of recontamination of clean linen.

Table 7.1 Examples of potential pathogens in fouled laundry

Body fluid	Potential pathogens
Faeces (esp. diarrhoea)	Salmonella Cryptosporidium Rotavirus Hepatitis A Clostridium difficile
Urine	Cytomegalovirus Coliforms
Blood	HIV Hepatitis B Hepatitis C
Wound exudate	MRSA Streptococcus group A Varicella

(Borton, 1995)

Handling used linen

The laundry process begins at the bedside when used linen is removed and sent off to the laundry. At this stage there is considerable risk of personal contamination, particularly if the linen is soiled or fouled with excreta and body fluids. Linen that is not visibly soiled will be contaminated with skin scales which have been shed into the bedclothes, and adhering to these squames are skin organisms that may be pathogenic in some circumstances, such as *Staphylococcus aureus* or methicillin-resistant *Staphylococcus aureus* (MRSA). Shaking the sheets, and other careless handling, will disseminate these micro-organisms into the air, and they may eventually come to rest on exposed wounds, or add to the layer of dust on horizontal surfaces such as curtain rails or bed frames. Overton (1988) demonstrated an increase in personal contamination during bedmaking by identifying 11/15 instances of finger contamination after contact with used linen for as little as 90 seconds.

For these reasons it is important to adopt simple rules during bedmaking (see Table 7.2).

Table 7.2 Rules to adopt during bedmaking

Action	Rationale
• Wear an apron	minimize contamination of clothing
• Wear disposable gloves if linen is soiled	minimize contamination of hands
• Never shake linen	prevent dissemination of squames
• Roll linen carefully	prevent dissemination of squames
• Do not place on floor or furniture	prevent contamination of environment
• Do not allow linen to touch uniform/clothing	prevent contamination of clothing
• Place directly into skip	prevent contamination of environment
• Sort linen in the laundry	prevent personal and environmental contamination (Borton, 1995)
• Handwash after handling	remove any micro-organisms acquired during bedmaking

Packaging of used linen

Those involved in packaging (bagging) of used linen must be aware of their duty of care to others who will be handling the linen at later stages, and ensure that no action or omission on their part will put others at risk. Consequently staff must always be vigilant in preventing concealed sharps and other extraneous items from being sent to the laundry with the linen.

The NHS Executive (1995) has published procedures to protect laundry workers, including a colour coding system. This system helps staff working in laundries which may be remote from the ward or nursing home etc. to identify whether the linen is high or low risk and handle it appropriately. The NHSE identified three categories of used linen (see Table 7.3).

Table 7.3 Categories of used linen

Category	Description	Colour code
1. Used linen	Linen which is soiled or fouled with excretions, but not considered to be infectious	White linen bags
2. Infected linen	Contaminated linen from those with a known or suspected communicable disease, e.g. salmonella, hepatitis A, B, C, HIV, chickenpox, shingles, etc.	Place in a water-soluble bag (or seam membrane) before dispatch
3. Heat labile linen	Linen which cannot withstand hot-water washing. This may require dry cleaning or low-temperature washing	White linen bag with an orange stripe

Duvets

Increasingly equipment such as duvets and pressure relieving-devices are being used in healthcare. These can become sources of infection if not kept clean (Croton, 1990), yet repeated laundering may damage the fabric. When purchasing such equipment it is important to check that it can withstand frequent laundering. Where possible such items should be protected with a washable cover to reduce the need for laundering (Webster et al., 1986).

Staff uniforms

Nurses' uniforms are not worn as protective clothing, therefore they should always be protected from gross contamination by a plastic apron (Brewer, 1996). Some employers will make arrangements for laundering uniforms, while others may expect the staff to make their own arrangements.

In many areas staff are permitted to wear their own clothes in order to make healthcare less clinical – for example for home deliveries and in community mental health units, etc. In these circumstances staff should wear clothes that are practical, clean and washable (Walker and Donaldson, 1993).

Laundering uniforms at home is acceptable because the risks of infection are slight. The clothing should be laundered separately at the highest temperature the fabric will withstand, then dried thoroughly and ironed. However, arrangements should be made for grossly contaminated uniforms to be laundered in the central laundry (Ayliffe and Collins, 1989).

Laundering procedures

The most effective method for ensuring that used linen is disinfected is by machine washing, otherwise known as thermal disinfection. Maurer (1985) experimented with different methods of disinfecting floor mops and showed that they remained heavily contaminated after handwashing in hot water and after soaking in a chemical disinfectant. Only machine laundering was effective. Steeping soiled linen in chemicals is a waste of time and money and may unnecessarily expose the laundry worker to potentially hazardous chemicals.

Washing machines

Hospital laundries use two main types of washing machine a) continuous batch tunnel washers and b) washer-extractors.

Continuous batch tunnel washers

These are used for general laundering of used, soiled and fouled linen. The linen is sorted by hand before or after the wash cycle, weighed and loaded into the machine in batches of a pre-determined weight. The batch proceeds through several compartments within the machine which subject the linen to pre-wash, disinfection and rinse cycles. Fresh water enters the machine at the rinse stage and moves through the compartments in the opposite direction to the linen. A proportion of the water and heat is re-used so these machines are very economical. The process is computerized, including the automatic addition of washing powders and other chemicals.

Washer-extractors

These have a much smaller capacity than continuous batch tunnel washers and fresh water is used for each wash and rinse cycle (Barrie, 1994). This type of machine is used for the laundering of infected linen, which should not be sorted prior to loading because of the increased risks of transmission of infection to the staff. The linen should be contained within a water-soluble bag which is placed directly into the washer-extractor and dissolves in the machine so that the laundry workers do not have to handle the linen. Unfortunately, the fact that the laundry is not sorted will increase the chances of extraneous items entering the machine unnoticed, and these may cause some damage.

Healthcare facilities may instal domestic washing machines in order to launder patients' personal clothing; however this should be the exception rather than the rule because of the risks of cross-contamination. It is preferable to send the laundry home to be laundered or to ensure that any commercial contract includes this service. Where washing machines are installed, an industrial-type washing machine with a sluice cycle is ideal and there should be agreed procedures for arrangements in the event of an outbreak, especially if the personal items cannot be thermally disinfected (Ayliffe et al., 1992).

Even in small units, laundering procedures and recommended temperatures should be clearly specified and a system of planned preventive maintenance in place to ensure that correct temperatures are reached and filters are changed, etc.

Temperatures and holding times

Standard disinfection temperatures and holding times have been specified by the NHS Executive (1995) (see Table 7.4).

Additional holding times must be added to take account of mixing, dependent on the weight of the load.

The unreliability of chemical disinfection means that heat-labile fabrics which have been contaminated with potentially infectious substances may not be adequately disinfected by dry cleaning or low-temperature washing. In most circumstances it is unlikely that the addition of sodium hypochlorite will be possible. In addition, personal clothing and flameproofed fabrics may be damaged by the chemicals. Therefore heat-labile fabrics should be avoided when purchasing items such as soft furnishings, curtains, etc.

Table 7.4 Temperatures and holding times for disinfection of linen

Type of linen	Temperature	Holding times
General linen	65°C 71°C	10 minutes 3 minutes
Heat-labile linen	40°C	5 minutes + 150 ppm sodium hypochlorite added to penultimate rinse

Quality control

Quality control in commercial or hospital laundries is maintained by adhering to the thermal disinfection procedures and through quality checks. Microbiological testing of linen is not usually of any value, except perhaps in the event of an outbreak if there is reason to suspect the linen as a possible source of the infection (Ayliffe et al., 1992).

A number of design features should be built into the laundry and washing machines to prevent aerosol contamination of the environment and of the clean linen, and to ensure thermal disinfection. These include:

- The calibration and testing of the machines on at least a 6-weekly basis
- Retention and analysis of records of the temperatures and holding times
- Rinse sections should be thermally disinfected at the start of each working day and if the machines are shut down for more than 3 hours
- Emergency procedures should be in place to manage breakdowns
- Open drains and sumps must be covered
- Pipe-work must be vented to the outside of the building
- The flow of the laundry should be from dirty to clean
- Machines, conveyors and other surfaces must be kept clean and free from algae and lint
- Planned preventive maintenance programmes.

(NHS Executive, 1995)

Transportation of linen

Careful carriage and the separation of used and clean linen is an important part of reducing infection risks (Garner and Favero, 1985). The dirty linen may be placed within linen skips, or linen baskets in community settings. If overfilled, the linen skips may present a manual handling problem and the surplus linen will need to be decanted into another container. Therefore containers should never be more than two-thirds full.

Clean and dirty linen should be transported separately or separated by a barrier. If the same container (basket, trolley or vehicle) is used for carrying clean linen after it has carried dirty linen, the container should be cleaned thoroughly between uses (NHS Executive, 1995). To accomplish this standard, commercial laundry vehicles may deliver clean linen to a site, or series of sites, before retracing the route to collect the dirty load. Alternatively two vehicles may be used, one for the clean load and a second for the dirty load. If there is a spillage of dirty linen, the contaminated surfaces must be cleaned thoroughly; some local policies recommend the use of a disinfectant.

Prevention of cross-contamination

Cross-contamination can occur at all stages of the laundering process if procedures are not followed. As previously mentioned, care must be taken to prevent this in the handling, packaging and transportation of linen. Clean linen can be contaminated if stored on the floor or touching the ceiling; if stored on dirty shelving; if over-stocked shelves allow dust to gather; or if stored near to sinks and slop hoppers, etc. Items must be sent back for re-washing if the linen has become contaminated in any way (Borton, 1995).

Procedures within the laundry are also of great importance. The linen should proceed in one direction only, from delivery of soiled linen through the washing, drying, pressing and packaging section, to the dispatch of the finished products. In smaller laundries and launderettes, the area of work is smaller than in commercial laundries and there are fewer defined procedures and quality systems. Therefore things may go wrong more easily, although the outcome of such problems will be on a smaller scale. In these facilities clean linen must be kept separate from soiled linen, and dried quickly after washing. The room must be kept clean, dry and lint-free and any spillages cleaned up quickly. Use of water-soluble bags can prevent personal and environmental contamination even in nursing homes and community homes.

Standaert et al. (1994) described an outbreak of salmonella gastroenteritis in a nursing home in which 32/222 residents and 8/244 staff had positive stool cultures. The residents had been infected by food which none of the staff had consumed. Symptoms in the staff began 7–10 days after the residents had been infected. Four nurses, 3 laundry workers and 1 cook were affected. The laundry workers had had no direct contact with the affected patients, other than handling diarrhoea-soaked linen. It was later found that the laundry workers ate their meals in the laundry room, they were inconsistent in their use of gloves and there was no regular cleaning of the laundry room.

Staff health

Managers and employers must ensure that the occupational health and safety of staff is maintained by the institution of good hygienic procedures; provision of personal protective clothing and enforcement of its use; the inoculation of staff against infection such as hepatitis B; and there should be good facilities for handwashing (NHS Executive, 1995; Barrie, 1994). Sometimes local procedures will need to be translated into other languages or accompanied by illustrations. Procedures for preventing inoculation injury should be enforced and there should be an inoculation injury procedure (Barrie, 1994). Staff must also receive training in all aspects on the policy and procedures (NHS Executive, 1995; Murdoch, 1992).

Management arrangements

When reviewing laundry facilities a multi-disciplinary approach should be adopted to ensure that all aspects of the required service are considered. The working group should include, as appropriate to the service, the laundry manager, finance manager, supplies manager, sterile supplies manager, theatre manager, service users and infection control specialists.

Facilities should conform to current guidelines and off-site facilities should be visited by the group to check that the required systems

Table 7.5 Laundry audit checklist

Standard	Compliance	Comments

Infection control issues in laundry

Protective clothing is worn when soiled linen
is handled:
   a) rubber gloves
   b) apron/overall
Handwash basin, soap, paper towels are available
in laundry and toilets
There is a system for handling and reporting/
returning extraneous items
Sharps containers are available
There is an Occupational Health Service
Staff are offered hepatitis B vaccine
There is an inoculation injury policy
There is a regular cleaning schedule for high and
low surfaces
Clean linen is stored in clean, dry containers
Vehicles are cleaned and dried:
   a) after any spillage
   b) after transporting foul laundry, if clean linen
     is to be carried next
   c) at least weekly
Containers for additives are clean and never
re-filled
Clean linen is kept separate from soiled linen
Clean linen is kept off the floor

Disinfection processes

Laundry bags are laundered after each use
A sluice cycle is incorporated into the washing
machines
Wash temperatures and mixing times comply with
current guidance (see text)
Infected linen is not sorted by hand
Infected linen is not washed in a continuous batch
washing machine
Machines are clean inside and out
Machines have heat sensors which are tested at last
6-weekly (records kept)
Thermal disinfection cycles are under electronic
control
Audit of the processes is carried out annually

are in place, standards are met and the laundry can cope with the workload. It is useful to develop a checklist to help managers make the best use of their visit and do not forget to observe any critical element. See Table 7.5, Laundry audit checklist.

There should be clear communication channels and a designated manager who will manage contract reviews and complaints and problems. A user group may also be helpful in identifying and solving problems and improving communications.

References

Ayliffe GAJ, Lowbury EJL, Geddes AM Control of Hospital Infection. London: Chapman and Hall Medical, 1992.

Ayliffe GAJ, Collins B Laundering of nurses dresses at home. Journal of Hospital Infection 1989; 13: 91–4.

Barrie D, Wilson JA, Hoffman PN, Kramer JM Bacillus cereus meningitis in two neurosurgical patients: an investigation into the source of the organism. Journal of Hospital Infection 1992; 25: 291–7.

Barrie D How hospital linen and laundry services are provided. Journal of Hospital Infection 1994; 27: 219–35.

Borton D How to safely handle linen. Nursing 1995; 16 December.

Brewer S No infection risk from home wash uniforms (letter). Nursing Standard 1996; 10 (6): 42.

Croton C Duvets on trial. Nursing Times 1990; 86 (26): 63–7.

Garner JS, Favero MS CDC Guidelines for the prevention and control of nosocomial infections. American Journal of Infection Control 1985; 14 (3): 110–29.

Maurer I Hospital Hygiene, 3rd edition. London: Edward Arnold Publishers Ltd, 1985.

Murdoch S A safe environment for care. Professional Nurse 1992; 519–22 May.

NHS Executive. Hospital Laundry Arrangements for Used and Infected Linen (HSG(95)18). London: NHSE, 1995.

Overton E Bedmaking and bacteria. Nursing Times Mar 2 1988; 84 (9): 69–71.

Standaert SM, Hutcheson RH, Schaffner W Nosocomial transmission of Salmonella gastro-enteritis to laundry workers in a nursing home. Infection Control Hospital Epidemiology 1994; 15 (1): 22–6 Jan.

Walker A, Donaldson B Infection control: dressing for protection. Nursing Times 1993; 89: (2) 60–62.

Webster O, Cowan M, Allen J Dirty linen. Nursing Times Oct 29 1986; 36–7.

Chapter 8
Food hygiene

LAUREN TEW

Introduction

The principles of safe food handling to be described in this chapter are applicable to any setting where food is prepared, and they provide the framework for the development of a food hygiene policy. In some settings risks to food, from micro-biological contamination for example, may be higher than others.

As the many who have suffered will vouch, gastroenteritis is no laughing matter. Symptoms include diarrhoea, vomiting, abdominal pain and fever and the extent of the problem is tremendous. From their analysis of infectious intestinal disease in the elderly, researchers estimate that 3555 new episodes of this 'largely preventable' illness are seen by general practitioners every week in people over 65 years of age alone (Djuretic et al., 1996). They comment that appropriate food hygiene and infection control measures could reduce this total. Education is the key.

In this chapter the principles of food hygiene will be examined, including the statutory duty of analysing hazards that might make food unsafe. This model of risk assessment will be useful to all who prepare food whatever the situation. The characteristics of the commonest foodborne illnesses, together with the implications of these illnesses for fitness to work, will be described briefly. Local situations need to be considered when writing a food policy. The next part of this chapter will provide guidance to those responsible for writing such a policy. The final section will deal with recommendations for training in food handling, the level of training being relevant to the worker's activities.

124

Before progressing further it may be useful to examine the definition of 'food handler' to be used in this chapter:

Food handler – any person involved in a food business who handles or prepares food whether open (unwrapped) or packaged. (Food includes drink and ice).
(Food Safety and Hygiene Working Group 1995, p. 10).

This definition will include many people who may not have considered themselves to be 'food handlers' and emphasizes the need for food hygiene education on a large scale. Later in this chapter a strategy for such training will be suggested.

Foodborne illness

Whilst this topic will be discussed fully in the chapter concerning gastrointestinal illness, it has direct relevance in this chapter, putting into context the importance of food hygiene. The term foodborne illness will be used throughout to include gastrointestinal infectious illness and food poisoning.

Given the risk of food handlers spreading foodborne disease, there may be occasions when they need to be excluded from work. Table 8.1 identifies those groups of people at special risk of spreading foodborne illness in a variety of settings.

The Department of Health Expert Working Group (1995), which reported on food handlers' fitness for work, recommends that anyone with diarrhoea and/or vomiting must report to their manager immediately and leave the food handling area. Food in the environment where a food handler has vomited must be discarded. Diarrhoea (loose stools passed more frequently than usual) can cause hands to be contaminated with huge numbers of micro-organisms during the acute stages of foodborne illness, increasing the risk of transmission from a food handler.

Food handlers must be excluded from work if they have been in contact with enteric fevers caused by *Salmonella typhi* (typhoid fever) or *Salmonella paratyphi* (paratyphoid fever) (Department of Health Expert Working Group, 1995). Table 8.2 lists the main clinical features of foodborne illness, possible causes and criteria for exclusion from work.

Table 8.1 Groups of people at special risk of spreading infection

---

Group 1: food handlers whose work involves touching unwrapped foods to be consumed raw or without further cooking. Food handlers who do not touch food in this way are not considered to pose a special risk.

Group 2: healthcare, nursery or other staff who have direct contact, or contact through serving food, with highly susceptible patients or persons in whom an intestinal infection would have particularly serious consequences.

Group 3: children less than five years attending nurseries, playgroups, nursery schools, or similar groups.

Group 4: older children or adults who are unable to implement good standards of personal hygiene, e.g. the mentally ill or handicapped or the infirm aged, and those in circumstances where hygienic arrangements may be unreliable, e.g. temporary camps housing displaced persons. Children in infants' schools may be considered under exceptional circumstances to fall into this group.

(Department of Health Working Group, 1994)

Outbreaks of foodborne illness are generally associated with catering establishments and institutions. However, catering for large numbers in the domestic environment has been shown to be particularly associated with the use of raw shell eggs where Department of Health guidelines recommend pasteurized, the limited cooling facilities of domestic fridges, cross-contamination in confined spaces and lack of food hygiene knowledge. Many instances of food poisoning arising in the domestic setting are not reported or investigated (Ryan et al., 1996).

Principles of food hygiene in practice

The practical application of food hygiene principles ensures that food, when served to consumers, is safe and will cause them no harmful effects. If these principles are not adhered to, the results can be disastrous. For example, in 1984, nineteen residents of Stanley Royde Hospital for the mentally ill died as a result of eating food that had not been stored correctly, allowing contaminating micro-organisms to multiply. In total 450 residents and staff were infected (Wilson, 1995). This outbreak was in part responsible for the

Table 8.2 Main clinical features of foodborne illness and possible causes

Incubation period	Typical symptoms	Duration of illness (approx)	Possible cause	Exclusion criteria
1–5 hr	Vomiting, nausea	24–36 hr	*Bacillus cereus*	*
2–6 hr	Vomiting, abdominal cramps, diarrhoea	12–48 hr	*Staphylococcus aureus*	Group 1 food handlers with septic lesions until treated successfully; nasal carriers if implicated in an outbreak
8–16 hr	Diarrhoea, abdominal pain		*B. cereus*	*
8–18 hr	Diarrhoea, abdominal pain	24 hr	*Clostridium perfringens*	*
9–12 hr	Vomiting, diarrhoea	Up to 14 days in infants	Enteropathogenic *Escherichia coli* (EPEC)	Isolate cases & room contacts until 3 negative samples, at 24-hr intervals
12–24 hr	Nausea, vomiting, diarrhoea for 1–2 days	2 days or less	Small round structured virus	*
12–48 hr	Diarrhoea, fever, abdominal pain for several days	Up to 3 weeks	*Salmonella* spp. excluding *S. typhi* & *S. paratyphi*	*
12–60 hr	From mild to bloody diarrhoea, kidney damage in young children (15% left with chronic kidney disease, 5% mortality rate)	Variable	Verocytotoxin-producing *E. coli* (VTEC)	Exclude until bowel habit normal for 48 hr and 2 negative samples, taken 48 hr apart
1–3 days	Diarrhoea (blood, abdominal pain & fever sometimes)	Up to 14 days	*Shigella sonnei/flexneri* (*Shigella boydii* and *dysenteriae* from abroad)	*

(contd)

Table 8.2 (contd)

Incubation period	Typical symptoms	Duration of illness (approx)	Possible cause	Exclusion criteria
2–3 days	Profuse watery diarrhoea	Up to 7 days	*Vibrio cholerae*	*
2–5 days	Diarrhoea (sometimes bloody), abdominal pain, fever	2–7 days	*Campylobacter* spp	*
4–25 days	Diarrhoea	Variable, may relapse	*Giardia lamblia*	*
1–2 weeks	Diarrhoea, bloating	Up to 3 weeks	*Cryptosporidium*	Unnecessary if cases/contacts have no diarrhoea
12–20 days	Fever, generalized symptoms of fever	10–14 days (sometimes asymptomatic lifelong carriage)	*Salmonella typhi / paratyphi*	Undertake individual case/contact assessment of risk; follow Department of Health guidelines (1995)
2–4 weeks	Jaundice, malaise	Less than 1 month	Hepatitis A	Exclude cases from school/work until 7 days after onset of jaundice or until recovery
1–10 weeks	Mild 'flu-like symptoms meningitis, encephalitis	Variable	*Listeria monocytogenes*	Not necessary

*Once symptoms of gastrointestinal illness are over, risk of transmission is greatly reduced. The following criteria should be met before returning to work/school: no vomiting for 48 hr; bowel habit normal for 48 hr; good hygiene, esp. hand hygiene, practised at all times. Department of Health Working Group (1994); Department of Health Expert Working Group (1995). Should an outbreak of foodborne illness arise it should be dealt with following the principles outlined in a previous chapter. Food poisoning is described as: 'Any disease of an infectious or toxic nature caused by, or thought to be caused by, the consumption of food or water' (Chief Medical Officer, 1992). An outbreak of infection or other foodborne illness is defined as either two or more linked cases of the same illness, or the situation when the observed number of cases unaccountably exceeds the expected number. (Department of Health Working Group, 1994).

removal of Crown Immunity from hospital kitchens in 1987. Like other food premises, hospital kitchens then became subject to the scrutiny of the environmental health departments of Local Authorities. Environmental health officers (EHOs) are empowered to inspect kitchens and enforce the Food Safety Act (1990) wherever food is stored, prepared and handled. They have right of entry to enforce the regulations (Wilson, 1995).

There are many Acts of Parliament, Regulations and European Community Directives pertaining to food hygiene and safety. The most relevant to this context are the Food Safety Act (1990), the Food Safety (General Food Hygiene) Regulations (1995) and the Food Safety (Temperature Control) Regulations (1995). Other legislation deals with related topics such as sale of food, water supply, Health and Safety at Work, and food labelling.

The Food Safety (General Food Hygiene) Regulations 1995, Industry Guide to Good Hygiene Practice: Catering Guide gives advice on compliance with the regulations. It explains how the activities critical to food safety can be analysed (Hazard Analysis Critical Control Point) so that procedures to implement, maintain and review the food process can be undertaken. This is a legal requirement relevant to a wide variety of food operations such as clubs, institutions, schools, healthcare establishments, mobile snack vehicles, takeaway and fast food restaurants. Each caterer must apply the principles of hazard analysis to their own environment and may find its documentation helpful if evidence of compliance with the regulation is required by an EHO. The key steps in food hygiene which must be considered are:

a) Purchase and delivery
b) Storage
c) Preparation
d) Cooking
e) Cooling
f) Chilled storage
g) Reheating
h) Hot holding and service
i) Cold service

Purchase and delivery

Only reputable suppliers of food should be used whose food is fresh and of good quality. It should be transported in vehicles that are kept in a clean and well-maintained condition that prevents contamination (Chartered Institute of Environmental Health, 1998).

On arrival the food quality should be checked and any unsatisfactory food discarded immediately, ensuring that no damaged food or blown tins, for example, can be re-sold or used for human consumption. Sometimes there may be little evidence that the food has been contaminated, so food should be checked carefully. Should birds have pecked through the foil on a bottle of milk on the doorstep, the entire bottleful must be thrown away.

Checking at this stage may include taking thermometer readings to ensure that temperature control has been maintained during transit. Electronic probe thermometers can be cleaned with an alcohol-impregnated wipe after use.

When purchasing food for domestic use a 'cool bag' can be very useful to preserve the temperature of frozen or chilled foods on the journey home from the shops. 'Use by' dates should also always be checked and adhered to.

Storage

By reducing the opportunities for food spoilage, correct storage can contribute substantially to food hygiene (CIEH, 1998). Storage areas should be designed to facilitate cleaning as crumbs and debris will encourage pests. Food should never be stored on the floor where pests such as mice and rats could damage it. Different food types (raw, cooked, high-risk) should be stored separately to avoid cross-contamination. Stock should be stored at the correct temperature (see also Chilled storage, below) and rotated to ensure that the products with the shortest lifespan are used first.

Preparation

The design and layout of a food preparation area will contribute not only to more efficient working but to safer practice in food handling by making the essential cleaning of the food preparation area easier (Sprenger, 1999). Washing food preparation areas with hot water and detergent will remove the vast majority of potentially contaminating micro-organisms (Ridgwell, 1996).

To prevent cross-contamination in commercial or healthcare kitchens, high- and low-risk foods should be prepared in different areas of the kitchen; a sink should be designated for vegetable washing only, another for washing up dirty dishes, another for hand hygiene; waste should be contained in foot-operated, lidded bins, and should be removed from the kitchen at regular intervals. Staff should not carry the waste through the area designated for high-risk foods.

In domestic kitchens where surfaces have a variety of uses, they must be cleaned thoroughly with hot soapy water between uses. Chopping boards for specific purposes, such as vegetables or meat only, must also be thoroughly washed between use. All equipment must be clean. 'Clean as you go!' is an excellent motto applicable to food preparation areas.

Humphrey et al. (1994) investigated the contamination of hands and work surfaces with *Salmonella enteritidis* Phage Type 4 (PT4) and illustrated just how easily cross-contamination can occur. They found that not only were fingers contaminated with *Salmonella enteritidis* PT4 after cracking an egg, so was the work surface more than 40 cm from a mixing bowl following preparation of batter. The bacterium survived for 24 hours in the thin film splashed from the bowl on to the worktop, much of which might be invisible to the naked eye.

Preparation of raw and salad vegetables should take place in an area designated for that purpose alone. In large organizations this may even be a separate room. Salad vegetables should be washed thoroughly twice under running water to remove the environmental organisms present on them, not only from the soil in which they grew, but also from irrigation with water which may have been contaminated.

Staff should maintain their personal hygiene at the highest level. A statutory duty for food handlers under the Food Safety (General Food Hygiene) Regulations 1995 is a requirement to inform their employer when they know or suspect they are suffering from or are a carrier of any illness or condition likely to result in contamination of food. Cuts and minor injuries must be covered with a brightly coloured plaster. Clean, suitable and, where necessary protective, clothing must be worn.

Cooking

One of the main purposes of cooking is to make it safe for consumption (Sprenger, 1999). All meat and poultry must be thoroughly cooked until juices run clear (PHMEG, 1996). A food thermometer can be used to ensure internal temperatures reach a satisfactory level – 75°C.

Where internal temperatures are inadequate, micro-organisms may remain and may cause illness. Evans et al. (1995) investigated only the second documented outbreak of illness implicating microwave ovens and caused by *Salmonella enteritidis* PT4. Five (out of 6) guests and their host developed symptoms after eating rice salad at a small domestic function, several of the ingredients of which tested positive for salmonella. The authors conclude that the outbreak resulted from uneven microwave heating of insufficient duration for adequate cooking.

Other micro-organisms may survive microwave cooking such as *Toxoplasma gondii* (Lunden and Uggla, 1992) and *Listeria monocytogenes* (Coote et al., 1991). Again the use of a thermometer to monitor internal temperatures will help reduce the risk of undercooking, as will following manufacturers' instructions to the letter (whether they are the instructions of the microwave manufacturer or the food manufacturer).

Cooling

Cooked food should be cooled to 10°C within 90 minutes (Sprenger, 1999) so that food is held in the 'danger zone' (between 8°C and 63°C when micro-organisms will multiply rapidly) for the minimum period of time. Placing hot food in the fridge may raise the temperature within the fridge, risking the safe storage of its entire contents. Preparing food in smaller or individual portions and cooling dishes in iced water, for example, will hasten cooling. Any cooling process must be consistent with food safety.

Chilled storage

Organisms are not killed by refrigeration but they do not usually multiply at low temperatures, making chilled storage an essential aid to food safety. However, *Listeria monocytogenes* and some strains of *Salmonella* spp. will grow slowly at 4°C, starting to multiply at 8°C (CIEH, 1999).

The Food Safety (Temperature Control) Regulations (1995) specify:

> Subject to certain exemptions, food which is likely to support the growth of pathogenic micro-organisms or the formation of toxins must not be kept at a temperature above 8°C.

This requirement relates to the temperature of the food, not the air in the storage facility.

Eggs should always be refrigerated in case they are contaminated with *Salmonella* spp., which would multiply at ambient temperatures. Wherever possible pasteurized eggs should be used (PHMEG, 1996), especially in institutions.

Where large volumes of food are prepared, it may be necessary to have a thawing cabinet (CIEH, 1999). Poultry, joints and large items must be completely defrosted before cooking. Defrosting foods should be so positioned in the fridge to prevent any dripping of fluid on to other food. Whilst stored in the fridge, food should be covered or wrapped and, as with all stored food, stock should be rotated. Raw and cooked foods should be stored separately to prevent cross-contamination.

Central kitchens preparing food for widespread distribution have, in some cases, changed to the Cook-Chill system of food preparation. Maintaining the cold chain is essential if these foods are not to present a health hazard to consumers. In 1989 the Department of Health issued guidelines on this system (Barrie, 1996).

An infection control nurse surveyed the ward fridges in the hospital where she worked (Smith, 1991). She found only three where the temperature was less than 10°C; there were *no* thermometers available in any fridge she examined; and many needed defrosting. Given the importance of ensuring that there is no possibility of hospital-acquired infection from inadequate refrigeration, she recommended:

- clear identification of responsibilities for food hygiene
- weekly cleaning and defrosting

- clear labelling, with date of refrigeration and 'best before' dates
- prompt reporting of malfunctions
- thermometers in every fridge, recording the statutory safe temperature
- new purchases of fridges should be made in consultation with the Infection Control Team.

Reheating, hot holding and service

> Food which has been cooked or reheated and needs to be kept hot to control the growth of pathogenic micro-organisms or the formation of toxins must be kept at a temperature at or above 63°C.
> The Food Safety (Temperature Control) Regulations 1995.

Using clean equipment and keeping it covered, food for service or display should be held at this temperature for no more than 2 hours.

Cold service

The Food Safety (Temperature Control) Regulations, 1995 dictate that food can be 'kept for service or on display' for a single period of up to 4 hours. The food should be covered wherever possible and all equipment used to serve it must be clean.

Other important food hygiene issues

Ice-making machines

There is no doubt that most drinking water tastes better when cooled by ice. This is especially true for those who may be unable to eat or who are simply 'off their food'. Unfortunately the unwell, and in particular those whose immunity is low, are at risk from contaminated ice-making machines.

A number of immunocompromised patients who were given ice to suck or drinks cooled with ice suffered septicaemia as a result of infection with *Xanthomonas maltophilia* which was contaminating the storage cabinet of a ward ice-making machine (Communicable Disease Report, 1993). As a result the Medical Devices Directorate issued a Hazard Notice (Medical Devices Directorate, 1993). Problems with ice may arise from contaminated water supply, the time lag between ice-making and consumption, contamination of ice by users, poor connection and maintenance, therefore Wilson (1995) has recommended that immunocompromised patients should not use ice from these machines. Commercially prepared ice is available.

Utensils used with ice-making machines should be durable and not become brittle at low temperatures (Food Safety and Hygiene Working Group, 1995). Ice containers and utensils should be washed regularly using a dish washer (wherever possible) or hot water and detergent. Ice should not be removed by hand (Wilson, 1995), but a vessel such as a clean teacup could be used once only, ensuring that the remaining ice is not contaminated in the process.

Pets

Pets can very often increase an individual's quality of life. However, there are times when extra care has to be taken to prevent the pet from posing a risk to the very people it is intended to help as they may carry a number of diseases, including campylobacter. The Guidelines on the Control of Infection in Residential and Nursing Homes (PHMEG, 1996) offer a number of points to be considered regarding pets:

- a member of staff should be designated as responsible for care of the pet
- handwashing should always follow handling the pet
- the pet should have a clean feeding space, away from the kitchen or food preparation area, and its own dishes that are washed separately
- the pet should be checked regularly for signs of infection and taken to a vet promptly if unwell. It should have all the relevant inoculations and dogs should be wormed every 6 months
- it should not lick or jump up on residents and staff
- claws should be trimmed regularly
- open containers of food, purchased from a commercial enterprise, should be stored separately from human food
- the pet should be allowed 20 minutes to eat its food, after which it should be discarded
- the pet should be exercised before meeting residents

- bedding and the animal's coat (especially cats and dogs) should be cleaned regularly. Insecticides may be necessary for both the pet and its environment to prevent infestation with fleas
- litter boxes should be cleaned on a daily basis, by healthy staff who are not pregnant. They should wear protective clothing for the procedure. Washing litter trays with hot water and detergent every week will remove most germs.

Pests

Infestation of food premises is a common but undesirable problem (Barrie, 1996). Pests can be classified into four main groups, all of which may pose a threat to food hygiene:

- insects – ants, flies, cockroaches, fleas, silverfish
- rodents – rats and mice
- birds – pigeons and sparrows
- feral cats and foxes (**PHMEG**, 1996)

Whilst their role in hospital-acquired infection is unclear, it is possible that salmonella could be transmitted by some pests (Barrie, 1996).

The Food Safety (General Food Hygiene) Regulations 1995 insist that 'adequate procedures must be in place to ensure pests are controlled'.

Such procedures include:

- preventing pests from gaining entry to food areas
- looking for evidence, e.g. droppings
- using a competent pest control contractor who liaises with a designated member of staff
- rotating dry goods stock
- promptly discarding contaminated food and waste
- maintaining a clean, crumb and debris-free environment.

Between visits by the pest control contractor, food handlers may become aware of evidence of infestation. By reporting suspicions at an early stage it may be much easier to eradicate the infesting pest.

Waste disposal

Disposal of waste from a food handling area will reduce risks of contamination of fresh foodstuffs. Where possible a food disposal unit should be installed to deal with waste food. If this is not available, food waste should be contained in a small, lidded, easy-to-clean swill bin, used only for this purpose and removed from the area three times a day (Philpott-Howard and Casewell, 1994). Prior to collection waste should be stored in a designated area away from food production which can be easily cleaned to deter pests. Handwashing *must* follow handling of waste, whether the food is produced for mass consumption or for the family.

Enteral feeding

Enteral feeding provides those who cannot take food by mouth with the means of maintaining the necessary intake of nutrients to remain as healthy as possible. The routes chosen include nasogastric, gastrostomy or jejunostomy.

The favourable medium for microbial multiplication provided by the food product, which is often hanging around at room temperature for several hours, and the opportunities for contamination that exist, mean food hygiene in this context has to be even more rigorous than usual (Wilson, 1995). Fernandez-Crehuet Navajas et al. (1992) investigated the bacterial contamination of enteral feeds and found that more than 25% of the feeds they investigated were contaminated. Contamination can occur at various stages. These are listed in Table 8.3, with interventions to reduce the risk of contamination.

Ward et al. (1997) described clinical guidelines for the prevention of infection associated with nasogastric tubes. The British Association of Parenteral and Enteral Nutrition (1994) estimates that between 3000 and 4000 patients are receiving enteral nutrition at home. Together, infection control nurses and nutrition nurse specialists can advise and teach carers to perform the necessary techniques safely (Fawcett, 1991).

Assisting with feeding

Those who help others with their feeding need to be aware of food hygiene responsibilities in order that risk of infection is minimized. The following principles need emphasizing here:

Table 8.3 Bacterial contamination of enteral feeds

Source of contamination	Intervention
Preparation of feed	Exemplary hygiene precautions under controlled conditions
Storage of feed	Refrigeration until use Discard after 24 hours in use
Administration of feed	Use pre-filled, commercially prepared, ready-to-use administration reservoirs rather than attempting decontamination Use non-touch technique when assembling and handling Wear clean disposable gloves
At home	Thorough education of carers

Fernandez-Crehuet Navajas et al., 1992; Wilson, 1995; Aneiros and Rollins, 1996.

- Hands must always be washed before any contact with food
- All equipment and utensils must be clean
- Leftover food must be discarded promptly
- The food serving area must be left in a clean condition
- It may be necessary to clean the mouth after feeding. Xavier (2000) emphasized the importance of mouth care to prevent oral infections.
- Dentures should be cleaned regularly with the patient's preferred product (Griffiths-Jones and Ward, 1995).

Development of a food hygiene policy

The Food Safety (General Food Hygiene) Regulations, 1995, do not contain an explicit requirement for documentation or record keeping. It is pointed out, however, that a defence of 'due diligence' may be upheld if, when faced with an enforcement notice under the regulations, a caterer can supply written policies and records of routine checks. 'A list of Codes of Practice applicable to foods' is available from the Institute of Food Science and Technology which provides more detailed information.

When writing a food hygiene policy local considerations should be taken into account when translating the legislation into a useful document that staff will find user-friendly. Some policies will be more succinct than others. Planning the policy with a multi-disciplinary team will ensure its relevance to the widest range of staff necessary. Taking extra care in consultation at this stage will pay dividends as all those involved will be 'singing the same tune' in the final document. By contributing early on they will be committed to the final document and will promote compliance.

As there is such a huge amount of legislation pertaining to food hygiene it may be helpful to divide the workload by asking sub-groups of the working party to examine the relevance of particular documents. This will help to ensure no statutory document is overlooked. Several drafts may be drawn up before the final, clearly written policy emerges which is easy to use and understand. The Hospital Caterers Association (1997) published guidelines for standards of food service at ward level, which draws relevant legislation together and describes its practical application in healthcare settings. It provides a useful framework, both for policy and for an educational programme.

Education should precede the introduction of a new policy wherever possible, to make sure staff actually understand the policy contents. If so, they will be much more likely to comply with it. Creative methods may be employed to encourage learning and compliance with the policy, for example competitions and puzzles, perhaps rewarded with relevant prizes. Davis-Beattie and de Wit (1996) have devised some unusual methods of raising knowledge of and compliance with their infection control policies which others would do well to emulate.

Using the standards laid down in the policy, an audit tool to assess compliance can be created and later administered by staff on a regular basis. This will clarify difficulties in turning the written word of the policy into practice and will highlight target groups and priorities for education.

Education and training

The Food Safety (General Food Hygiene) Regulations (Department of Health, 1995) have placed a new duty on proprietors in the food business to: 'ensure that food handlers engaged in the food business are supervised and instructed and/or trained in food hygiene matters commensurate with their work activities'.

Given the variety of tasks performed by food handlers they will need different levels of information. The regulations describe three categories of food handlers who *must* be supervised and instructed and/or trained in relation to the job they do:

- All food handlers, including those who handle low-risk or wrapped food only, must receive written or verbal instruction in the essentials of food hygiene before being allowed to start work and, as soon as possible after induction, hygiene awareness instruction.
- Food handlers who prepare open, 'high-risk' foods and those who also have a supervisory role should, within three months, receive formal training to develop understanding of the basic principles of food handling.
- Further levels of formal training, including more detail about food hygiene and management issues, should be provided as a matter of good practice according to the food handler's supervisory responsibilities.

The Food Safety (General Food Hygiene) Regulations 1995 – Industry Guide to Good Hygiene Practice: Catering Advice (Food Safety & Hygiene Working Group 1995) includes details of the subject matter that should be taught in this training scheme. The instructions on 'Essentials of Food Hygiene', which must be given verbally or in writing to any food handler *prior* to starting work, are as follows:

- Keep yourself clean and wear clean clothing.
- Always wash your hands thoroughly: before handling food, after using the toilet, after handling raw foods or waste, before starting work, after every break, after blowing your nose.
- Tell your supervisor, before starting work, of any skin, nose, throat, stomach or bowel trouble or infected wound. You are breaking the law if you do not.
- Cover cuts and sores with a waterproof, high-visibility dressing.
- Avoid unnecessary handling of food.
- Do not smoke, eat or drink in a food handling room.
- If you see something wrong, tell your supervisor.
- Do not prepare food too far in advance of service.
- Keep perishable food either refrigerated or piping hot.
- Keep the preparation of raw and cooked food strictly separate.

- When reheating food ensure it gets piping hot.
- Clean as you go. Keep all equipment and surfaces clean.
- Follow any food safety instructions either in food packaging or from your supervisor.

These points can be amended to suit each business. Some points may not be relevant to some businesses.

References

Aneiros S, Rollins H. Home enteral tube feeding. Community Nurse, 1996; 28–33 April.

Barrie D. The provision of food and catering services in hospital. Journal of Hospital Infection 1996; 33: 13–33.

Chartered Institute of Environmental Health. Food Safety for Supervisors. Chadwick House Group Ltd, 1998.

Chief Medical Officer. Definition of Food Poisoning. (PL/CMO (92) 144). London: Department of Health, 1992.

Communicable Disease Report Ice as a source of infection acquired in hospital. CDR Weekly 3 (53) 31 December 1993; 241.

Coote PJ, Holyoak CD, Cole MB Thermal inactivation of Listeria monocytogenes during a process simulating temperatures achieved during microwave heating. Journal of Applied Bacteriology 1991; 70, 489–94. Cited in Evans, Parry and Ribeiro (1995).

Davis-Beattie M, De Wit Creative infection control and adult learning. Journal of Hospital Infection, 1996; 32: 85–97.

Department of Health. Food Safety Act. London: HMSO, 1990.

Department of Health.. The Food Safety (General Food Hygiene) Regulations. London: Department of Health, 1995a.

Department of Health. The Food Safety (Temperature Control) Regulations. London: Department of Health, 1995b.

Department of Health Expert Working Group. Food Handlers: Fitness to Work. London: Department of Health, 1995.

Department of Health Working Group. Management of Outbreaks of Foodborne Illness. London: Department of Health, 1994.

Djuretic T, Ryan MJ, Fleming DM, Wall PG Infectious intestinal disease in elderly people. Communicable Disease Report 1996; 6 (8): R107–R112.

Elia M Enteral and Parenteral Nutrition in the Community. British Association for Parenteral and Enteral Nutrition, Maidenhead, 1994. Cited in Aneiros and Rollins, 1996.

Evans MR, Parry SM, Ribeiro CD Salmonella outbreak from microwave cooked food. Epidemiology & Infection 1995; 115 (2): 227–30.

Fawcett H A new specialist for nutritional care. Professional Nurse, 1991; 246–50 February.

Fernandez-Crehuet Navajas M, Jurado Chacon D, Guillen Solvas JF, Galvez Vargas R Bacterial contamination of enteral feeds as a possible risk of nosocomial infection. Journal of Hospital Infection 1992; 21: 111–20.

Food Safety and Hygiene Working Group. Food Safety (General Food Hygiene) Regulations 1995 – Guide to Compliance by Caterers. London: HMSO, 1995.

Griffiths-Jones A, Ward K Principles of Infection Control Practice. London: Scutari Press, 1995.

Hospital Caterers Association. Good Practice Guide: Food Service Standards at Ward Level. Hospital Caterers Association, 1997.

Humphrey TJ, Martin KW, Whitehead A Contamination of hands & work surfaces with Salmonella enterititis PT4 during the preparation of egg dishes. Epidemiology & Infection 1994; 113: 403–9.

Institute of Food Science and Technology. A list of Codes of Practice Applicable to Foods. ISBN 0 905 367 12X.

Lunden A, Uggla A Infectivity of Toxoplasma gondii in mutton following curing, smoking, freezing or microwave cooking. International Journal of Food Microbiology 1992; 15: 357–63. Cited in Evans, Parry and Ribeiro (1995).

Medical Devices Directorate. Infection Caused By Xanthomonas maltophilia. Hazard (93) December 1993; 42: 16.

Philpott-Howard J, Casewell M Hospital Infection Control. Policies & Practical Procedures. London: WB Saunders Co Ltd, 1994.

PHMEG (Public Health Medicine Environment Group). Guidelines on the Control of Infection in Residential & Nursing Homes. London: Department of Health, 1996.

Ryan M, Wall P, Gilbert R, Griffin M, Rowe B Risk factors for outbreaks of infectious intestinal disease linked to domestic catering. Communicable Disease Report December 6 1996; 6 (13): R179–R183.

Ridgwell J Food Hygiene. Microsoft (R) Encarta (R) 96 Encyclopedia. Microsoft Corporation, 1996.

Smith F. Looking into the refrigerator. Nursing Times, 1991; 87 (38): 61–2 September 18.

Sprenger R Hygiene for Management. A Textbook for Food Hygiene Courses. London: Highfield Publications, 1999.

Ward V, Wilson J, Taylor L, Cookson B, Glynn A Preventing Hospital Acquired Infection: Clinical Guidelines. London: PHLS, 1997.

Wilson J Infection Control in Clinical Practice. London: Baillière Tindall, 1995.

Xavier G The importance of mouth care in preventing infection. Nursing Standard, 2000; 14(18): 47–51 January 19.

Chapter 9
Decontamination

LESLY FINN

Introduction

The role of decontamination procedures as part of the essential measures for the prevention and control of infection is now well accepted. Changes in decontamination methods over the years have included the development of sophisticated sterilizing equipment utilizing steam and/or chemicals, hot water disinfectors and a burgeoning market in new or modified chemical disinfectants.

Sadly, numerous studies have indicated that knowledge and practice of safe decontamination is often less than satisfactory in many healthcare settings, including hospitals (Gardiner, 1995; Fleming, 1993; Taylor et al, 1994) and health authority clinics and general practice (Farrow et al.; 1988, Foy et al.; 1990, Hoffman et al., 1988; Morgan et al.; 1990, Finn and McCulloch, 1996).

However, the advent of HIV and new variant Creutzfeldt-Jakob disease (vCJD) infection, together with concern regarding MRSA and the appearance of multi-resistant organisms in hospitals, has resulted in increased awareness amongst healthcare professionals and the general public of the need for safe and reliable decontamination procedures. In addition, employers are required under Health and Safety legislation to evaluate and control the risks to health of patients and employees posed by hazardous substances, including both chemicals and pathogenic micro-organisms (Health and Safety Executive, 1999a, b; Advisory Committee on Dangerous Pathogens, 1998).

Employers and employees need to be aware of their legal obligations as set out in the Control of Substances Hazardous to Health (COSHH) regulations (Health & Safety Executive, 1994). These include risk assessment of any process involving a hazardous substance and taking action to reduce the risk to a minimum. The regulations also require constant review of any process and the documentation of risk assessments, together with monitoring and health records, which should be kept for 30 years. Employers must provide information and training and consult workers on health and safety measures. Employees are required to take steps to ensure their own health and safety. Chief executives are required to ensure that current guidance on decontamination is implemented (NHS Executive, 1999b).

Problems may arise in all areas of the decontamination process, while the choice of method will depend on many factors including the nature of the contamination, the time required for processing, the heat, pressure, moisture and chemical tolerance of the object and the quality and risks associated with the decontamination method (Department of Health, 1993a).

Definition of terms

Clarification and understanding of terms is the first step in the development of a decontamination policy. The following terms are adapted from Department of Health, 1993a.

Contamination

The soiling or pollution of inanimate or living material with harmful, potentially infectious or other unwanted substances. Examples include organic matter, micro-organisms, dust, chemical residues, radioactive material and degradation products. Such contamination may have an adverse effect on the function of the inanimate object or may be transferred to a susceptible host during use, subsequent processing or storage.

Decontamination

A process which removes or destroys contamination thus preventing micro-organisms or other contaminants reaching a susceptible site in sufficient quantities to cause infection or other harmful response.

Cleaning

Physical removal of contaminants which does not necessarily destroy micro-organisms. The reduction in microbial contamination cannot be defined and will depend on many factors including the efficiency of the cleaning process.

Disinfection

A process which reduces the number of viable micro-organisms but is not necessarily effective against bacterial spores or some viruses.

Disinfectant

A chemical agent which under defined conditions is capable of disinfection.

Sterilization

A process used to render an object free from viable micro-organisms, including bacterial spores and viruses.

Methods of decontamination

Cleaning

This is the first level of decontamination and may be all that is required for certain items. Cleaning is also an essential prerequisite for disinfection or sterilization as the presence of any organic matter may render these higher levels of decontamination ineffective (HSE, 1999a).

Method

1. Protective gloves and apron should be worn for all cleaning activities. Masks and protective eyewear may be necessary when cleaning some items if splash or spray is likely, e.g. surgical instruments, endoscopes. The use of an ultrasonic washer for cleaning prior to sterilization eliminates the need for stages 3 and 4, thus reducing the risks of operator exposure to contaminants. The ultrasonic washer should itself be cleaned and dried after use and regularly maintained.
2. If appropriate the item should be dismantled prior to cleaning.
3. The item should be carefully submerged in a deep sink (not a hand washbasin), or a suitably sized receptacle, containing a solution of warm water and simple detergent and carefully washed on all surfaces. Care must be taken to prevent contamination of self and the environment.

4. Where immersion in water is impracticable or inappropriate the item should be washed with a disposable cloth/paper substitute wrung out in a solution of warm water and detergent. The cloth should be rinsed in the solution and wrung out at frequent intervals.

5. The item should be rinsed with hot water and dried. Drying is an important part of the cleaning process as many Gram-negative organisms are able to flourish in wet residues. Drying can be achieved by physical drying with disposable paper towels/clean cloth, by allowing the item to drain or air dry naturally, or through the use of a drying cabinet.

6. Disposable cloths, or a paper substitute, should be used for wet cleaning. Any other cleaning equipment, e.g. brushes, should be washed in hot water and detergent and allowed to dry between uses. All cleaning equipment should be discarded or disinfected by heat at least daily.

7. Protective clothing must be discarded and the hands thoroughly washed after any cleaning procedure.

Disinfection

Disinfection can be achieved through the use of heat or chemicals.

Disinfection by chemicals

Chemical disinfection is not a substitute for sterilization and is not as effective as disinfection by heat. It must not be used where these methods, or the use of single-use items, would be more appropriate and should not be regarded as a routine 'housekeeping' procedure (Department of Health, 1993a).

The main disadvantages of chemical disinfection are set out in Table 9.1. Certain chemicals, e.g. glutaraldehyde, can achieve high-level disinfection but their use must be strictly controlled due their irritant and sensitizing properties. Alternative high-level disinfectants include peracetic acid (NuCidex, Steris) and chlorine dioxide (Tristel, Dexit), both of which are highly effective in destroying micro-organisms and act more rapidly than glutaraldehyde. However, they are far more expensive and are also more damaging to instrument and processor components. Their long-term effects on both users and the environment are unknown at present. A peroxygen compound (Virkon) and a quaternary compound (Dettox, Sactimed Sinald) are also available but these have been shown to be ineffective against some mycobacteria and enteroviruses (Babb and Bradley, 1995).

Ethyl alcohol (ethanol) 70% and 60–70% isopropyl alcohol are rapid and effective disinfectants but can only be used on clean surfaces and are highly flammable. They are ineffective against spores and their action is variable against viruses. Chlorine-releasing agents are cheap and effective disinfectants but are unstable in at-use dilutions, are inactivated by organic matter and can damage many materials. Although non-toxic at low dilutions, and therefore safe for babies' feeding bottles and food preparation areas, their use at higher concentrations is not without risk. They are corrosive and may also produce free chlorine gas when in contact with acidic body fluids such as urine (Ayliffe et al., 1992).

Disinfection of endoscopes

The transmission of pathogens to immunocompromised or generally frail patients via contaminated endoscopes is possible during routine gastrointestinal endoscopy, but the greatest risks are associated with bronchoscopy. There has been one report of hepatitis B transmission via a gastroscope, and *Serratia marcescens*, pseudomonas, borrelia, tuberculosis and non-tuberculous mycobacteria have all been transmitted during bronchoscopy, occasionally with fatal results (Taylor et al., 1994).

Rigid endoscopes inserted into sterile body cavities at laparoscopy, arthroscopy or cystoscopy must be sterilized. High-level disinfection is necessary for the flexible endoscopes used for gastrointestinal and bronchoscopic examination. Autoclaving would be the method of choice but the heat-sensitive nature of the flexible equipment requires the employment of alternative methods such as ethylene oxide, low-temperature steam or chemical disinfection.

Glutaraldehyde remains the disinfectant of choice for flexible endoscopes in the majority of hospitals. However, it is a toxic poison, a teratogen and mutagen which can damage DNA. It is highly irritant to the upper respiratory tract and an allergic response may lead to occupational asthma. Non-specific symptoms as a result of exposure include headache, nausea, vomiting, skin discoloration and change in taste.

Table 9.1 Disadvantages of chemical disinfection

1. Does not guarantee a sterile product. While most disinfectants are capable of eliminating Gram-negative and Gram-positive bacteria and enveloped viruses, very few
   are effective against non-enveloped viruses, myocobacteria, protozoal cysts and
   bacterial spores. Even if a particular disinfectant has been shown to be capable of
   killing a specific organism in laboratory tests, this does not mean it will do so in all
   circumstances.
2. The chemical may be toxic, e.g. via contact with skin or mucous membranes or
   vapour inhalation, corrosive and/or flammable.
3. It may be inactivated by chemical or physico-chemical reactions. For example,
   blood or other body fluids, incompatibly charged detergents, wood, cork, plastics,
   rubber and some inorganic chemicals can neutralize detergents.
4. A residue of blood or certain other organic substances will hamper penetration of
   any disinfectant. Some disinfectants will coagulate proteins hampering their own
   penetration.
5. Disinfectants can decay and lose efficacy, e.g. during storage, on dilution, at elevated
   temperatures. The presence of impurities can initiate and accelerate decay.
6. The time required for a disinfectant to work will be affected by a combination of its
   speed of action and required concentration, plus the amount of neutralization and
   protection of target organisms by extraneous matter.

The maximum exposure limit in the UK is 0.05 parts per
million (HSE, 2000). Where glutaraldehyde is used employers have a
legal duty to provide health surveillance for workers exposed to it
and individual health records and demographic data should be kept
(Taylor et al, 1994). In a questionnaire survey of 216 endoscopy units
in the UK, Wicks (1994) found that, although 98.6% were using
glutaraldehyde, 63.9% used open systems, 56% had no policy of
regular health checks for staff, 40.3% had no fume extraction system
and 57.4% did not have a policy for regular measurement of
glutaraldehyde limits.

Use of glutaraldehyde should be restricted to properly equipped
units with specifically trained and experienced staff. Strategies to
reduce the risks to staff and patients associated with decontamination of flexible endoscopes are set out in Table 9.2. Comprehensive
guidance on the safe decontamination of endoscopes has been
published by the Medical Devices Agency (Medical Devices Agency,
1996).

Table 9.2 Risk reduction in the decontamination of flexible endoscopes

- All endoscopes must be cleaned manually prior to disinfection
- Change to disposable accessories where possible, or purchase enough accessories to enable a Sterile Supplies Department to be used
- Ensure that control measures are used and that all equipment is properly maintained and records retained
- Aldehyde systems should be enclosed and sited away from the patient area
- A local exhaust system is essential. It should be tested regularly and maintenance records kept
- Automated chemical washer/disinfectors provide a standardized, timed process and reduce staff contact but may also require extract ventilation and must be maintained in accordance with HTM 2030
- Machines should be cleaned/disinfected daily prior to use
- Training programmes should include risk assessment, safe working methods, the role of ventilation, use of protective clothing, management of spillage, health surveillance arrangements and symptoms of exposure.

Disinfection by heat

This is the preferred method for those items that must be rendered safe to use but do not need to be sterile, e.g. linen, crockery/cutlery, re-usable bedpans. The process involves the use of a washer-disinfector which, at the correct time/temperature setting, will inactivate all micro-organisms except bacterial spores and some heat-resistant viruses.

Dishwashing machines

Crockery and cutlery should be washed on a cycle with a minimum temperature of 60°C and a final rinse of at least 80°C. This achieves the higher quality which is required in clinical settings, so washing up by hand should be avoided if at all possible. The filter of the machine should be inspected and cleaned regularly. Particular attention should be paid to the door edges and seals where dirt and grease tends to accumulate. The machine should be maintained on a regular contract.

Cabinet washer-disinfectors

Cabinet washer-disinfectors are designed to process a wide range of materials for immediate use in patient treatment areas. The most familiar type to nursing staff is the bedpan washer-disinfector. Some machines incorporate a mechanism which will empty the container contents before processing.

Washer-disinfectors should not be used for items intended for single-use only or for any hollow or porous items where the hot water cannot penetrate the internal lumen adequately. Some machines may have special adaptors to enable hollow and lumen items to be processed satisfactorily (Department of Health, 1993a). The machine should have a phase of the cycle that achieves a temperature of at least 71°C for 3 minutes, 80°C for one minute or 90°C for one second in all parts of the load – this is usually on the final rinse.

Washer-disinfectors, including chemical washer-disinfectors and ultrasonic washers, must be managed and maintained in accordance with Health Technical Memorandum (HTM) 2030. 'Management' is defined as the owner, occupier, employer, general manager, chief executive or other person who is ultimately accountable for the sole operation of the premises. HTM 2030 defines the test, maintenance and reporting procedures required for good practice in the use of washer-disinfectors and requires that training be given to the users in the correct use of the machine. In addition, an identified user must be invested with the responsibility for seeing that the washer-disinfector is operated safely and efficiently (Department of Health, NHS Estates, 1996).

Disinfection with boiling water

Disinfection using a hot water boiler can only be carried out on clean items which can withstand immersion in water at a temperature of 100°C for more than 5 minutes. It should not be used if a better method is available as there is no independent method of checking efficiency and no means of indicating a failed process. The process requires careful attention to detail and, following disinfection, the articles are wet, unfit for storage and may readily become recontaminated (Department of Health, 1993a).

Sterilization

This is most commonly achieved by the use of steam under pressure or dry heat. The process may be carried out centrally by a Sterile Supplies Unit (SSU) or through the use of a benchtop steam sterilizer or dry heat sterilizer, e.g. in laboratories, surgeries/health clinics and certain hospital wards and departments.

The use of SSU, or of single-use disposables, is the safest option as this reduces the risk of process error, and/or operator exposure, to a minimum. The SSU may also safely sterilize heat-sensitive items through alternative methods such as the use of ethylene oxide or low-temperature steam with formaldehyde.

The current main British Standards for sterilizers are BS3970 for clinical sterilizers and BS2645 for laboratory sterilizers. European standards on sterilization will be more extensive and will specify not only design, construction, performance and safety requirements, but will also require the operation of a quality system by the operator to include validation and routine testing of the process.

Maintenance schedules, routine commissioning and performance tests are necessary for *all* sterilizing equipment under Health Technical Memorandum (HTM) 2010, which has been designed to conform broadly with draft European standards (Department of Health NHS Estates, 1994).

Dry heat (hot air) sterilizers

Dry heat sterilizers are used to process medicinal products or devices. The process should not be used for aqueous fluids or materials that are denatured or damaged at 160°C. The process is inefficient compared to moist heat sterilization.

The heat-up time varies widely according to the load volume and the type of material. The heat-up process is slow and sterilization times are long. Loads should be designed to contain items of the same size and nature and these should be arranged to allow free circulation of air. If mixed loads are used, extreme care must be taken to ensure that the sterilization time is long enough for the slowest to heat items.

The recommended holding time/temperature combinations for dry heat sterilization are 160°C for 120 minutes, 170°C for 60 minutes or 180°C for 30 minutes (Department of Health, 1993a).

Sterilizers for unwrapped instruments and utensils

These machines can be used to sterilize unwrapped, nonporous items only because air removal is by displacement with steam. This means that direct steam contact with all surfaces cannot take place if the item is wrapped. This type of sterilizer must not be used for items with lumens such as catheters, hollow-bore needles, trocars, etc.

Transportable sterilizers for unwrapped instruments and utensils should conform with BS3970: Parts 1 & 4 together with the safety specifications in EN 61010: Part 2-041. A European standard is under development and will supersede BS3970 in the future (Department of Health NHS Estates, 1994).

The recommended holding time/temperature combinations for steam sterilization are 134°C for 3 minutes or 121°C for 15 minutes. The higher temperature is preferred for items which will withstand this temperature and associated pressure (Department of Health, 1993a). Because the sterilized items are exposed to the air on being removed from the chamber they are susceptible to rapid recontamination. The items should be covered immediately with a sterile paper towel or sterile cloth and should be re-sterilized if not used within 3 hours.

Benchtop steam sterilizers with vacuum extraction are now becoming available. These are designed to enable the processing of wrapped instruments and must conform to BS3970 and EN61010: Part 2-041. They should be used strictly in accordance with the manufacturer's instructions and the user must be sure that all wrappings are dry on completion of the cycle if the items are not to be used immediately. Detailed guidance has been published by the Medical Devices Agency (1997, 1998).

Instruments used for minor surgery

For minor surgery in general practice settings disposable instruments should be used wherever possible and sufficient instruments should be purchased to enable separate sets to be made up and sterilized individually before each procedure. Alternatively, the use of a sterile supply service represents optimum practice, reducing contamination risks and operator time.

Instruments and appliances used in the vagina and cervix

Because of the potential danger of cross-infection in relation to human papilloma virus, herpes, hepatitis B, HIV and chlamydiae, all items used in the vagina and cervix must be either sterilized or disinfected by heat between patients in accordance with Safety Action Bulletin 108, SAB(94)22 – chemical disinfection should not be used (Department of Health NHS Estates, 1994).

Risk assessment for decontamination methods

Protection of patients/clients and staff from exposure to infection from medical devices and other equipment requires the adoption of safe systems of work. This includes risk assessment and the implementation of appropriate decontamination methods to render the item(s) safe for subsequent handling or use. All medical and other equipment can be categorized according to its potential infection risk to the patient. The following method of risk assessment and selection of appropriate decontamination methods can be applied across all care settings and situations.

High-risk items

These can be classified as those items that come into contact with a break in the skin or mucous membranes or enter a body cavity or organ. High-risk items must be *sterile*.

Examples: Surgical instruments, urinary catheters, cardiac catheters, wound dressings, arthroscopes, intravenous/intra-arterial devices, all respiratory equipment.

Medium-risk items

These are those items that come into contact with intact mucous membranes. Medium-risk items must be cleaned then disinfected – preferably by heat.

Examples: Re-usable bedpans/urinals, re-usable face-masks, cutlery/crockery, bed linen, oral/rectal thermometers, auriscope ear pieces.

Decontamination of the majority of medium-risk items has already been discussed. Certain heat-sensitive items, e.g. glass thermometers and some auriscope ear pieces, can be safely decontaminated by washing in a solution of cold water and detergent, dried thoroughly then soaked in fresh 70% alcohol for 10 minutes and drained dry.

Low-risk items

These are those items that do not come into direct contact with the patient, or only come into contact with healthy, intact skin. Low-risk items must be physically cleaned and dried.

Examples: *Equipment* – drip stands, monitors, blood pressure cuffs, mattresses, examination couches, bath hoists, bed cradles, washbowls, suction machines, disposable bedpan holders, commodes.

Environment – furniture, floors and floor coverings, soft furnishings, fixtures and fittings.

Low-risk does not mean no risk, as any low-risk item may become a source or vehicle of infection if it becomes contaminated with pathogenic micro-organisms. For example, following two cases of infection caused by vancomycin-resistant enterococci (VRE) on a paediatric oncology ward, 14 other children were found to be colonized on screening and the environment was found to be extensively contaminated. VRE was recovered from bed-rails, chairs, toilet seats, telephones and a clothes-dryer (Murphy, 1996).

Other examples have included the widespread distribution of Group A streptococci, isolated from carpets and soft furnishings, in a nursing home during investigation of 5 residents with skin lesions infected with this organism (Sarangi and Rowsell, 1995), and methicillin-resistant *Staphylococcus aureus* infections linked to environmental contamination of shelving and an ultrasound machine in a urology treatment room (Finn, 1995) (see Chapter 4, example 4).

General cleaning

If the general environment (floor, furniture, low-risk equipment, walls) is kept physically clean and dry it is unlikely to pose an infection risk. Dust represents a hazard as it is largely made up of skin scales, which are constantly being shed into the environment, each one of which may be covered in micro-organisms. The more people there are within a given area, and the greater the activity levels, the more dust will be produced. The removal of dust is therefore an important control measure, particularly in clinical and treatment areas.

Training and supervision of domestic staff is usually the responsibility of the domestic services manager within hospitals or the owner or manager in other premises. Routine cleaning schedules must be agreed and should include floors, toilets, baths, sinks, basins, locker tops, shelving, beds, bed tables and other furniture. Cleaning schedules should specify the method, frequency, timing, together with the equipment to be used, and should be agreed with infection control staff where possible (Ayliffe et al., 1992). Standards of hygiene have been developed and adopted by the Department of Health (ICNA/ADM, 1999).

In most situations a solution of neutral detergent and hot water is adequate for damp-dusting of furniture, equipment and horizontal surfaces, together with the wet-cleaning of floors. The solution used should be freshly made up and to the correct concentration. Bathroom, sluice room and toilet floors should be wet-cleaned daily. A cream cleanser can be used for baths, basins and other sanitary ware. Disposable cleaning cloths should be used and changed at least daily. Mopheads and non-disposable cloths should be sent for laundering daily. Cloths and equipment used in kitchens and food-preparation areas should be colour-coded and kept separately from those used elsewhere.

Gram-negative organisms can quickly contaminate solutions and wet residues. If spray cleaners are used it is important that solutions are freshly prepared and spray bottles are emptied and stored dry when not in use. All equipment used for wet cleaning should be washed and allowed to dry between uses, with bowls, buckets and other receptacles stored inverted.

Dry dusting and sweeping with brooms re-disperses dust and bacteria into the air and should not be carried out in patient, service or food preparation areas. Dry cleaning of floors can best be achieved by using an anti-static mop or a vacuum cleaner. All electrical equipment must be cleaned after use and maintained according to the manufacturer's instructions.

Bed curtains in patient areas should be changed six-monthly, when visibly soiled and after use by a patient with a communicable disease. Carpets should be vacuumed at least twice weekly and will require steam-cleaning following contamination with blood, body fluid or excreta.

Low-risk medical equipment

The responsibility for the cleaning of low-risk medical equipment should be clarified between domestic services and care staff. Nursing and other care staff need to be alerted to the importance of maintaining medical equipment in a clean condition and instructed in safe cleaning methods.

Spillages

Any spillage should be dealt with immediately. Cleaning with detergent and water is adequate for the majority of spillages. Gloves and a protective plastic apron should be worn when dealing with excreta or blood spills. National guidelines recommend that blood spillage is first covered by a granular chlorine-releasing agent, or covered by paper towels which are then treated with 10,000 ppm sodium hypochlorite solution, and left for at least two minutes before clearing away (Advisory Committee on Dangerous Pathogens (ACDP), 1995; UK Health Departments, 1998). At these concentrations chlorine-releasing concentrations are both toxic and corrosive and this method is no longer used in some areas because of the potential risk to staff from the chemical itself. Provided that care is taken, protective gloves and an apron are worn and the hands thoroughly washed afterwards, soaking up the spill with absorbent material followed by thorough cleaning with detergent and water should be sufficient.

Decontamination of equipment prior to inspection, service or repair

The Department of Health continues to receive complaints regarding medical or laboratory devices sent for inspection, service or repair without the necessary accompanying documentation indicating their contamination status (Department of Health, 1993b). Items should be appropriately treated to remove or minimize the risk of infection to anyone who may subsequently handle them and full details of the item, its contamination status (i.e. what it has been used for and what it may have been contaminated with), plus the method of decontamination used, should be available to the person inspecting or receiving the item. This declaration must be signed by the person authorizing/sending the equipment.

If decontamination of the item is not possible for any reason, this information must be communicated to the recipient prior to receipt or clearly stated on the label so that its status can be determined before it is handled. Any packaging should be sufficiently robust to withstand damage in transit and should ensure that the inner packing does not contaminate the outer one. Advice on reporting incidents involving medical devices to the Medical Devices Agency is available in Safety Notice SN9601 (1996). In order to assist those responsible for implementing best practice the Department of Health has provided Chief Executives of NHS Trusts and Health Authorities with a CD-ROM entitled 'Decontamination Guidance'. This draws together existing guidelines and copies are available from Publications, NHS Estates, 1 Trevelyan Square, Boar Lane, Leeds LS1 6AE (HSE, 1999b).

Re-use of single-use only items

The re-use and re-processing of medical devices intended for single use involves a number of potential hazards. Organizations and individuals need to be sure that any reprocessing method has been validated, to prove the safety of both the process and the end product, before such an item is used on a patient. Re-use has legal, technical and economical implications for the user and may render them liable to prosecution unless the stringent validation criteria are satisfactorily met (Medical Devices Agency, 1995).

References

Advisory Committee on Dangerous Pathogens (ACDP. Protection Against Blood-borne Infections in the Workplace: HIV and Hepatitis. London: HMSO, 1995.

Advisory Committee on Dangerous Pathogens (ACDP) and Spongiform Encephalopathy Advisory Committee (SEAC). Transmissible Spongiform Encephalopathy Agents: Safe Working and the Prevention of Infection. London: HMSO, 1998.

Ayliffe GAJ, Lowbury EJL, Geddes AM, Williams JD Control of Hospital Infection, 3rd edition. London: Chapman and Hall, 1992.

Babb J, Bradley CR A review of glutaraldehyde alternatives. British Journal of Theatre Nursing 1995; 5 (7): 20–24.

Department of Health. HSG(93)26 Decontamination of Equipment Prior to Inspection, Servicing or Repair. London: DoH, 1993a.

Department of Health. Sterilization, Disinfection and Cleaning of Medical Equipment: Guidance on Decontamination from the Microbiology Advisory Committee to the Department of Health, Medical Devices Directorate, Parts 1 & 2. London: DoH, 1993b.

Department of Health, NHS Estates. Health Technical Memorandum 2010 (HTM 2010). London: HMSO, 1994.

Department of Health, NHS Estates. Health Technical Memorandum 2030 (HTM 2030). London: HMSO, 1996.

Department of Health. SN 9601 Reporting Adverse Incidents Relating to Medical Devices. London: DoH, 1996.

Department of Health, Scottish Office Home and Health Department, Welsh Office, DHSS (Northern Ireland). Safety Action Bulletin 108: SAB(94)22. Instruments and Appliances Used in the Vagina and Cervix: Recommended Methods for Decontamination. London: DoH, 1994.

Farrow SC, Kaul S, Littlepage BC Disinfection methods in general practice and health authority clinics: a telephone survey. Journal of the Royal College of General Practitioners 1988; 38: 447–9.

Finn LF (1995) An outbreak of Methicillin resistant *Staphylococcus aureus* on a urology ward – the role of the environment. Free Paper. Infection Control Nurses Association National Conference (York). ICNA, 1995.

Finn LF, McCulloch J Infection control in GP surgeries: safe practices? British Journal of Nursing 1996; 5 (6): 341–8.

Fleming F Unhygienic Practices. Journal of Infection Control Nursing, (suppl.) Nursing Times 1993; 20 (5): 70–74.

Foy C, Gallagher M, Rhodes T, Setters J, Phillips P, Donaldson C, Bond J, Moore M, Naji S HIV – measures to control infection in general practice. British Medical Journal 1990; 300: 1048–9.

Gardiner A Knowledge of disinfection. Journal of Infection Control Nursing, (suppl.) Nursing Times 1995; 91 (20): 59–64.

Health and Safety Executive. Control of Substances Hazardous to Health Regulations. London: HMSO, 1994.

Health and Safety Executive. Health Service Circular 1999/178 Variant Creutzfeldt-Jacob Disease (vCJD): Minimising the Risk of Transmission. London: HMSO, 1999a.

Health and Safety Executive. Health Service Circular 1999/179 Controls Assurance in Infection Control: Decontamination of Medical Devices. London: HMSO, 1999b.

Health and Safety Executive EH40 Occupational Exposure Limits. Sudbury: HSE, 2000.

Hoffman PN, Cooke EM, Larkin DP, Southgate LJ, Mayon-White RT, Pether JVS, Wright AE, Keelyside D Control of infection in general practice: a survey and recommendations. British Medical Journal 1988; 297: 34–7.

Infection Control Nurses Association/Association of Domestic Manager.s Standards for Environmental Cleanliness in Hospitals. Northumberland: ADM/ICNA, 1999.

Medical Devices Agency, DB 9501. The Re-use of Medical Devices Supplied for Single Use Only. London: MDA, 1995.

Medical Devices Agency. Decontamination of Endoscopes DB 9607. London: MDA, 1996.

Medical Devices Agency. The Purchase, Operation and Maintenance of Benchtop Steam Sterilizers MDA DB 9605. London: MDA, 1997.

Medical Devices Agency. The Validation and Periodic Testing of Benchtop Vacuum Steam Sterilisers MDA DB 9804. London: MDA, 1998.

Morgan DR, Lamont TJ, Dawson J, Booth C Decontamination of instruments and control of cross infection in general practice. British Medical Journal 1990; 300: 1379–80.

Murphy H Control of Spread of Vancomycin Resistant Enterococci (VRE): Back to Basics. Paper. The Fourth International Conference and Exhibition on Infection Control (Dublin). ICNA, 1996.

Sarangi J, Rowsell R A nursing home outbreak of Group A streptococcal infection: case control study of environmental contamination. (Letter). Journal of Hospital Infection 1995; 30 (2): 162–4.

Taylor EW, Mehtar S, Cowan RE, Feneley RCI Endoscopy: disinfectants and health – Report of a meeting held at the Royal College of Surgeons of England, February 1993. Journal of Hospital Infection 1994; 28: 5–14.

UK Health Department. Guidance for Clinical Health Care Workers: Protection Against Infection with Blood-borne Viruses. London: Department of Health, 1998.

Wicks J Handle with care Nursing Times 1994; 90 (13) suppl: 67–70.

Chapter 10
Standard setting and audit

JANE BARNETT

Introduction

Since the publication of the government's White Paper on the National Health Service (Working for Patients, 1989), more attention has been directed not only towards the service provided by hospitals but the quality and performance of that service. This is becoming increasingly relevant to infection control services, with some authors suggesting that infection control is an area in which quality standards may be established and monitored, and qualitative improvements made (Horton, 1993; Chaudhuri, 1993; Millward et al., 1993).

Despite these assertions by experts in the field, infection control is often regarded as an 'extra' which can be optional when clinical staff are busy and time is limited. However, it should be incorporated into all practitioners' education as an essential skill which, if omitted, can lead to devastating consequences for patients. Not only should infection control skills be taught and practised but minimum standards of these need to be observed in order for them to be of any value. A handwash is worth little if the skin is merely moistened by running water and soap is not used! Hence, if the profile of infection control is to be raised, then quality standards should be drawn up, built into contracting arrangements and monitored both by the providers and the purchasers of healthcare.

Clinical healthcare staff must play an active role in this process, and this chapter will set out the terminology that is often used in relation to quality issues, as well as some examples of how quality in infection control may be maintained and monitored.

Changes in the National Health Service

Both economic and political pressures have contributed to significant changes in the National Health Service (NHS) during the 1990s. The Patients' Charter (1992) drew attention to minimum quality standards, thus increasing expectations by those receiving care. Reorganization of the NHS and the introduction of contracting for healthcare, which resulted from the NHS and Community Care Act (1990), led to the setting up of contracts which specified what is to be provided; at what cost; to whom and with what guarantees of quality.

In addition, the White Paper entitled 'A First Class Service' (Department of Health, 1998) has indicated the importance of clinical governance in healthcare. With the increase in demand and parallel increase in expectations among patients, there is more emphasis upon value for money and cost effectiveness. Alongside this, there is a need to ensure that standards are upheld and resources are used effectively, enforcing accountability amongst professionals and managers.

Donabedian (1988) distinguishes between 'maximum' and 'optimum' standards of care. The former ignore costs and define highest quality of care as that which should achieve the best improvement in health; the latter excludes care that is deemed to be too expensive in relation to possible outcomes. There are three dimensions to health service quality outlined by Ovretveit (1992):

Client: what the client wants from the service.
Professional: whether the service meets the needs and whether it correctly carries out techniques and procedures.
Management: most efficient and productive use of resources within limits and directives set by higher authorities/purchasers.

Quality and quality assurance

Whilst it is difficult to find a consensus on a definition of quality, the Department of Health (1993) has issued some very specific requirements about quality in NHS establishments:

> NHS Authorities and Trusts should demonstrate an organization-wide approach to quality through the development of quality improvement

strategies which should be made explicit in business plans, specify continuously renewable standards for services, and require changes arising from audit to be implemented.

This, in effect, sets out a recognized format for the *quality assurance process* (that is, the means of ensuring a guaranteed minimum acceptable standard) which involves the following stages (Luthert and Robinson, 1993). (See Table 10.1 and Figure 10.1).

Table 10.1 Components of the quality/audit cycle

Define a level/degree of excellence to be achieved
(standard setting)

Measurements of this level
(audit standards)

Implement change

If achieved:	If not achieved:
Check defined level of excellence set was appropriate (can target be moved?)	Identify deficits, problems or difficulties which make level unattainable
If level to remain the same (i.e. it is appropriate) continue measurement	If change is considered possible, implement change and continue measurement
	If change is not possible, redefine level of excellence

Standard setting

Standard setting is a central focus in quality assurance. The standards may be unique to a particular organization or profession, adapted from existing standards or a combination of both. Standard setting should be achieved through a consensus among those involved in the area of practice and should be based upon well-researched principles and published protocols. Definitions need to be unambiguous and definitions of clinical terms agreed and adopted.

Professional bodies have always been involved to some degree in standard setting, with guidelines for practice and the codes of

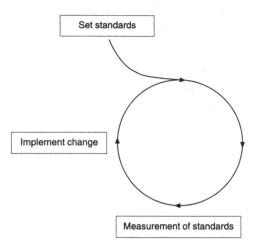

Figure 10.1 The Quality/Audit Cycle

conduct, below which minimum standards should not fall. In response to the demand for quality mechanisms and standard setting, professional groups developed systems to evaluate care, such as the Dynamic Standard Setting System (RCN, 1990). Although this system takes the form of a review, giving guidance on each stage of the quality assurance process, its main emphasis is on the setting of standards and criteria and it is closely bound to Donabedian's (1966) structure, process and outcome triad. This system of organizing healthcare into resources (structure), actions (process) and results (outcomes), has had a profound effect on the development of quality assurance methods (RCN, 1989). Within the framework for quality devised by the RCN there is an emphasis on shared objective setting (across multi-disciplinary boundaries), and on setting achievable standards of care (see Figure 10.2).

One means of achieving consensus on areas for standard setting may be the creation of a quality circle; this is designed to maximize staff involvement in quality activities and to foster the development of a quality culture. It usually involves a small group of people from a common background whose purpose is the implementation of quality in a specialized area of care. The task of such a group is to identify and select problems for attention (Ellis and Whittington, 1993).

Standard setting in infection control has been helped by the efforts of a multi-disciplinary working party, which formulated a

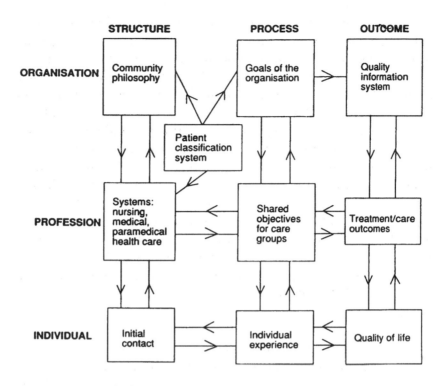

Figure 10.2 Framework for quality assurance in healthcare

range of infection control standards, including standards relating to the management structure and responsibilities in infection control, policies and procedures, the microbiology service, surveillance and education (Infection Control Standards Working Party, 1993). These standards may be useful in assessing the activities of the infection control team, but they do not assist with the setting of clinical standards. Clinical standards have been developed by Millward et al. (1993), based upon recognized good practice and research into infection control. An infection control audit tool was subsequently published; it will be discussed later.

Audit

According to the dictionary definition, audit is the 'official examination', usually of financial accounts (Shorter Oxford English

Dictionary, 1983). It is now commonly used to describe the *measurement* of quality standards and is therefore one stage in the quality process. Once the measurement of quality standards has taken place, the necessary information is available to determine whether improvements in practice are required. A broadened definition of audit has recently developed in the context of medical audit (i.e. carried out by the medical profession). In this case audit incorporates two stages of the audit quality cycle, i.e. measurement and improvement when required (Norman and Redfern, 1995). Medical audit became mandatory in the early 1990s (Department of Health, 1991), but since then there has been a move towards multi-disciplinary audit. This has been actively encouraged by the government, with the aim of integrating professional expertise and approaches and developing the wider concept of the 'clinical audit'.

To achieve this, the Department of Health (1994) recommends that successful clinical audit must be patient-focused and involve the following:

- It should be carried out at healthcare team level
- It should make links between health and social services
- It should encourage contributions from individual healthcare professionals
- It should link any uni-professional audit activity with overall patient care by the multi-professional team.

The use of audit as a means of measuring the standards of clinical practice in infection control was evaluated by Millward et al. in 1993. These authors devised an infection control audit tool, and measured its effectiveness in three different districts. The objectivity of this tool was later measured in a study involving 22 hospitals in the UK (Millward et al., 1995), which demonstrated that the audit tool was a useful means of measuring infection control standards. Examples of the standards and audit tool are shown in Appendix 1.

Feedback of results

Feedback of the outcomes of audit is essential if change is to be implemented where necessary. This completes the quality/audit cycle. The forms which feedback may take can vary between verbal, written or both. Immediate feedback can be provided verbally at the time of the audit, then followed by a written report with clear recommendations for improved practice. Table 10.2 shows an example of a format for the provision of written feedback.

Table 10.2 Format for provision of written feedback of audit results

Area	Problem	Recommendation	Action taken	Sign/date
Sharps disposal	Container not assembled correctly and not labelled	All staff to be aware of how to assemble containers correctly and why this is important. Containers must be labelled before dispatch.		

Surveillance

Where the term 'audit' can be applied to the measurement of clinical practice quality standards and associated outcomes, the term surveillance is more commonly used in relation to the measuring of data on infections. This usually involves 'the collection ... analysis and dissemination of resulting information to those who need to know so that appropriate action can be the result' (Hospital Infection Control: guidance on the control of infection in hospitals – Department of Health, 1995).

The above advisory document defines the objectives of surveillance as:

- The prevention and early detection of outbreaks in order to allow timely investigation and control
- The assessment of infection levels over time in order to detect the need for, and measure the effect of, prevention and control measures.

The Senic Report (Study into the Efficacy of Infection Control) carried out by Haley et al. (1985) concluded that carrying out surveillance can be effective in reducing hospital-acquired infection by up to one-third. However, despite the apparent benefits of surveillance in terms of avoiding preventable infections and achieving cost savings as a result, it does have implications in terms of the demands on the infection control team's time, and the need for follow-up in the community. Both Law et al. (1990) and Molyneux (1991) found that follow-up in the community was important in identifying patients with infection, who would otherwise not have been included in the postoperative surveillance data. This aspect is particularly important in the light of the increasing use of day surgery and early postoperative discharge from hospital.

Larson et al. (1988) suggest that there are at least two factors, other than quality of care, which have important influences on hospital-acquired infection rates. These are i) intrinsic patient factors, and ii) variations in recognition of infection and hence infection rates.

It is because of these variables that Ayliffe, as long ago as 1986, suggested that the 'multifactorial nature of hospital-acquired infection leads to the assumption of an irreducible minimum level'. Larson et al. (1988) suggest that in order to use hospital-acquired infection rates as an outcome measure it is necessary to ensure that variables are accounted for, and to adopt standard methods for defining and detecting infections.

Bowell (1990) describes those intrinsic risk factors that could be significant in the development of infection, but concludes that there is not a decisive means of measuring these and assessing possible outcomes. Rogers (1993) goes one step further with the development of a tool to assess patient intrinsic risk factors. Because it is based on other nursing assessment tools, this tool appears to be more user-friendly than the mathematical model devised by Bibby et al. (1986). The steering group of the second national prevalence survey (1993) has gone some way towards standardizing definitions of infection which may be used by infection control staff. It is because of some of the difficulties concerning standardization that the Department of Health (1995) advised purchasers to be cautious in their expectations and use of surveillance data.

Nevertheless, most infection control teams recognize that there should be a selective approach to data collection, and suggested formats include:

Alert organism surveillance

This consists of the reporting of clinically important isolates to the infection control team on a regular (usually daily) basis, so that control measures may be put in place to prevent spread. An example of an 'alert organism' would be an antibiotic-resistant strain that may cause serious clinical infection, e.g. epidemic MRSA. See Table 10.3.

Table 10.3 Example of an 'alert' organisms report

Ward	Jan	Feb	Mar	Apr	May	Jun	Jul
Ward 1							
C. difficile	1		1			1	
MRSA		1	2	1			
WARD 2							
Salmonella	1						
MRSA	1			1			2
Ward 3							
Rotavirus	4	3	1				
Strep. gp A				1			

This is most commonly carried out as a routine part of the infection control team's activities but it is dependent upon the clinical staff sending good quality specimens to the laboratory at an appropriate time, e.g. prior to commencement of antimicrobial therapy.

Incidence studies

This type of surveillance is a comprehensive form of data collection that depends upon the case finding on the ward as well as upon laboratory results, i.e. it is not dependent solely upon the specimens being sent as mentioned above. Once a defined caseload has been agreed, all patients who fall within that definition during a period of time are followed up in order to determine whether or not they developed infection. This requires the following:

- Review of medical and nursing notes and charts of all patients in a chosen ward/speciality
- Review of all microbiology results (positive and negative)
- Discussion with staff about any patients who they consider to be infected

This review is repeated several times weekly, depending on the speed of turnover.

To undertake such comprehensive surveillance to detect all infections in a given group of patients or speciality, it has been estimated that six wards of a general hospital would require 18 hours a week of infection control nurse time per 100 beds (Glenister et al., 1992).

Prevalence studies

Where an incidence study measures the number of patients in a defined caseload who become infected, a prevalence study measures the proportion of patients infected at the time during which the survey is carried out, i.e. a 'snapshot'. Infected patients tend to remain in hospital longer than uninfected ones, and consequently prevalence rates are higher than incidence rates (Department of Health, 1995). An important prevalence study was carried out by Meers et al. (1981) involving 43 hospitals in the UK and over 18,000 patients. This work indicated that 9.2% of patients who came into hospital developed an infection. Although this national survey has been repeated (Emmerson et al., 1995), the results are not entirely comparable because of the many changes in medical practice and patient mix that have occurred since the original survey. Hospital stays are much shorter and technical advances have altered the nature of surgery. However, repeated prevalence studies in an individual hospital may give useful information on infection trends and the efficacy of infection control measures. French et al. (1989) recommend the use of repeated prevalence studies as a means of measuring infection control activities and to aid quality assurance.

Research

Whereas audit and surveillance aim to measure outcomes of practice in terms of measurable data, research aims to discover new and better practice where this is lacking (Gaunt, 1993). The research process begins with a question, which is followed by the process of answering that question in an objective and reliable way. It is not simply a search for existing information, as in a literature search, but it is a rigorous search for new knowledge. Although research is usually carried out by a few, its results can and should be utilized by many professionals. Good research which is well validated can contribute to the quality process by assisting healthcare workers to set and review standards.

Conclusions

This chapter has attempted to provide an insight into aspects of quality, standard setting and audit and how these principles can be applied to infection control. It is essential that a quality approach is adopted by all those who work in healthcare so that there is a mechanism for monitoring and improving standards. Absence of good infection control can have a negative effect on the outcome of care for many patients and so it is essential that this receives high-profile treatment in all healthcare settings. A positive outcome of the recent changes in healthcare has been that the expectations of patients have been raised, which encompasses good standards in staff practices and in the hygiene of their environment.

Audit of clinical practice and surveillance of hospital-acquired infections are two means of measuring outcome of infection control activity. However, before either of these can be initiated, education of staff is essential in order to highlight the infection control standards that need to be met, and why they are important. It is not feasible for individual infection control practitioners to carry out the infection control practices themselves. They advise and educate others about how they can do it properly! Therefore all healthcare workers must take responsibility for setting their own standards and continually improving their practice and outcomes. Good compliance with infection control is an important contribution to the quality of healthcare.

References

Ayliffe G Nosocomial infection – the irreducible minimum. Infection Control 1986; 7 (2): 92–5.

Bibby B, Collins B, Ayliffe G A mathematical model for assessing risk of postoperative wound infection. Journal of Hospital Infection 1986; 8: 31–9.

Bowell B In Applied Microbiology, Caddow P (ed). London, Scutari Press, 1990.

Chaudhuri A Infection control in hospitals: has its quality enhancing and cost effective role been appreciated? Journal of Hospital Infection 1993; 25: 1–6.

Department of Health. National Health Service and Community Care Act (1990). London: HMSO, 1990.

Department of Health. HC(91)2: Medical audit in the Hospital and Community Health Services. London: HMSO, 1991.

Department of Health. Achieving an Organisation Wide Approach to Quality: EL (3) 116. London: HMSO, 1993.

Department of Health. The Evolution of Clinical Audit. Leeds: NHS Executive, 1994.

Department of Health. Hospital Infection Control – guidance on the control of infection in hospitals. Public Health Laboratory Service, 1995.

Department of Health. A First Class Service. London: DoH, 1998.

Donabedian A Evaluating the quality of medical care. Milbank Memorial Fund Quarterly 1966; 44 (2): 166–206.

Donabedian A The quality of care: how can it be assessed? Journal of the American Medical Association 1988; 260 (12): 1743–8.

Ellis R, Whittington D Quality Assurance in Health Care. London: Edward Arnold Publishers Ltd, 1993.

Emmerson A, Enstone J, Kelsey M The Second National Prevalence Survey of infection in hospitals: methodology. Journal of Hospital Infection 1995; 30: 7–29.

French G, Cheng A, Wong S, Donnan S Repeated prevalence surveys for monitoring the effectiveness of hospital infection control. The Lancet 1989; 1021–3 October 28.

Gaunt P Audit in infection control – data analysis and infections in the intensive care unit. Journal of Hospital Infection 1993; 24: 291–300.

Glenister H, Taylor L, Cooke E, Bartlett C A Study of Surveillance Methods for Detecting Hospital Infection. London: Public Health Laboratory Service, 1992.

Haley R, Culver D, White J et al. The efficacy of infection surveillance and control programmes in preventing nosocomial infections in US hospitals. American Journal of Epidemiology 1985; 121: 182–205.

Horton R Introducing high quality infection control in a hospital setting. British Journal of Nursing 1993; 2 (15): 746–54.

Infection Control Standards Working Party. Standards in Infection Control in Hospitals. Southampton: Hobbs, 1993.

Larson E, Oram L, Hedrick E Nosocomial infection rates as an indicator of quality. Medical Care 1988; 26 (7): 676–84.

Law D, Mishriki S, Jeffery P The importance of surveillance after discharge from hospital in the diagnosis of post-operative wound infection. Annals of the Royal College of Surgeons of England 1990; 72: 207–9.

Luthert J, Robinson L (eds) Manual of Standards of Care. Oxford: Blackwell Scientific Publications, 1993.

Meers P, Ayliffe G, Emmerson AM, Leigh D, Mayon-White R, Mackintosh C, Stronge J Survey of Infections in Hospitals. Journal of Hospital Infection 1981; 2 (suppl.): 1–49.

Millward S, Barnett J, Thomlinson D A clinical infection control audit programme: evaluation of an audit used by infection control nurses to monitor standards and assess effective staff training. Journal of Hospital Infection 1993; 24: 219–32.

Millward S, Barnett J, Thomlinson D Evaluation of the objectivity of an infection control audit tool. Journal of Hospital Infection 1995; 31: 229–33.

Molyneux R Assessing surgical wound infections. Nursing Times 1991; 87 (24): 67–70.

Norman I, Redfern S In Kogan M, Redfern S (eds) Making Use of Clinical Audit – a guide to practice in the health professions. Buckingham: Open University Press, 1995.

Ovretveit J Health Service Quality – an introduction to quality methods for Health Services. Oxford: Blackwell Scientific Publications, 1992.

Patients Charter. London: HMSO, 1992.

Rogers F Quality initiative. Nursing Times 1993; (Infection Control supplement) 89 (45): xii–xiii.

Royal College of Nursing (RCN). Standards of Care: a Framework for Quality. London: Royal College of Nursing, 1989.

Royal College of Nursing. Dynamic Standard Setting System. London: Royal College of Nursing, 1990.

Shorter Oxford English Dictionary, 3rd Edition, Vol. 1. Oxford: Oxford University Press, 1983.

Steering Group of the Second National Prevalence Survey. National prevalence survey of hospital-acquired infection: definitions. Journal of Hospital Infection 1993; 24: 69–76.

Working for Patients (White Paper). London, HMSO, 1989.

Chapter 11
Immunosuppressed patients

JANE BARNETT

Introduction

Due to the nature of hospitals, where patients are admitted for the treatment of a variety of conditions and are in contact with many staff, as well as undergoing invasive procedures, there will always be a susceptible population. However, the risk to patients is increased when their immune system is not functioning normally, thus making them even more vulnerable to infection. This may be due to a variety of reasons such as the immaturity of a newborn's immune system, the presence of disease such as leukaemia or as a result of specific drugs or treatments (Bowell, 1992).

This chapter will discuss how this group of patients may acquire infection and some of the means by which we can avoid this.

Endogenous infection

Infections may arise from the patient's own microflora, generally termed 'commensal organisms' which under normal conditions live on or in the body with no ill effects. However, in a state of immunosuppression, these commensals have the potential to become pathogenic, that is, cause infection. When this occurs the infection is termed *endogenous* (see Figure 11.1). Kibbler and Prentice (1994) suggest that the majority of infections which occur in the immunosuppressed bone marrow transplant patients are caused by endogenous infection. Wade and Schimpff (1989) describe the microbial shift that can occur in immunosuppressed individuals which may allow colonization of susceptible sites such as the lungs or gastrointestinal tract with organisms which may in turn go on to cause infections. In particular, these authors cite Gram-negative organisms or

172

fungal infections such as *Candida albicans* as the main problems. The main causes of this microbial shift are given as the underlying disease itself, invasive techniques, and the use of antibiotics.

Exogenous infection

Another means of introducing infection to a susceptible host is via an external source, that is *exogenous* infection. This may be the hands of personnel with whom the patient has had close physical contact, or, potentially, via contaminated equipment. Recognized pathogens include *Staphylococcus aureus*, which can cause serious wound and systemic infections and may be particularly difficult to treat, especially if the strain exhibits multiple resistance. Another potentially important exogenous organism may be *Aspergillus* species which, although present in abundance in the outside air, can cause infections in seriously immunosuppressed patients if allowed to enter a hospital environment. This is discussed in more detail later.

The extent to which either of the above means of acquiring infection go on to cause clinical sepsis is dependent upon the level of immunosuppression in the patient.

Microorganisms originate from the patient's own body

Microorganisms originate from other people or inanimate objects

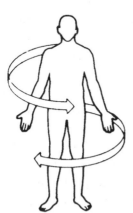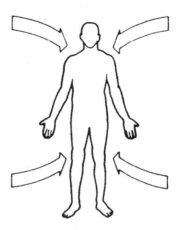

Figure 11.1 Endogenous and exogenous infections

Prevention of infection

Although there are many practices associated with the care of patients who are immunosuppressed, many of these do not seem to be supported by research but have developed over many years. Several authors raise questions about the validity of such procedures, which have evolved in specialist centres caring for immunocompromised patients (Kibbler and Prentice, 1994; Mooney et al., 1993; Poe et al., 1994).

It would seem sensible to rationalize procedures depending on the level of immunosuppression being experienced by the patient. A higher level of intervention may be required for those patients undergoing bone marrow transplantation than those undergoing less suppressive therapy.

Intervention may be necessary to minimize infection risks when the levels of granulocytes (of which neutrophils account for the largest proportion) in the blood fall below $0.5 \times 10^9/1$ (Wilson, 1995). The more severe infections and Gram-negative bacteraemia are more likely to occur when the count falls below $0.1 \times 10^9/1$ (Wade and Schimpff, 1989). These authors suggest that the level of neutropenia can be a reliable indicator of infection risk.

Protective isolation

Isolation of patients in order to prevent them acquiring infection may be detrimental to the overall wellbeing of the person. Knowles (1993) showed through her qualitative study involving the interviewing of patients with infectious conditions in isolation that this can have a negative effect. Terms such as loneliness, boredom and feeling stigmatized were highlighted in this work. It is therefore essential that patients receive support and information about their condition and the reasons for the isolation. However, it has been suggested in earlier work that patients who are protectively isolated tend to be more involved in the decision-making processes and are therefore more likely to be prepared and able to cope with the experience (Collins et al., 1989).

Indeed, Lesko et al. (1984) in the review of the literature, discuss the 'specialist status' experienced by patients in protective isolation units who often resented being moved out from their 'germ free' environment when their condition improved. However, both Collins et al. (1989) and Lesko et al. (1984) found that the stresses of the disease and sometimes painful treatment processes were difficult to separate out from the pressures of being in protective isolation.

Nauseef and Maki (1981) compared two groups of severely neutropenic patients, one of which received simple protective isolation and the other standard hospital care. These authors concluded that neither survival nor response to antileukaemic therapy was improved by isolation measures and that less expensive measures, such as good handwashing before patient contact, avoidance of invasive devices where possible and the use of prophylactic antibiotics alone, may be sufficient to protect this group of patients. However, Wilson (1995) suggests that when a patient is isolated in a single room, this alone acts as a reminder to staff and visitors of the importance of the simple hygiene measures necessary.

It is essential that information is given to visitors and relatives, who may be overwhelmed by the processes involved in caring for their loved one. Visitors should be advised not to visit if they have an infection, even a common cold, as this may place the patient at risk. Hands should be washed before entering and unless relatives are actively involved in the giving of care, there is little evidence that the donning of protective clothing is either useful or cost effective.

Filtered air

Although infections acquired via an air ventilation system are relatively uncommon in the immunocompromised host (Wilson, 1995) outbreaks of infection caused by *Aspergillus*, an environmental fungus, have been reported (Barnes and Rogers, 1989). Many units have HEPA (high efficiency particulate air) filters which remove 99.97% of particles 0.3 micron in diameter (Ayliffe et al., 1992) and air is pushed into the room through the filters under positive pressure. However, Nauseef and Maki (1981) suggest that Aspergillus is an infrequent pathogen in most studies of the protective environment, even amongst those receiving care in a ward rather than a single room. These authors suggest that the introduction of filters into a unit needs to be carefully assessed in light of the risk to the population to be cared for, as well as the quality of the air in the hospital environment. Such filtration systems can be costly to maintain and install, and for this reason, should only be considered in units where severely immunocompromised patients will be nursed, for example, liver and bone marrow transplant units (Ayliffe et al., 1992). Mooney et al. (1993) set down guidelines for the monitoring of the air quality in units where HEPA filtration is installed; this should include the following periodic sampling:

- before opening a newly constructed unit
- thereafter, depending on the levels of fungal disease in a hospital
- as part of an outbreak investigation.

Handwashing

This is probably the most important part of the care of a patient who is immunocompromised and should be carried out using a good technique both before and after contact with a patient (Wilson, 1995). Soap and water is adequate for use in protective isolation environments; there is no evidence to suggest that providing a good handwash technique is used, it is any less effective than an antiseptic. However, in the event of a cluster of infections in a unit caring for immunosuppressed patients, an antiseptic may be introduced to avoid transient carriage of organisms on the hands. Alcohol handrub is a useful addition to basic hand hygiene, which can be readily available at the bedside to disinfect hands before direct contact with vulnerable sites, for example invasive devices.

Protective clothing

Gloves and aprons are the only two items of protective clothing that should be worn in the context of protective isolation. Gloves should be worn when in contact with wounds, blood or body fluids in accordance with universal precautions (Advisory Committee on Dangerous Pathogens, 1995), although Mooney et al. (1993) suggest the wearing of non-sterile gloves for all direct patient contact in particularly vulnerable units.

Aprons should be donned when carrying out close physical care. There is no evidence that masks are useful in reducing infection risks to patients (Kibbler and Prentice, 1994), especially if the patient is being nursed in a room with HEPA filtration; masks may contribute to the anxiety felt by patients and visitors during a period of isolation.

Although some authors suggest the wearing of masks when staff have a respiratory infection or herpetic lesions on the mouth (Mooney et al., 1993), it would be better practice to redeploy such staff to other areas rather than rely on the questionable efficacy of a face mask.

Cleaning

General cleaning is essential to keep levels of dust to a minimum and reduce surface contamination risks from equipment. Detergent and water are adequate in the protective isolation room. However, a disinfectant may be appropriate if there has been a spillage of body fluids. It may also be necessary for the removal of any mould that may be growing on windows or in bathrooms.

Decontamination of equipment

There appears to be little evidence supporting the use of sterile equipment such as linen and utensils for patients in protective isolation. All equipment should be cleaned with detergent and water following use; if there is any doubt whether this will be done then higher risk items such as commodes, which are more readily contaminated, should be allocated for single-patient use (Wilson, 1995). The only equipment which is required to be sterile is that used for invasive procedures.

Food

Due to the potential contamination of raw or uncooked food such as salads with potentially harmful pathogens such as *Listeria monocytogenes*, it is preferable to give immunosuppressed patients only food that has been cooked thoroughly. Although some infections have been associated with ice-making machines, this can be easily avoided by regular and thorough cleaning of this equipment (Newsom, 1968; CDR, 1993; Stout et al., 1985). Only in units with very severely immunosuppressed patients should the provision of sterile drinking water be considered necessary.

Selective gut decontamination

Selective gut decontamination aims to suppress potentially pathogenic Gram-negative organisms present in the gut via the administration of oral, non absorbed antibiotics. Although Wade and Schimpff (1989) cite various studies that demonstrate apparent benefits for the use of such antibiotics, there are a number of real and potential disadvantages associated with this therapy. Sensitivity reactions may occur following some antibiotics, and there may be an increased risk of fungal infections unless an antifungal substance is given concurrently. Another potential problem is the possibility of development of resistant organisms. However, despite these difficulties, Wade and Schimpff (1989) suggest that for patients with acute immunosuppression, who may be undergoing prolonged periods of neutropenia, such prophylaxis may be beneficial.

References

Advisory Committee on Dangerous Pathogens. Protection Against Blood-borne Infections in the Workplace: HIV and Hepatitis. London: HMSO, 1995.

Ayliffe G, Lowbury E, Geddes A, Williams J Control of Hospital Infection – A Practical Handbook, 3rd Edition. London: Chapman and Hall Medical, 1992.

Barnes R, Rogers T Control of an outbreak of nosocomial aspergillosis by laminar air flow isolation. Journal of Hospital Infection 1989; 14: 89–94.

Bowell B Protecting the patient at risk. Nursing Times, 1992; 88 (3): 32–5.

CDR. Ice as a source of infection acquired in hospital. CDR Weekly 1993; 3 (53): 241.

Collins C, Upright C, Aleksich Reverse isolation: what patients perceive. Oncology Nursing Forum 1989; 16 (5): 675–9.

Kibbler C, Prentice H Infection Control aspects of bone marrow transplantation. Current Opinion in Infectious Diseases 1994; 7: 427–9.

Knowles H The experience of infectious patients in isolation. Nursing Times 1993; 89 (30): 53–6.

Lesko L, Kern J, Hawkins D Psychological aspects of patients in germ free isolation: a review of child, adult and patient management literature. Medical and Paediatric Oncology 1984; 12: 43–9.

Mooney B, Reeves S, Larson E Infection control and bone marrow transplantation. American Journal of Infection Control 1993; 21 (3): 131–8.

Nauseef W, Maki D A study of the value of simple protective isolation in patients with granulocytopenia. New England Journal of Medicine 1981; 304 (8): 448–53.

Newsom SWB Hospital infection from contaminated ice. Lancet 2 Sept 1968; 14: 620–22.

Poe S, Larson E, McGuire D, Krumm S A national survey of infection prevention practices on bone marrow transplant units. Oncology Nursing Forum 1994; 21 (10): 1687–94.

Stout JE, Victor LY, Mucara P Isolation of Legionella pneumophila from the cold water of hospital ice machines: implications for the origin and transmission of the organism. Infection Control 1985; 6 (4): 141–6.

Wade J, Schimpff S Epidemiology and prevention of infection in the compromised host. In Clinical Approaches to Infection in the Compromised Host, 2nd Edition. Ed: Rubin R, Young L. New York and London: Plenum Medical Book Co, 1989.

Wilson J Infection Control in Clinical Practice. London: Bailliere Tindall, 1995.

Chapter 12
Mother and child infections

LAUREN TEW

Introduction

Increasing standards of public health have been clearly demonstrated in the improved welfare of mothers and their children. Infant mortality figures (a recognized measure of maternal health) are falling all over the globe although there is wide variation in these figures around the world. The infant mortality rate in most of Africa is four times that in Europe (Peters, 1991). Basic facilities such as clean water, which have a major impact on infection rates, are still not available to all.

The micro-organisms that caused 10–20% of women to die in childbirth in the seventeenth to nineteenth centuries are ever-present, remaining a substantial clinical problem (Gantz et al., 1991). One of the developments that led to the reduction in maternal mortality and morbidity, antibiotic therapy, has paved the way for a new threat – the evolution of micro-organisms resistant to many of the chemotherapeutic agents.

This chapter will examine infection control issues through the stages of pregnancy and childbirth, and on to childhood.

Infection during pregnancy

Control of infection in maternity care has been described as 'complicated' (Tew, 1990). It is integral to all systems related to patient care (Bowell, 1992), including maternity care, in order to maintain a safe environment for mother and baby. Until deteriorating social conditions brought about 'lying-in' wards in hospitals, babies were born at home and cross-infection was a domestic problem (Selwyn, 1991). The hospitalization of maternity care has led to infection risks for the mother, baby and the staff in attendance.

Infection risks to the mother

Awareness of infection risks to the mother can ensure that interventions are planned to reduce the risk. These interventions often start with the mother's first attendance for antenatal care. At the first antenatal appointment blood samples are taken to assess blood group, rubella status, presence of Rhesus antibodies and antibodies indicating infection with syphilis.

The midwife can use the booking appointment and further antenatal visits to educate the mother about safe food handling and hygiene measures she can take to reduce the likelihood of certain infections, such as *Listeria monocytogenes* or *Toxoplasma gondii* (Department of Health, 1992). An assessment of the risk of occupational exposure to infection should take place at an early stage in pregnancy. Employers should refer to the guidelines on protecting new and expectant mothers, in order to prevent and control infection risks under health and safety legislation (Advisory Committee on Dangerous Pathogens, 1997).

At all stages of pregnancy the mother is at risk of infection, which may have devastating results such as miscarriage, premature labour, perinatal or congenital infection of the baby. The immunological relationship between the mother and foetus has prompted much research but many questions remain to be answered (Stirratt, 1990). Whilst mothers' sera contain antibodies to paternally derived tissue in the foetus, the major deviations from the immunological norm elude clarification yet permit the 'most amazing sequence of events which involve the rapid but totally controlled invasion of maternal tissues by a semi-alien parasite' (Stirratt, 1990).

Stirratt (1990) suggests that the placenta may act as an immuno-absorbent sponge for potentially harmful antibodies, thus protecting foetal material.

In early pregnancy viral infections (for example, rubella, influenza, mumps) can cause a miscarriage. Bacterial infections rarely have this result, with the exception of *Listeria monocytogenes*, which can also cause stillbirth. Protozoal infections are rarely seen in Britain, toxoplasmosis being the most relevant. Up to the early 1960s septic abortions were a result of infection with *Clostridium perfringens* and other anaerobes (Shanson, 1989).

Maternal viral infections during pregnancy can cause congenital malformations. The earlier in the pregnancy the infection occurs, the more severe the likely malformation. *Toxoplasma gondii*, rubella, cytomegalovirus and *Herpes simplex* infections (TORCH) may have serious effects on the foetus's development (see Table 12.1).

Asymptomatic bacteriuria has been found in up to 5% of antenatal attenders (Shanson, 1999). If untreated, this can lead to severe pyelitis but some areas are no longer screening routinely.

Intrauterine infection (chorio-amnionitis) complicates 20% of cases of premature rupture of membranes and is caused by ascending potential pathogens found in the normal vagina, such as anaerobic streptococci and Gram-negative bacilli (Llewellyn-Jones, 1990). There is a high risk of premature birth or still birth in these cases (Shanson, 1999).

Infection risks to the baby

During pregnancy the baby is well protected from the outside world as long as the membranes surrounding the foetus in utero remain intact. If premature rupture of the membranes occurs, micro-organisms have access to the foetus and the liquor amnii (Ayliffe et al., 1992). Ascending infection can cause amnionitis. Transplacental transfer of infection from the mother is the more likely cause of congenital infection. Table 12.1 gives details of the most important congenital infections and the effects on mother and baby. It also outlines methods of preventing spread of infection.

Infection risks to the staff

The blood and body fluids to which modern-day birth attendants are exposed may place them at risk of infection (Hart, 1991). Hepatitis B and C and the HIV virus are invisible but real threats; obstetric staff will inevitably sustain blood and amniotic fluid contact during deliveries if protective clothing is not worn. The avoidance of needlestick injury (McKeown, 1992) and adoption of universal precautions (Hart, 1991) will protect staff. Hart (1991) lists prevention of inoculation incidents, prevention of contamination, use of protective clothing, waterproof covering to skin lesions and efficient hand washing as the means by which staff can achieve this. For further information see Chapter 15 and Health Departments, UK, 1998.

Table 12.1 Congenital infections

Organism	Effects on mother	Effects on baby	Specific prevention
Chlamydia trachomatis	Cervicitis, urethritis, Bartholinitis, pelvic inflammatory disease, salpingitis	Ophthalmia, pneumonia, otitis media, bronchiolitis, gastroenteritis	Sexual health education for public and health professionals; investigate parents of ophthalmia neonatorum cases in GUM clinic. Screen all women receiving antenatal care.
Cytomegalovirus (CMV)	Subclinical infection in 95% of women; 5% have mild flu-like illness	Intrauterine growth retardation, thrombocytopaenia, hepatitis, chorioretinitis, cerebral palsy, deafness (10%). Occurs in 0.3% live births, 10% have serious handicap	Handwashing of caring staff; immuno-compromised children to receive CMV negative blood products. Screening not appropriate. No known effective maternal treatment.
Hepatitis B	Chronic liver disease	Asymptomatic or minimal symptoms	Screen mothers antenatally; health promotion; bath baby soon after birth; accelerated vaccination programme for babies, starting within 24 hours of birth.
Herpes simplex virus (HSV)	Genital vesicles, fever and malaise	Abortion, stillbirth and neonatal death; 1 in 50,000 newborn babies in UK have clinically significant infection; local infection of skin, eyes and mouth, encephalitis, pneumonia and hepatitis	Swab vesicular fluid if current infection in mother; if active lesion late in pregnancy, deliver by LSCS; screen baby if normal delivery follows recently healed lesion.

Organism	Effects on mother	Effects on baby	Specific prevention
HIV	Initial infection may be asymptomatic. No effect of pregnancy on disease progression.	Signs of infection rare at birth; early serology testing difficult due to mother's IgG; 20% of infected babies will develop AIDS or die in first year.	Access to information and guidance for all sexually active women; antenatal HIV testing for all pregnant women; advice, treatment and interventions to reduce vertical transmission; high level of compliance with universal precautions by staff.
Listeria monocytogenes	Influenza-like illness; asymptomatic vaginal, faecal and urine carriage; amnionitis.	Stillbirth; septicaemic illness within 48 hours of birth; meningitis; pneumonia.	Pregnant women should avoid: pate, unwashed salads; unpasteurized dairy products; ensure adequate reheating of prepackaged meals; avoid working with silage. Well maintained domestic fridges.
Neisseria gonorrhoeae (Gonorrhoea)	Vaginal discharge, dysuria, urinary frequency, cervicitis, salpingitis, PID	Ophthalmia neonatorum within 2 days of birth. Without treatment blindness may ensue.	Investigation and treatment of mother by GUM specialist
Parvovirus	50% of infections are asymptomatic; mild systemic upset with fever and rash; arthropathy.	Increased risk of hydrops fetalis, foetal death and spontaneous abortion in 2nd and 3rd trimesters.	Source of infection often not traced
Rubella	Subclinical infection is common; mild febrile illness, rash, arthralgia.	Foetal effects depend on timing of infection; risk of defects high until 17 weeks' gestation; deafness, cardiac malformation, cataract, chorioretinitis, micro-ophthalmia.	Screen female attenders for pre-conceptual counselling and immunize if necessary; advise seronegative mothers at booking to avoid children and adults with rashes during pregnancy and to be immunized after birth; infected infant should avoid contact with pregnant women for its first year while excreting virus.

(contd)

Table 12.1 (contd)

Organism	Effects on mother	Effects on baby	Specific prevention
Streptococcus agalactiae (Group B streptococcus)	Asymptomatic carriage in vagina of 30% of women.	Neonatal septicemia and meningitis.	High standards of hygiene and handwashing; compliance with infection control procedures and policies.
Toxoplasma gondii	Asymptomatic, mild 'flu. If first infection happens during pregnancy, transplacental transmission occurs in 30–40% of cases.	Miscarriage, stillbirth; hydrocephalus, epilepsy, partial sight or blindness, mental retardation.	No current screening programme; early detection in pregnancy; avoidance of undercooked meat, unwashed vegetables and fruit, soil contaminated with cat faeces, unpasteurized goats' milk and dairy products.
Treponema pallidum (Syphilis)	Miscarriage, fetal death, stillbirth.	Intrauterine growth retardation, preterm delivery.	Each pregnancy should be routinely screened antenatally for syphilis.
Varicella (Chickenpox)	Risk of primary maternal infection in pregnancy is 1–3 per 1000 pregnancies; itchy vesicular rash, pneumonitis; 3% spontaneous abortion rate if infection at less than 16 weeks' gestation.	Less than 1% affected pregnancies result in congenital varicella syndrome. Maternal primary infection just before birth can result in disseminated chickenpox, rash, fever, pneumonitis and encephalitis with 5% mortality.	Check for VZV antibodies if susceptible pregnant woman is in contact with chickenpox; if seronegative seek specialist advice. Exclude susceptible staff (history and anti-VZV negative) from working with vulnerable patients from 8–21 days after exposure.

Sources: Alexander J, Levy V, Roch S (eds) (1990); Ayliffe GAJ, Lowbury EJL, Geddes AM, Williams JD (eds) (1992); Balows A (ed) (1991); Cooper J, Morrison T (1995); Graham Davies E, Elliman D, Anthony Hart C, Nicoll A, Rudd P (1995); Howe J (1996); Pendleton E, Coussey C, Sanger S (1996); Quintanilla K (1996); Stucke V (1993); Waters J (1996); NHSE (1999).

Infection risks from the environment

The maternity ward environment must be maintained at a high level of cleanliness to reduce the risks from contaminated dust and wet residues harbouring Gram-positive or Gram-negative organisms respectively. Ndawula and Brown (1991) found mattresses in a poor state of repair. An outbreak of an epidemic strain of methicillin-resistant *Staphylococcus aureus* was not controlled until all the mattresses had been replaced. Window and bed curtains and mattresses in labour rooms have been found soiled with body fluids. A systematically planned housekeeping routine, organized through liaison between midwifery staff, the infection control nurse and the Hospital Services Department, will reduce environmental risks to a minimum. It is also important to purchase easily laundered soft furnishings and heat-sealed mattresses and pillows.

Infection risks during childbirth

In the mid-nineteenth century birth at home was far safer than in hospital, where the risk of death from puerperal fever was great. The reduction in infection rates at the end of the nineteenth century was not due to medical treatments, but to improvements in public health, although understanding of the causes and modes of transmission of infections had advanced (Tew, 1990).

Aseptic technique must be employed by caring staff attending the delivery. Puerperal sepsis is usually caused by *Streptococcus pyogenes*, known today as beta-haemolytic streptococcus Group A (Philpott-Howard and Casewell, 1994). This micro-organism may cause a post-partum endometritis or wound infection. Investigation of surgical and obstetric staff may be necessary.

Congenital infections may occur as the baby passes through the birth canal. In some cases, such as active *Herpes simplex* infection, the baby may be delivered by Caesarean section to avoid infection (Table 12.1).

Infection after birth

Postnatal infection

Puerperal sepsis continued to be the greatest single cause of maternal death as the twentieth century progressed, and it made up nearly half of the direct causes of maternal mortality into the 1950s (Tew, 1990). The 'conquest of sepsis' was the greatest single cause of the decline in maternal mortality. This was due to better standards of living and diet, with the consequent health benefits, as well as to the introduction of antibiotics, which brought about a rapid and steep decline in maternal deaths from puerperal sepsis (Tew, 1990) caused in the most part by Group B streptococci (Selwyn, 1991).

Endometritis is the most common postnatal infection, its incidence increasing sharply if rupture of membranes occurs more than six hours prior to delivery (Shanson, 1999). Gantz et al. (1991) confirm that neither the number of vaginal examinations, use of an internal foetal monitor, anaemia nor obesity enhance susceptibility to infection. Occasionally there will be a dramatic onset of symptoms when infection is caused by Group A or B haemolytic streptococci, *E. coli* or anaerobes such as clostridium or bacteroides. This will occur within 12 hours of delivery and needs prompt antibiotic therapy for both anaerobes and aerobes. Gantz et al. (1991) point out that wound infection following Caesarean section, urinary tract infection and breast abscess will also cause a puerperal fever. *E. coli*, *Staphylococcus aureus*, haemolytic streptococci and anaerobic bacteria are the most commonly isolated organisms from abdominal incisions. *E. coli* causes 80–90% of urinary tract infections whereas *Staphylococcus aureus* causes 95% of breast abscesses (Gantz et al., 1991).

Neonatal infection

The mother or staff may be the source of minor neonatal sepsis, frequently caused by *Staphylococcus aureus*. Outbreaks are now less common than they were 30–40 years ago. Skin pustules, sticky eyes, umbilical infections and breast abscesses are the results of staphylococcal infection. Scalded skin syndrome, in which toxins split the epidermis, is a rare but serious disease of neonates with a high mortality rate (Shanson, 1999).

Low birth weight babies are most likely to succumb to Group B haemolytic streptococcus and Gram-negative organisms (such as *E. coli*, *Klebsiella aerogenes* and *Pseudomonas aeruginosa*), which may be associated with the prescribing of broad-spectrum antibiotics to the mother. These organisms cause more sepsis and deaths in low birth weight infants during their first week of life than any other organism (Shanson, 1999).

Babies are susceptible to infections with organisms that may not cause problems to adults (Line, 1992). Breast pumps (Moloney et al., 1987; Gransden et al., 1986; Blenkarn, 1989), milk kitchens (Ayliffe et al., 1970) and feeding utensils have been incriminated in outbreaks of infection in neonates, mostly due to inadequate decontamination of equipment and also poor hand hygiene. Inadequate handwashing by personnel is the most common means of transmission of organisms to babies.

There is much debate concerning the need for prophylaxis against staphylococcal colonization of infants. 30% of babies are colonized with this organism within their first week of life (Shanson, 1999).

A frequent maternal complication following colonization of a baby's nostrils with staphylococci is entry of the organism through the broken skin of a sore nipple, resulting in a breast abscess (Ayliffe et al., 1992), 90% of which are indeed caused by staphylococci (Llewellyn-Jones, 1990). The Cochrane review of ten studies of cord care (Zupan and Garner, 1999) concluded that in institutions in developed countries, "simply keeping the cord clean appears to be as effective and safe as using antibiotics or antiseptics" (p. 1) where there may be greater risk of infection, for example preterm babies, babies in neonatal units, or where bacterial contamination is more likely, the use of antiseptics is unlikely to do any harm. Any intervention that prolongs the time until cord separation and increases the number of visits by the midwife will have profound effects on the midwives' workload (Mugford et al., 1986). In their survey of cord care in 93 English Health Districts, Mugford et al. (1986) estimated that current cord treatment policies were costing the NHS 45,000 midwife hours a year. However, the decision to stop anti-staphylococcal prophylaxis should not be taken by any maternity professional unilaterally, but following multi-disciplinary liaison with the infection control team, paediatricians, obstetricians and midwives.

Preventing transmission of infection

Llewellyn-Jones (1990) identifies four main areas of practice that will promote good infection control measures. Firstly, the design of the maternity unit, properly equipped and with sufficient single accommodation; and staff with an inflamed throat (caused by streptococci in 30% of cases; Thomas, 1988) should not come to work; thirdly, the prompt treatment of any septic foci antenatally. Finally, he states that labour should be carried out with surgical asepsis, that vaginal examinations should only be performed wearing sterile gloves on scrupulously cleaned hands and that repair of vaginal tears should be performed aseptically. Good handwashing and aseptic techniques are supported by Shanson (1999).

Observation of the mother postnatally will ensure that fever (more than 38°C) will be recognized promptly, although many mothers have a transient low-grade pyrexia postnatally (Gantz et al., 1991). Regular observation of mother and baby is a means of detecting infection (Llewellyn-Jones, 1990).

Staff need access to up-to-date information regarding infection control (Sarosi and East, 1991). Practising universal precautions, avoiding needlestick injury and using protective clothing will reduce risks to staff from potentially infectious body fluids (Hart, 1991).

Teaching mothers about hygiene for their baby is often included in the plan of postnatal care. A checklist will record aspects of the baby's progress, for example, skin spots, discharging eyes, mouth and umbilical infection.

In order to reduce the number of babies infected with HIV, Health Authorities must ensure that all pregnant women are offered HIV testing, by the end of 2000. The use of anti retroviral drugs, Caesarean section and bottle feeding can reduce the risk of vertical transmission from 25% to less than 5% (NHSE, 1999). All pregnant women are offered antenatal screening for hepatitis B. Appropriate immunization will reduce the risk of the baby becoming a carrier by more than 90% (NHSE, 1998). Dearden (1990) recommends the reinforcement of infection control policies and procedures, emphasizing basic infection control principles relating to the transmission of infection as a means to reduce neonatal infections.

Ayliffe et al. (1992), Llewellyn-Jones (1990) and Shanson (1989) recommend prompt isolation of any infant or mother showing signs of sepsis. Shanson (1989) cites the delivery of a full-term baby of normal weight as the optimum way to reduce risks of infection in babies. He also recommends good standards of hygiene, uncrowded nurseries and aseptic techniques of hand decontamination. Careful caring techniques and rooming-in of babies with their mother are promoted.

Compared with the appalling maternal death rates from sepsis of the not too far distant past, immense improvements have been made in providing a safe environment for mother and baby.

Immunization

> It is every child's right to be protected against infectious disease
> (Department of Health, 1996 p.19).

Two hundred years ago Edward Jenner demonstrated the success of vaccination to protect against smallpox. 170 years later, in May 1980, the World Health Organization (WHO) was able to announce that smallpox had been eradicated. Vigorous immunization programmes across the globe have reduced the scourge of many infectious diseases. The WHO is now aiming for eradication of poliomyelitis throughout the world by the year 2000.

In order to protect the population as a whole from an infectious disease, a high proportion of susceptible individuals must be immunized. This is known as 'herd immunity'. In the 1970s and 1980s children died of whooping cough when immunization levels fell as a result of fears about vaccination. (See Table 12.2 for a list of conditions which are *not contraindications to immunization*.) In 1994 a campaign was organized to vaccinate school children against measles as there was a serious risk of an epidemic in this group (Nurse Prescriber, 1996). In the UK coverage for most vaccines is 95%. Were this figure to fall, diseases no longer seen would reappear (Salisbury, 1996).

In the UK a comprehensive vaccination programme has been in place for many years. The programme is reviewed regularly and changes made in the light of advances in epidemiological and scientific knowledge (Salisbury, 1996). For example, the 'Green Book' (Department of Health, 1996) notes changes in immunization against diphtheria, measles, mumps and rubella (MMR) and the use of Hib and BCG vaccine. There have been some reports in the media concerning the administration of the MMR vaccine and possible links with Crohn's disease and autistic spectrum disorders.

Table 12.2 Conditions that are *not* contraindications to immunization

---

a. Family history of any adverse reactions following immunization.
b. Previous history of pertussis, measles, rubella or mumps infection.
c. Prematurity: immunization should not be postponed.
d. Stable neurological conditions such as cerebral palsy and Down's syndrome.
e. Contact with an infectious disease.
f. Asthma, eczema, hay fever or 'snuffles'.
g. Treatment with antibiotics or locally acting (i.e. topical or inhaled) steroids.
h. Child's mother is pregnant.
i. Child is being breast fed.
j. History of jaundice after birth.
k. Under a certain weight.
l. Over the age recommended in the immunization schedule.
m. 'Replacement' corticosteroids.

Department of Health. Immunisation Against Infectious Disease. London: HMSO, 1996.

However the Department of Health investigated relevant literature and concluded that there are no such links and that children should continue to receive the vaccine as usual and there is no need to receive the vaccines separately (Department of Health, 1998).

The 'Green Book' includes essential information about the whole immunization process, for example consent, storage of vaccines, immunization procedures, indications and contraindications. It is beyond the remit of this chapter to cover these topics in any detail. The reader is therefore referred to the Department of Health's text for comprehensive guidance.

Table 12.3 shows the currently recommended immunization schedule.

Attending school

Once a child is old enough to mix with others it is at risk of picking up infectious diseases from its playmates. Nowadays more children are attending day care facilities from an early age, whilst an increasing proportion of mothers go out to work. The principles of infection control can be applied to such caring facilities, ensuring the safety of the children attending (Ross, 1994). The principles outlined by Ross (1994) include:

Table 12.3 Immunization schedule

Vaccine	Age	Notes
D/T/P and Hib/ Polio	1st dose 2 months	Primary course
Meningococcal C conjugate vaccine	2nd dose 3 months	
	3rd dose 4 months	
Measles/mumps/rubella (MMR)	12–15 months	Can be given at any age over 12 months
Booster DT and polio	3–5 years	Three years after completion of primary course
2nd dose MMR		
BCG	10–14 years, or in infancy	
Booster tetanus, diphtheria and polio	13–18 years	

Children should therefore have received the following:

Adults should receive the following:

By 6 months	3 doses of DTP, Hib and polio	Women, sero-negative for rubella — Rubella
By 15 months	MMR	Unimmunized individuals — Polio
		Tetanus
By school entry	4th dose DT and polio	Diphtheria
		Hepatiis B
		Hepatiis A
		Individuals in high-risk groups — Influenza
		Pneumococcal
Between 10 & 14 years	BCG	vaccine
Before leaving school	5th polio and Td	

From Department of Health (1996)

DTP = diphtheria/tetanus/pertussis; Hib = *Haemophilus influenzae b* vaccine

Td = tetanus and diphtheria reinforcing dose; DT = diphtheria and tetanus booster

- **Handwashing**: young children need to be supervised when handwashing; they need to be taught how and when to wash their hands. Hands must always be washed after using the toilet and before eating or drinking. Staff must wash hands after nappy changing. The number of wash handbasins and toilets (1 for 10 children) should be adequate.

- **Nappy changing**: should take place in a designated area away from food preparation. Surfaces should be impervious and easy to clean. A wash handbasin should be nearby.

- **Food hygiene**: staff preparing food should receive training for this role. A wash handbasin must be available in the kitchen (see Chapter 8). Staff dealing with children with enteric symptoms should not serve food. Feeding bottles should be decontaminated in individual tanks of cold disinfectant for each child (see Chapter 9).

- **Laundry**: soiled clothes should be rinsed then placed in a plastic bag for parents to take home. Washing machines should be in an area separate from the kitchen. Soft toys and bedding should be washed at 60°C on a weekly basis or when soiled.

- **Health promotion**: managers of daycare centres should ensure their staff are aware of hygienic and infection control practice. There may be opportunities for providing parents with information about infectious diseases, etc.

- **Exclusion**: each daycare facility should have explicit policies for the exclusion of children with infectious diseases. Children with a fever and other signs and symptoms may need to be excluded, but each case should receive individual consideration.

These principles can be applied to children throughout their school career and into adulthood. Comprehensive guidelines for the control of common infections in schools and nurseries are available (Department of Health, 1999). Handwashing is the most important activity in the control of infection, not only in hospital but also in general life. Whilst the wonders of modern life and science have reduced the influence of infection on the population, particularly in the developed nations, there is still a major part we can all play in reducing the effects further. By following a healthy lifestyle that keeps our immune systems fighting fit and by maintaining hygienic standards of living we can all play our own part in the control of infection in our lives.

References

Advisory Committee on Dangerous Pathogens. Infection Risks to New and Expectant Mothers in the Workplace. HSE Books, 1997.

Alexander J, Levy V, Roch S (eds) Intrapartum Care: a research-based approach. London: Macmillan Educational Ltd, 1990.

Ayliffe GAJ, Collins BJ, Pettit F Contamination of infant feeds in the Milton milk kitchen. The Lancet, March 14 1970; 559–60.

Ayliffe GAJ, Lowbury EJL, Geddes AM, Williams JD (eds) Control of Hospital Infection: A practical handbook, 3rd Edition. London: Chapman and Hall Medical, 1992.

Balows A (ed) Manual of Clinical Microbiology. Washington: American Society for Microbiology, 1991.

Blenkarn J Infection risks from electrically operated breast pumps. Journal of Hospital Infection 1989; 13: 27–31.

Bowell B Protecting the patient at risk. Nursing Times, 1992; 88 (3): 32–5 January 15.

Cooper J, Morrison T Congenital infections in pregnancy. Infections, 1995; 5–8 August.

Dearden D Neonatal infections. Nursing Times, May 9 1990; 86.

Department of Health. While you are Pregnant: Safe eating and how to avoid infection from food and animals. London: HMSO, 1992.

Department of Health. Immunisation Against Infectious Diseases. London: HMSO, 1996.

Department of Health. Measles, Mumps and Rubella (MMR) Vaccine, Crohn's Disease and Autism (PL/CMO/98/2). London: Department of Health, 1998.

Department of Health. Guidance on Infection Control in Schools and Nurseries. London: HMSO, 1999.

Gantz N, Gleckman R, Brown R, Esposito A Manual of Clinical Problems in Infectious Diseases. USA: Little, Brown & Co, 1991.

Graham Davies E, Elliman D, Anthony Hart C, Nicoll A, Rudd P Manual of Childhood Infections. London: WB Saunders Company Ltd, 1995.

Gransden WR, Webster M, French GL, Phillips I An outbreak of Serratia marcescens transmitted by contaminated breast pumps. Journal of Hospital Infection 1986; 7: 149–54.

Hart S Blood and body fluid precautions. Nursing Standard, March 13 1991; 5 (25): 25–7.

Health Departments, UK. Guidance for Clinical Health Care Workers: Protection Against Infection with Blood Borne Viruses. London: Department of Health, 1998.

Howe J Chlamydia trachomatis: symptoms and consequences. Nursing Standard 1996; 11 (10): 34–6.

Line S Sterilising feeding bottles in the home. Professional Care of Mother & Child, September 1992; 249–50.

Llewellyn-Jones D Fundamentals of Obstetrics and Gynaecology Volume 1: Obstetrics. London: Faber & Faber Ltd, 1990.

Moloney AC, Quoraishi AH, Parry P, Hall V A bacteriological examination of breast pumps. Journal of Hospital Infection 1987; 9: 169–74.

McKeown M Sharpening awareness. Nursing Times 1992; 88 (14): 66–8 April 1.

Mugford M, Somchiwong M, Waterhouse I Treatment of umbilical cords: a randomised trial to assess the treatment methods on work of midwives. Midwifery 1986; 2: 177–86.

Ndawula EM, Brown L Mattresses as reservoirs of epidemic Methicillin resistant Staphylococcus aureus. The Lancet 1991; 337: 448 Feb 23.

NHSE. Reducing mother to baby transmission of HIV. HSC 1999/183.

NHSE. Screening of pregnant women for hepatitis B and immunisation of babies at risk. HSC 1998/127.

Nurse Prescriber. Some basic facts on immunization. Nurse Prescriber/Community Nurse July 1996; 29.

Pendleton E, Coussey C, Sanger S Targetting groups at risk of hepatitis B. Nurse Prescriber/Community Nurse, 1996; 54 April.

Peters A Compact Peters Atlas of the World. UK: Longman, 1991.

Philpott-Howard J, Casewell M Hospital Infection Control. Policies & Practical Procedures. London: WB Saunders Co Ltd, 1994.

Quintanilla K Can HIV be transmitted through breast milk? Nursing Times, 1996; 92 (31): 35–7 July 13.

Ross S Infection Control in Childcare Facilities. In Worsley M, Ward K, Privett S, Parker L, Roberts J (eds) Infection Control: A Community Perspective. Infection Control Nurses' Association of the British Isles, 1994.

Salisbury D Nurses' most frequent questions on immunization. Nurse Prescriber/Community Nurse, July 1996; 30–32.

Sarosi L, East J Marketing infection control. Nursing Times June 12 1991; 87 (24): 72–5.

Selwyn S Hospital infection: the first 2,500 years. Journal of Hospital Infection 1991; 18, Supplement A: 5–64.

Shanson DC Microbiology in Clinical Practice, 3rd Edition. Sevenoaks: Wright and Sons, 1999.

Stark V, Harrison SP Staphylococcus aureus colonization of newborn in a Darlington hospital. Journal of Hospital Infection 1992; 21: 205–11.

Stirrat G Immunology of Pregnancy. In Studd J (ed). Progress in Obstetrics and Gynaecology 5: 3–21. London: Churchill Livingstone, 1990.

Stucke V Microbiology for Nurses. London: Baillière Tindall, 1993.

Tew M Safer Childbirth. London: Chapman & Hall Medical, 1990.

Thomas C Medical Microbiology. London: Baillière Tindall, 1988.

Waters J The hidden parasite. Nursing Times, 1996; 92 (47): 16–17 November 20.

Zupan J, Garner P Topical umbilical cord care at birth (Cochrane Review) in: The Cochrane Library, Issue 2, 1999. Oxford: Update Software.

Chapter 13
Sexually transmissible infections

PATRICIA MILLS

Introduction

Infection control in the field of sexually transmissible infections relies on access to accurate diagnosis and, if available, treatment through genito-urinary clinics or general practitioners. The accessibility of services and the attitudes of people working in these areas have effects on the uptake of care and support. A person's sexuality and how they express it is an individual matter and usually private. Risk assessment for sexually transmissible conditions is therefore affected by the secrecy which surrounds sexual activity and there may be a reluctance to discuss such matters even when a problem arises. Levels of knowledge about infections and lay beliefs may also affect how people view their risk of contracting a sexually transmissible infection (STI) (Howell 1996; McManus 1995; Peart et al., 1996).

Many of these infections have been recorded in literature throughout the ages (Hicks, 1994) and usually carry stigma due to the mode of transmission (Moreton, 1995). Although bacterial infections are now treatable, viral infections cannot yet be eradicated. However, management of these infections is improving with new drugs and increased knowledge. Many people feel distressed and uncomfortable when diagnosed with a sexually transmissible infection and the approach of nurses, doctors and health advisers working in this area must be professional, supportive and free from judgements (ENB, 1994). This will encourage people to attend for treatment and advice, which are important factors in the context of infection control.

Sexually transmissible infections are largely caused by two groups of organism, viruses or bacteria. Venereal diseases are those defined by the Venereal Diseases Regulations, which were first drawn up in 1917 and have been updated and amended periodically since then (Moreton, 1995). The diseases covered by the regulations are syphilis, gonorrhoea and chancroid. These regulations are the basis of the confidentiality offered by Genito-urinary Medicine (GUM) clinics which is one reason why people are prepared to use the service for examination and treatment. Confidentiality within clinics is a prime consideration and people may attend giving a false name if they wish (SHASTD, 1996). GUM clinics are one of the few services to which patients have direct access without going to their GP, and the patient is able to contact the clinic directly to make an appointment. The confidentiality offered under the National Health Services VD Regulations (1974) apply only to hospitals in the NHS and health authorities (Haigh and Harris, 1995). Examination and testing for a range of sexually transmissible infections, and many other laboratory tests, will be undertaken in the clinic. If required, treatment is arranged and is free.

In this chapter, venereal diseases and other infections most commonly seen in GUM clinics will be discussed, together with a brief description of the signs and symptoms, relevant tests and treatment. Sexual intercourse is not the only mode of transmission. In some cases auto-inoculation may be possible, e.g. with herpes simplex, and some infections such as candida and bacterial vaginosis occur in both sexually active and celibate women.

Viral infections

Genital warts

Organism: Human papilloma virus (HPV)

There are many sub-types of HPV. Numbers 16 and 11 are commonly associated with genital warts. Numbers 16, 18, 31, 33 and 34 are less common, but may be associated with malignant changes on the cervix in some women. There are likely to be other factors involved in malignant changes.

Indications: Bumps in the skin, or easily visible warty lesions, itching and/or soreness. Infection may be asymptomatic and painless. Lesions may appear from between 2 weeks to 2 years (or longer) after infection with the virus. In men warts may be found on shaft of the penis, urethral meatus, prepuce, perianal region and anal canal. In women they may be found at introitus, labia majora and minora, perineum, vagina or cervix (may be unnoticed if in vagina or on cervix).

Laboratory tests: HPV cannot be cultured, therefore diagnosis is made from observation of clinical features. The virus may be present subclinically, and may be infectious in this state.

Treatment: This is aimed at removing the wart lesions as the virus cannot be eradicated and remains in the body for life after the initial infection. Lesions may be painted with podophyllin, podophyllo-toxin or trichloracetic acid (self treatment is not recommended unless prescribed by a doctor). Cryotherapy or cautery of lesions may be used.

Complications: Recurrence of infection and possible changes on cervical smear in women. Warts may get very large in pregnancy and all patients with genital warts should be screened for other sexually transmissible infections. This is the commonest STI seen in British and American GUM clinics.

(Adler, 1998; Ferenczy, 1995; Herrington, 1995; Knox, 1995; Sims and Fairley, 1997)

Genital herpes

Organism: Herpes simplex virus (HSV) Type 2. Genital herpes may also result from infection with HSV Type 1 which usually causes facial herpes. Auto-inoculation is possible with herpes.

Indications: Vary from mild to severe and usually appear within 2–20 days of direct contact with virus, through either penetrative or oral sex. Other symptoms include itching, burning, blister formation at area of discomfort, flu-like illness, enlarged inguinal glands. If there is a blister on cervix, women may develop vaginal discharge or rarely retention of urine. When the blister bursts, a shallow painful ulcer is present before healing begins. Acquisition of the virus can occur without visible lesions appearing.

Laboratory test: Swab from the ulcer or fluid from blister. In ulcer-forming genital infections, syphilis must always be excluded.

Treatment: The virus remains in the body for life and may recur. Antiviral drugs are the best available therapy at present. This does not eradicate the virus but if given early may damage viral replication. Poor compliance with therapy, due to the frequency of medication, has been reported.

If recurrences are more frequent than once per month, antiviral therapy may be given for extended periods to suppress the virus. Painkillers are given for systemic effects, e.g. paracetamol or aspirin. Rest is important if an episode is severe.

Notify partner: Partner notification is advisable after diagnosis because infection may recur and it is possible to pass on the virus without clinical signs and symptoms being present (silent shedding), especially around the time of recurrence. If herpes lesions are present at the time of childbirth, a caesarian section may be performed.

(Adler, 1998; Knox, 1995; Hoffman and Schmitz, 1995; Woolley, 1995; Bowman, 1994; Clarke, Tatum and Noble, 1995; Milne, 1997; Herpes Virus Association; Horn, 2000)

Hepatitis

Organism: Several recognized viruses cause hepatitis and these may be transmitted in various ways. Hepatitis B is recognized as being sexually transmissible. Hepatitis C may be sexually transmissible but the evidence for this is not conclusive at present. Although hepatitis A is generally foodborne, it may also be sexually transmitted if there is oral–anal contact.

Indications: These are similar for all viral hepatitis infections and include tiredness, fatigue, fever, dark urine, anorexia and jaundice. In some people nothing may be noticed. Careful history-taking may suggest the likelihood of exposure to virus.

Laboratory tests: Specific serological test should be requested and tests for other sexually transmissible conditions should be considered, including offering an HIV test, depending on the risk.

Treatment: There is no effective cure for any of the viral hepatitis infections, therefore identifying risk activities and offering vaccination for hepatitis B is important. There is no vaccination for hepatitis C at present, although interferon, in combination with Ribavirin, may be effective in some people with confirmed infection.

Notify partner: This would need to be considered if the patient was a carrier of infection, identified by laboratory tests.

Complications: Rarely, chronic hepatitis (active or not) may develop, or a severe illness, such as cirrhosis of the liver or carcinoma. People with hepatitis C may develop chronic illness. Patients with active hepatitis disease require referral to gastro-enterologist, or a specialist unit for liver disease.

(Adler, 1998; Knox, 1995; Horn, 2000; British Liver Trust).

Human immunodeficiency virus (HIV)

Organism: Retrovirus, HIV 1 or HIV 2

Indications: At the time of infection usually none, though some people get a flu-like illness called a sero-conversion illness. After infection with HIV people usually remain symptom-free for a number of years, although they are infectious to others through blood and body fluids (semen and vaginal fluid and, in lactating women, breast milk). HIV can damage the immune system to the extent that people develop acquired immune deficiency syndrome (AIDS).

Laboratory tests: Specific serological test, HIV Antibody Test, with follow-up confirmatory test if positive. Viral load and CD4 counts if the antibody test is positive.

Treatment: Highly active antiretrovival therapy (HAART) can slow the progress of the disease, preventing opportunistic infections. The choice of drugs and time of commencement are discussed between the doctor and patient in partnership. Adherence to treatment is important, and requires regular monitoring and support. Currently drugs are required for years. There is as yet no cure for HIV.

Notify partner: Health Advisors or HIV Councillors work closely with HIV positive people to support and encourage them to notify current, past and future sexual partners of the potential risk. Improving treatments may encourage people to undertake testing. HIV is not a notifiable disease.

Complications: Damage to the immune system, weight loss, diarrhoea, AIDS-related illnesses, psychological effects of living with a life threatening illness, social and relationship consequences of living with a disease that may be transmitted to others. Some of the drug treatments have side effects such as nausea, diarrhoea and skin sensitivity.

(Adler, 1998; Knox, 1995; Alcorn, 1996; Hoffman and Schmitz, 1995; Alder et al., 1995; NAM, 1998; BHIVA, 2000)

Bacterial infections

Non-gonococcal urethritis (NGU)

Commonly referred to as NSU: non-specific urethritis.

Organism: This is not usually identified, but up to 30% of cases may be due to *Chlamydia trachomatis* (see below). *Mycoplasma genitalis* and *Ureaplasma urealyticum* may be implicated in some of the Chlamydia negative patients. *Trichomonas vaginalis* may also be rarely implicated and consideration may need to be given to intraurethral herpes simplex and syphilis. However, no infective agent is found in the majority of cases.

Indications: Urethral discharge or dysuria may also be asymptomatic.

Laboratory tests: A urethral smear is taken and examined microscopically in the GUM clinic to identify the presence of pus cells. Swabs are sent to the laboratory for culture for gonorrhoea and chlamydia. The urine may be examined for evidence of infection such as threads of pus.

It is important that male patients attending GUM clinics do not pass urine for 4 hours prior to the examination, or the exudate may be washed away, making diagnosis difficult.

Treatment: Broad-spectrum tetracycline or macrolide based antibiotics are usually prescribed for NGU, but if a specific infection is diagnosed on culture further treatment may be required. The patient is advised not to have sexual intercourse.

Notify partner: People with NGU should consult a health adviser or nurse specialist for information about safer sex practices. Sexual contacts are treated, if results of swabs indicate this is necessary.

Complications: Occasionally men develop a chronic and persistent urethritis or prostatitis.

Adler, 1998; Jafri, 1995; Knox, 1995; Horn, 2000; Woolley, 1994; Milne, 1997; Horner et al., 1993; McClean, 1997)

Chlamydia

Organism: *Chlamydia trachomatis*, intracellular bacteria.

Indications: Up to 70% of women and 30% of men have no signs and symptoms. If present, symptoms appear 7–21 days after infection and may be vague, e.g. slight vaginal discharge or discomfort in women and dysuria and urethral discharge in men. Women with untreated infections may develop pelvic inflammatory disease and experience lower abdominal pain with uterine tenderness, dysuria, dyspareunia, bleeding between periods and after sexual intercourse, heavy or irregular periods, mucopurulent cervicitis, vaginal discharge. Infections affecting the rectum or throat are usually symptomless.

Laboratory tests: *Women* require endocervical and urethral swabs; a high vaginal swab is not appropriate. Care should be taken not to contaminate the swab on the vaginal wall. The local laboratory should be consulted regarding the use of transport media as this may vary. A first voided urine test may be used. *Men* should provide a first voided urine specimen at the clinic after holding urine for 4 hours. A urethral swab from 5–6cms into the distal urethra may be required. People who receive anal sex will need to provide a rectal swab.

Treatment: Broad-spectrum tetracycline or macrolide based antibiotic. In pregnancy and in lactation, erythromycin. There are now single-dose treatments available. The patient is advised not to have sexual intercourse.

Notify partner: This is undertaken because of the possible severe sequelae of untreated infection in women, and the likelihood of reinfection if the partner is not notified and treated.

Complications: In women, chronic abdominal pain, pelvic inflammatory disease with increased risk of ectopic pregnancy and infertility. There may be transmission to the neonate if infection is present at time of delivery, causing eye and chest infections. Reiter's syndrome (rare in women).

In men, complications include epididymitis, Reiter's syndrome (reactive arthritis and conjunctivitis with urethral discharge). *Chlamydia trachomatis* can infect the rectum, conjunctiva and throat.

(Adler, 1998; Knox, 1995; Thin et al., 1995; Fitzgerald et al., 1998; Richey et al., 1999; Watt, 1997)

Gonorrhoea

Organism: *Neisseria gonorrhoea*, which infects the site of columnar epithelium especially in genital tract.

Indications: In men, these appear 2–14 days after infection. 90% of infected men have symptoms of dysuria, yellow or green urethral discharge. The rectum or throat may also be infected, when there may be few indications.

In women the infection affects the cervix and urethra, producing a profuse watery discharge, low abdominal pain and dysuria. Many women are asymptomatic. Women may develop gonorrhoea of the throat or rectum, but this is less common.

Laboratory tests: In men and women the infection may be diagnosed in the GUM clinic by microscopic examination of a Gram-stained smear of the discharge. In women, an endocervical, urethral smear is taken and examined as above. Microscopic examination alone is not sufficient to exclude gonorrhoea. Swabs required are: endocervical, urethral, throat and rectal for women and urethral and throat, plus rectal swab if recieving anal sex for men.

Treatment: Penicillin is the drug of choice, but care must be used in history-taking as penicillin-resistant strains are common in some parts of the world and would require alternative treatments (guidance on current treatment is available from microbiologists). Treatment is given as a stat dose in the clinic and the patient is followed up for two consecutive weeks to ensure treatment has been effective. The patient is advised not to have sexual intercourse.

Notify partner: This is undertaken under the NHS VD Regulations (1974). Because many people with gonorrhea have symptoms, the government has been able to use the reports of numbers of cases as an indicator of unsafe sexual activities.

Complications: In men, epididymo-orchitis and in women salpingitis, damage to fallopian tubes. Two rare complications are perihepatitis, and disseminated gonococcal infection. If present at delivery the eyes of the neonate may be infected.

(Adler, 1998; Knox, 1995; Horn, 2000; Sherrard and Bingham, 1995; Milne, 1996; Thin et al., 1995; Fitzgerald and Bedford, 1996)

Syphilis

Organism: *Treponema pallidum*.

Indications: Primary stage
Appears 9–90 days after infection. A painless, usually single, ulcer at site of inoculation develops, called a primary chancre, which may exude serous fluid. In men, chancre is usually on the shaft of the penis or glans penis, in women it appears on the vulva, cervix or vaginal walls. It may also appear on the anus, rectum or anywhere on body where inoculation occurred. Chancre can heal spontaneously within 2–3 weeks if untreated or may last into the secondary stage of disease and may even be unnoticed if not present on the genitals.

Secondary stage
This occurs 3–20 weeks after infection and the primary chancre may occasionally still be present. It is a generalized illness, consisting of headaches, malaise, sore throat, maculo-papular rash and mucosal ulceration, which will clear without treatment.

Latent stage
This occurs when the secondary systemic signs and symptoms have healed. Syphilis can then only be detected by serological tests.

Laboratory tests: If the affected person presents at a GUM clinic during the primary stage exudate from the chancre can be examined by darkground microscopy, to visualize the spirochaetes characteristic of syphilis. In the early stages this may be the only way to establish diagnosis because serological tests may be negative. Serological tests undertaken are VDRL (venereal diseases research laboratory test), TPHA (*Treponema pallidum* haemagglutination test). If any of the initial screening tests offered to pregnant women and people attending GU clinics prove positive, further tests, e.g. FTA (fluorescent treponemal antibody test) and ELISA test is undertaken. Other infections may give false positive results and guidance should be sought from a GU medicine consultant and microbiologist. Serological tests undertaken will be decided by local laboratory in conjunction with the GUM clinic and may vary in different parts of U.K.

Treatment: Penicillin is the drug of choice, given intra-muscularly. Tetracyclines or erythromycin may be used if the patient is sensitive to penicillin. Syphilis can be treated at any stage. Some of the serology tests always remain positive after treatment.

Notify partner: Syphilis is covered by NHS VD Regulations (1974), so contact tracing of all partners is undertaken by the health adviser working with the patient. In women this may include children, because syphilis can cross the placental barrier in pregnancy and a mother may also infect a child after the disease has ceased to be sexually transmissible. The disease is no longer sexually transmissible approximately 2 years after the initial infection.

Complications: There may an allergic reaction to penicillin.

At the secondary stage there may be involvement of the liver, kidneys or meninges (all rare). If untreated, syphilis may progress to a tertiary stage with neurological symptoms such as dementia, or GPI (generalized paralysis of the insane). These are extremely rare, however. There may also be cardiovascular involvement such as aortitis, or aortic aneurism. Damage to the cardiovascular and neurological systems will not be reversed by treatment. Many people with untreated syphilis develop no related health problems.

(Adler, 1998; Knox, 1995; Milne, 1996; McClean, 1997; Thin et al., 1995)

Chancroid

Organism: *Haemophilus ducreyi.*

Indications: Appear within 3–7 days. An inflamed papule develops at the site of entry of the organism, which erupts within 2–4 days forming a well-defined ulcer. Ulcers are often multiple and painless. The formation of abscess in inguinal lymph glands may occur. A GUM clinic referral is recommended for everyone with genital ulceration.

Laboratory tests: Swab from the ulcer is sent for culture.

Treatment: Antibiotic therapy is given after sensitivity has been determined by the laboratory, as drug-resistant strains may be a problem.

Notify partner: This should be undertaken under NHS VD Regulations (1974). However, chancroid is extremely rare in the U.K.

(Adler, 1998; McClean, 1997)

Trichomoniasis: A protozoal infection

Organism: *Trichomonas vaginalis.*

Indications: In women there will be a vaginal discharge which may smell offensive, soreness around vulva, dysuria, dyspareunia. In men, occasionally urethritis or dysuria. This infection may be asymptomatic, especially in men.

Laboratory tests: The live organism can usually be seen by microscopy in the GUM clinic, but may be difficult to isolate in males. Tests for other sexually transmissible conditions should be undertaken.

Treatment: Metronidazole, which in pregnancy should be used with caution.

Notify partner: Regular sexual partners are offered examination and treatment.

Complications: If present in pregnancy the infection may be associated with premature labour, and neonatal infections.

(Adler, 1998; Hicks, 1995; Jaffri, 1995; Knox, 1995)

Other genital infections

Sexual transmission is not the main mode of transmission in the following.

Bacterial vaginosis

Organism: No single causative organism, but may include *Gardnerella vaginalis*, or anaerobic bacteria such as bacteriodes, mobiluncus or pepto-streptococci.

Indications: Women experience a grey, runny discharge and there may be an unpleasant smell in genital area, often worse after sex. The vaginal area may be oedematous but not inflamed. However, many women are asymptomatic.

Laboratory tests: The pH of the vaginal discharge is higher than 4.5. A distinctive odour (fishy) develops on adding 10% potassium hydroxide to a sample of the discharge. Gram staining and microscopy would reveal absence of lactobaccilli and the presence of clue cells.

Treatment: Metronidazole, which should be used with caution during pregnancy or lactation.

Notify partner: Not usually undertaken.

Complications: If untreated, bacterial vaginosis in pregnancy may contribute to premature labour.

(Knox, 1995; Smith, 1994; Temple, 1994).

Genital candidosis

Organism: *Candida albicans*, which is an opportunistic pathogen commonly found in humans.

Indications: Local irritation and sometimes discharge.

Laboratory tests: Gram staining will show spores and hypae. Swabs may also be sent for culture.

Treatment: Antifungal agent, either in pessary form or orally.

Notify partner: This is not usually required. The infection is more common in women, both celibate and sexually active. Men may require treatment if candida is isolated.

Complications: Recurrence of infection may be frequent, causing distress, and requiring sympathetic handling by staff.

(Adler, 1998; Knox, 1995; Kennedy, 1995; Milne, 1997)

Infestations

The infestations which are most often seen in GUM departments are scabies and pubic lice. These are passed through direct bodily contact and can be easily treated and eradicated.

Molluscum contagiosum

This is a viral infection, which is treated by ablation of the viral body by cryo-therapy. Complete removal of the lesion is not necessary. More than one visit to the clinic may be needed if there are many lesions (Horn, 2000; Milne, 1996).

Health promotion

Prevention of infection through good education and appropriate contact tracing are the best methods of infection control and are particularly important in respect of HIV and other viral infections for which there is no definitive treatment.

Risk activities for STIs may be difficult for people to discuss, and health professionals involved in care have to grasp opportunities when they arise. An ability to talk freely and frankly using explicit language when necessary, is required for work in this area (Howell, 1996; Alcorn, 1996). Good communicating and listening skills can do much to put people at ease and can create a safe atmosphere for them to begin assessing their risk (Curtis et al., 1995). This needs to happen before people are able to examine their behaviour and make changes. Good quality information and a positive approach to safer sex are necessary aspects of infection prevention. Suggesting alternatives to penetrative sex, instruction in condom use and helping young people to talk to partners and use negotiating skills can empower people to break the chain of transmission.

Sexual health promotion is aimed at changing risky behaviours and targeting information towards people who practise high-risk activities. This has evolved as an effective way of reaching people and developed from the more general awareness-raising campaigns used, especially for HIV/AIDS in Britain (McManus, 1995; Markin, 1995; Darrow, 1997). Targeting information gives the opportunity to use methods such as leaflets, videos, role play, using language suitable for the group (Baggaley, 1991; Darrow, 1997). Health campaigns may link information to other activities that are known to put people at risk of infection from unprotected sex, for example highlighting the increased risk associated with summer holidays, drinking alcohol and moving away from home (Markin, 1995; Howell, 1996; Marion and Cox, 1996). Many nurses are well equipped to undertake this work in family planning clinics, GP practices and sexual health clinics and some people prefer to approach a nurse rather than a doctor.

Provision of free condoms through the GUM clinic, family planning services and gay men's projects, provides the chance to engage people in discussion about high- and low-risk activities. Feelings of powerlessness within relationships, cultural and religious beliefs, will impact on decisions about the use of barrier methods of contraception (Richey et al., 1999; Peart et al., 1996). Use of the oral contraceptive may lead women, including the young, divorced or separated, to believe that they do not also need to use a barrier method to prevent infection (Marion and Cox 1996), and nurses need to encourage people to consider carefully their risks.

There are a number of agencies where good quality information about HIV/AIDS can be obtained. These include drop-in centres for young people, specialist centres for young gay men and lesbian women, and people from ethnic groups. For information and treatment for other sexually transmissible conditions these agencies will often refer to local GUM clinics (Alcorn, 1996). Free and confidential HIV antibody testing is available through GUM clinics. General practitioners and agencies will usually advise people of this (Alcorn,

1996; Knox, 1995). The national AIDS helpline is available 24 hours a day every day of the year for information, including the availability of local facilities. HIV testing within GUM clinics is usually undertaken by the health adviser, as is partner notification or contact tracing. The health adviser is involved in education of patients, staff and the wider community through personal contact and teaching. For people with HIV, herpes or recurrent STIs the health adviser has an ongoing role to offer support and counselling as required.

Partner notification, whilst considered an effective method of disease control, has to be undertaken with sensitivity and due regard for the confidentiality of the person presenting with an infection (index patient). The health adviser will work closely with the index patient to explain the importance of contacting sexual partners, and this can be undertaken by the patient with support and information, or by the health adviser or a combination of both (see Figure 13.1).

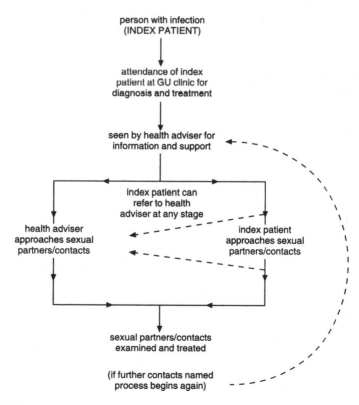

Figure 13.1 Contact tracing

The aim is to offer the person contacted an appointment for examination, testing and treatment if available (Hunter et al, 1980; SHASTD, 1996).

The expectation is that GUM clinic staff have the relevant training, knowledge and expertise to ensure that patients attending clinics are given the opportunity to assess their sexual health risk and receive treatment, support, advice or information. Raising the profile of GUM clinics can help to prevent the spread of infection by encouraging people to attend for tests. Open and honest communication can help to overcome the unease which people often feel when attending GUM clinics, thereby improving infection control and public health in this area of care.

References

Adler MW ABC of Sexually Transmitted Diseases, 4th Edition. London: BMJ Publishing Group, 1998.

Adler M, Fenton K, French R, Giesecke J, Howson J, Johnson A,. Petruckevitch A, Trotter S The HIV Partnership Notification Project. London: Department of Health, 1995.

Alcorn K (ed.) National AIDS Manual. London: NAM Publications, 1996.

Baggaley J Media Health Campaigns. In AIDS Prevention Through Health Promotion. Geneva: WHO, 1991.

BHIVA Writing Committee. British HIV Association guidelines for the treatment of HIV infected adults with antiretroviral therapy. HIV Medicine Vol 1 Issue 2 March 2000.

Bowman C Herpes virus infection. British Journal of Sexual Medicine 1994; 21 (2).

BNF British National Formulary. BMA & Royal Pharmaceutical Society of GB, 1995.

Clark JL, Tatum ND, Noble S Management of genital herpes. American Family Physician 1995; 51 (1): 175–82, 187–8.

Curtis H, Hoolaghan T, Jewitt C Sexual Health Promotion in General Practice. Oxford: Radcliffe Medical Press, 1995.

Darrow WW Health education and promotion for STD prevention: lessons for the next millennium. Genito Urinary Medicine 1997; 73 (2): 88–94.

ENB. Caring for People with Sexually Transmitted Disease Including HIV. London: ENB, 1994.

Ferenczy A Epidemiology and clinical patho-physiology of condylomata acuminata. American Journal of Obstetrics & Gynaecology 1995; 172 (4) pt 2.

Fitzgerald M, Bedford C The Clinical Management of Gonorrhoea. London: Central Audit Group in GU Medicine, 1996.

Fitzgerald MR, Welch J, Robinson AJ, Ahmed-Joshuf IH Clinical Guidelines and Standards for the Management of Uncomplicated Genital Chlamydial Infection. International Journal of STD and AIDS 1998; 9 (5): 253–62.

Haigh R, Harris D AIDS – A Guide to the Law. London: Routledge, 1995.

Herrington CS Human papilloma viruses and cervical neoplasia. Journal of Clinical Pathology 1995; 48

Hicks D A brief history of STDs. British Journal of Sexual Medicine July/August 1994.

Horn K Consultant GU Medicine, Royal United Hospital Bath NHS Trust. Personal Communication 2000.

Horner P, Gilroy C, Thomas B, Naidoo R, Taylor Robinson D Association of Mycoplasma genitalium with acute non-gonoccocal urethritis. Lancet 1993; 342 (8871): 582.

Howell K Safer Holiday Sex. Community Nurse 1996; 2 (4).

Hunter I, Jacobs J, Kinnell H, Satin A Handbook on Contact Tracing in Sexually Transmitted Diseases. London: The Health Education Council, 1980.

Jafri K Vaginal discharge. British Journal of Sexual Medicine 1995; 22 (2).

Kennedy R Vulvo vaginal candidiasis cures and diagnosis. British Journal of Sexual Medicine 1995; 22 (suppl.).

Knox H Sexplained; An Uncensored Guide to Sexual Health. London: Knox Publishing, 1995.

Martin J Advising travellers on health abroad. Nursing Standard July 12th 1995; 9 (42).

Marion LN, Cox LC Condom use and fertility among divorced and separated women. Nursing Research 1996; 45 (2).

McClean AN Consultant GU Medicine, Royal United Hospital Bath. Personal communication, 1997.

McManus J Promoting sexual health: the local government contribution. Health Education Journal 1995; 54: 251.

Milne D Consultant, GU Medicine, Bristol Royal Infirmary (retired). Personal communication, 1996.

Morcton R The development of Genito-Urinary Medicine services. British Journal of Sexual Medicine Jan/Feb 1995.

National AIDS Manual (NAM). HIV/AIDS Treatment Directory. London: NAM Publications, 1998.

National Health Service (Venereal Diseases) Regulations 1974.

Peart R, Rosenthal D, Moore S The heterosexual singles scene: putting danger into pleasure. AIDS Care 1996; 8 (3): 341.

Richey C, Macaluso M, Hook E Determinants of re-infection with Chlamydia trachomatis. Sexually Transmitted Diseases, 1999: 26(1).

Society of Health Advisers in Sexually Transmitted Diseases (SHASTD). Partner Notification Guidelines. London: MSF, 1996.

Sherrard JS, Bingham JS Gonorrhoea now. International Journal of STD and AIDS 1995; 6 (3): 162–6.

Sims I, Fairley CK Epidemiology of genital warts in England and Wales. Genito Urinary Medicine 1997; 75 (5): 365–7.

Smith T Diagnosing bacterial vaginosis. Journal of Community Nursing 1994; 7 (4): 9–10.

Temple CA Diagnosis and treatment of bacterial vaginosis. Nursing Times 1994; 90 (37) September 19.

Thin RN, Barlow D, Bingham C Investigation and management for sexually transmitted diseases (excluding HIV). International Journal of STDs & AIDS 1995; 6 (2): 130–36.

Watt P Safeguarding women's health. MRC News. Autumn 1997.
Woolley P The prevalence and transmission of H.S.V. British Journal of Sexual
    Medicine 1995; 22 (3): 5–8.

Chapter 14
Gastrointestinal infections

LESLY FINN

Gastrointestinal infection follows the ingestion of sufficient numbers of a pathogen to cause illness. Exposure to the organism can occur through contaminated food or water, or through secondary spread via the faecal-oral route. People may become infected on an individual basis (sporadic cases), with other members of a household, or as part of a wider outbreak depending on the nature of the infection and its source.

The term 'food poisoning' has been defined by the Advisory Committee on the Microbiological Safety of Food (ACMSF) as follows:

> 'any disease of an infectious or toxic nature caused by, or thought to be caused by, the consumption of food or water'
> (Department of Health, 1994a).

All doctors in clinical practice have a statutory duty to notify the proper officer of the local authority of cases, or suspected cases, of certain infectious diseases and food poisoning. Between 1992 and 1994 the gastrointestinal pathogens listed in Table 14.1 represented 45% of all laboratory reports received by the PHLS Communicable Disease Surveillance Centre (CDSC) (Wall et al., 1996):

However, this total represents only the tip of a very large iceberg. This figure does not include isolates from cases of gastrointestinal infection caused by ingestion of other pathogens, for example *Giardia lamblia*, *Bacillus* spp., hepatitis A virus, *Staphylococcus aureus*, or positive cultures or toxin detection in cases of diarrhoea caused by *Clostridium difficile*. In addition, laboratory reports of confirmed gastrointestinal

pathogens represent only a fraction of their true incidence for the
following reasons:

a) a proportion of those affected have only mild symptoms or are
    asymptomatic;
b) not all those who are ill seek medical attention;
c) clinicians do not always arrange for specimens to be obtained
    and sent for investigation;
d) not all specimens tested yield a pathogen;
e) not all pathogens are reported to CDSC.

Gastrointestinal infections are a growing problem and, although
the majority of such infections are of short duration and are self-limiting, the costs in terms of working days lost, clinical investigations and
treatment, not to mention human discomfort, is considerable. It must
also be remembered that these infections are largely preventable.

Table 14.1 Infectious disease cases reported 1992–94 for the following pathogens:

Campylobacter	122,250
All salmonellas	92,416
Rotavirus	47,463
Shigella sonnei	29,080
Cryptosporidium	14,454
SRSV	4,020
Clostridium perfringens	1,813
Escherichia coli 0157	1,266
Total	313,064

Factors involved in gastrointestinal infection

There are many factors involved in the possible development of
gastrointestinal infection following exposure to an infecting organism.
These include microbial factors, host defences and social factors.

Microbial factors

Infecting dose

This refers to the number of micro-organisms that need to be
ingested in order to produce disease. For example, a healthy person
would need to ingest a large amount of *Salmonella* spp. before becom-

ing ill whereas only one oocyte may need to be swallowed for cryptosporidiosis to develop.

Hardiness

Organisms vary in their ability to survive extremes of cold, heat or drying. For example, *Campylobacter* spp. prefer cooler, moister conditions, although they do not survive freezing, drying or heat. *Listeria monocytogenes* also prefers cooler temperatures and is able to multiply rapidly in foods chilled for long periods. Although *Salmonella* spp. are able to survive freezing and multiply rapidly at room temperature, the spores of *Clostridium difficile* tolerate drying and survive in the environment for extended periods of time.

Toxin production

Many pathogens produce powerful toxins which affect different types of body cell:

Neurotoxins – e.g. botulism (*Cl. botulinum*), *Staphylococcus aureus*
Enterotoxins – e.g. cholera, enterotoxigenic *E. coli* (ETEC)
Cytotoxins – e.g. *Clostridium difficile*

Clinical syndromes

The presentation of symptoms vary according to the properties of the infecting organism:

Febrile/septicaemic   –   Penetrating infections, e.g. *S. typhi*, listeriosis
Neurological   –   Toxin-mediated, e.g. botulism, paralytic shellfish poisoning (PSP)
Diarrhoeal   –   Non-inflammatory/secretory, e.g. cholera, rotavirus
    –   Inflammatory/colitic, e.g. *Salmonella* spp., *Campylobacter* spp., *Shigella* spp.

Host defences

Susceptibility to infection varies according to affected individuals' defence mechanisms, which include gastric acidity, intestinal motility, enteric microflora, specific immunity and intestinal receptors. Age and immune status are important risk factors for gastrointestinal infection, with the very young, the elderly and the immunocompromised being at particular risk (Evans and Maguire, 1996; Djuretic et al, 1996).

Social factors

Hygiene – particularly handwashing practice and environmental cleanliness in toilets and food preparation areas

Housing – person-to-person spread of infection is more likely in overcrowded conditions or in communal settings such as residential/nursing homes, schools, hospitals, hotels, cruise liners

Food production – standards in animal husbandry, e.g. 'factory' farming methods

EU – movement of foods between countries

Eating habits – increase in 'eating out', fast food outlets, snack foods, cook-chill, increased consumption of shellfish and raw molluscs

Affluence – use of freezers and microwaves

Travel – rapid travel within and between countries; increasing numbers of people taking foreign and 'exotic' holidays

Social activities – watersports, swimming, farm visits, pets

Iatrogenic – antibiotic-associated e.g. *Cl. difficile* Vancomycin-resistant enteroccal (VRE) infections in hospitals. Widespread use of antibiotics in veterinary and human medicine has resulted in antibiotic resistance in *Salmonella typhimurium*.

Clinical features of gastrointestinal infection

The clinical features of different gastrointestinal infections, including the causative organism and incubation period are set out in Chapter 8, Table 8.2.

Groups which pose an increased risk of person-to-person spread

In its guidelines for the prevention of human transmission of gastrointestinal infections, infestations, and bacterial intoxications a working party of the PHLS Salmonella Committee (1995) identifies four groups of persons who pose an increased risk of spreading infection:

Group 1: Food handlers whose work involves touching unwrapped foods to be consumed raw or without further cooking.

The role of infected food handlers in the transmission of infection is often difficult to establish because they may be victims rather than the source. However, food handlers who are ill at the time of food preparation are more likely to contribute to an outbreak. For example, in 12 outbreaks caused by small round structured viruses (SRSVs) food handlers either admitted to suffering from an illness with typical symptoms prior to the outbreak, or had laboratory evidence of SRSV infection (Viral Gastro-enteritis Sub-Committee of the PHLS Virology Committee, 1993).

Under the Food Safety (General Food Hygiene) Regulations 1995, food business proprietors have a duty to ensure that they operate a safe food-producing and handling system. They are now under a legal obligation to 'exclude' workers from any food-handling area if they know them to be suffering from a specified medical condition which makes them likely to contaminate food. Guidance for food businesses, enforcement officers and health professionals on food handlers' fitness for work has been published by the Department of Health (1995a).

Group 2: Staff employed to work in healthcare facilities who have direct contact, or contact through serving food, with susceptible patients or persons in whom an intestinal infection would have particularly serious consequences.

Foodborne outbreaks have occured in healthcare facilities and outbreaks, such as those associated with SRSVs, can affect patients, residents and staff alike in the relatively enclosed environments of hospital wards and nursing or residential homes. For example, the attack rate from SRSV-associated infection over a period of 7–14 days may exceed 50%, with the possibility of wider spread as the virus is transmitted by patient and staff movement (Working Party of the PHLS Salmonella Committee, 1995). Pressure of work and staff shortages may lead to symptomatic staff continuing to work, thus contributing to the spread of infection.

Group 3: Children aged less than 5 years who attend nurseries, nursery schools, playgroups, or other similar groups.
Outbreaks in schools and nurseries accounted for 7% (90) of all general outbreaks of infectious intestinal disease reported in England and Wales from 1 January 1992 to 31 December 1994, with the majority occurring in nurseries and infant schools. The main pathogens responsible were salmonellas (31%), shigellas (18%) and SRSV (16%) and accounted for 2,119 cases in total (Evans and Maguire, 1996). Unlike general outbreaks, in which foodborne spread is the most common mode of transmission, person-to-person spread predominates in school and nursery settings. Poor handwashing practice and/or poor toilet facilities have been identified as factors in transmission.

Group 4: Older children and adults who may find it difficult to implement good standards of personal hygiene (for example, those with learning disabilities or special needs); and in circumstances where hygienic arragements may be unreliable (for example temporary camps housing displaced persons). Under exceptional circumstances children in infant schools may be considered to fall into this group.
Outbreaks of SRSVs have occurred in schools catering for special needs (Evans and Maguire, 1996) and homes for the elderly seem to be frequently affected by outbreaks of infective diarrhoea (Djuretic et al., 1996; Ryan et al., 1997). Within hospitals *Cl. difficile* infection is particularly prevalent in debilitated patients, e.g. oncology and renal patients, and in the over 65s (Department of Health, 1994b), many of whom may find it difficult to implement good standards of personal hygiene without the assistance of care staff. In addition, 10–20% of elderly patients in hospital are asymptomatic carriers of the organism (Wilcox, 1995) and will therefore be likely to develop symptoms of infection during antibiotic therapy. The organism has also been isolated from the hands of care workers treating patients with *Cl. difficile* and this is a likely route of spread.

The spores of *Cl. difficile* have been found in the environments of symptomatic patients, on commodes, toilets, wheelchairs, sinks and linen. They may persist on fomites and surfaces for five months or longer and may also survive heat disinfection. Infected patients may excrete up to 10^9 organisms per gram of faeces and the explosive nature of the diarrhoea contributes to spread through contamination of the environment and also possibly through transmission of the organism and its spores by aerosol (Department of Health, 1994b).

Methods of preventing spread of gastrointestinal infection

Early recognition and identification

Although the symptoms of diarrhoea and vomiting may have many non-infective causes, all cases of gastroenteritis should be regarded as potentially infectious. Appropriate measures should be taken, whether in the home or elsewhere, to prevent spread of organisms from liquid stools or vomit by instituting the enteric precautions described below. Asymptomatic carriage and excretion can occur, but transmission is unlikely provided that personal hygiene is good.

Faecal specimens should be taken from all sporadic cases and from as many cases as possible in outbreaks. It may be necessary to take specimens from contacts, or others exposed to a suspected source, in order to establish the route and extent of infection. Specimens need to be obtained within 48 hours from the start of symptoms if a viral cause of illness is to be identified.

In all cases, details of symptoms and date of onset, together with other relevant details, for example recent travel abroad, contact with farm/domestic animals and possible association with food, etc., should be given. These details assist in surveillance activities and the early identification of outbreaks. In hospital wards, and in other care settings, awareness of the 'background' incidence of diarrhoea and/or vomiting can assist staff to recognize when the observed number of cases exceeds the number expected, indicating the possiblity of an outbreak situation.

Enteric precautions

The aim of enteric precautions is to minimise exposure of people and the environment to contamination from faeces, thereby reducing the risk of person-to-person spread of infection.

Handwashing

Thorough handwashing with soap in warm running water followed by careful drying, preferably using disposable paper towels or a hot-air hand drier in settings outside the home, is the most important factor in preventing the spread of gastrointestinal infections.

- Everyone should wash their hands after handling affected persons, their bedding, clothing or sickroom equipment.
- Patients and carers should always wash their hands after defecation or urination, and before eating, drinking or smoking.
- Everyone should wash their hands before preparing or serving food or drinks.
- In clinical settings the use of an alcohol-based handrub, applied after washing the hands thoroughly, can reduce the number of residual organisms remaining on the hands following faecal soiling.

Isolating the infection

- People in Groups 1 to 4 should be excluded from returning to school or work until 48 hours after any symptoms of gastrointestinal illness have ceased and they are passing formed stools.
- Special measures are required for any food-handler infected with verocytotoxin-producing *Escherichia coli* (VTEC) or hepatitis A, or who is suffering from, or is a contact of a case or carrier of, enteric fever (i.e. typhoid or paratyphoid) (Department of Health, 1995).
- People not in Groups 1 to 4 may return to work or school once clinically well and when stools are formed. However, in the case of certain serious infections e.g., enteric fever or VTEC infection, microbiological clearance may be required.
- Anyone suffering from acute vomiting should be encouraged to stay away from others.
- In hospital settings anyone with vomiting, or who has diarrhoea and is unable to look after his/her own toilet requirements, should be nursed in a single room, preferably with an en-suite toilet. Where several cases occur at the same time, and if side-rooms are unavailable, symptomatic patients should be nursed together (cohorted) in one bay or ward.

Disposal of excreta and soiled materials

- Patients at home should use a flush toilet wherever possible.
- In communal settings the affected person(s) should be allocated a WC and washbasin which should not be used by those who are well.
- Similarly, potties, bedpans and commodes used for affected persons should be kept separate from those used by others.
- If vomit bowls, urinals, bedpans or potties are used, attendants should wear disposable gloves and protective disposable aprons when handling the items and wash their hands thoroughly after attending the ill person.
- In the home, and in residential settings without an industrial washing machine with a sluicing cycle, soiled clothing and bed linen should be washed in a domestic washing machine on the hottest cycle that the fabric will withstand. Where heavy soiling has occurred, as much solid matter as possible should be removed by wiping with tissues or rinsing, into the toilet bowl if possible, taking great care to prevent personal and environmental contamination.
- In clinical settings, linen which is soiled with diarrhoea should be placed in an alginate bag before laundering, regardless of whether or not the patient is known to have an enteric infection.

Decontamination

- Particular attention should be paid to the cleaning of toilet seats, flush handles, taps and door handles, which should be cleaned several times per day with a solution of household detergent and hot water.
- Alcohol wipes may be used on toilet seats and hard surfaces if not visibly soiled. If soiled, they should be washed as above.
- In the home potties, urinals or bedpans, etc., should be emptied down the toilet then thoroughly cleaned in very hot water and household detergent, preferably while wearing disposable gloves for protection. Cleaning should not be undertaken in an area where food is prepared.
- The sickroom, bay or ward should be frequently damp-dusted

and vacuumed. Soiled carpets will need to be shampooed, or even steam-cleaned, in some circumstances.

- In clinical settings bedpans, etc., should either be disposable or heat-disinfected using a washer/disinfector.
- Certain local policies may recommend the use of hypochlorite solution, particularly during outbreaks of viral gastroenteritis.

Education

- Verbal and written information with regard to hygiene and food storage and preparation, etc., is required for the general public, care staff, patients and their contacts.
- Guidance regarding the need for supervision of toilet hygiene for children, people with learning difficulties and the debilitated or infirm is required for staff and managers of the relevant agencies.
- Advice on how to avoid illness during foreign travel is also very useful and may include information on food and water safety, hand hygiene, and treatment of infection.

References

Department of Health. Management of Outbreaks of Foodborne Illness: Guidance Produced by the DoH Working Group. London: Department of Health, 1994a.

Department of Health/Public Health Laboratory Service Joint Working Group Report. Clostridium difficile Infection – Prevention and Management. London: Department of Health, 1994b.

Department of Health. Food Handlers' Fitness to Work: Guidance for Food Businesses, Enforcement Officers and Health Professionals. Prepared by an Expert Working Group convened by the Department of Health. London: Department of Health, 1995a.

Department of Health. Food Safety (General Food Hygiene) Regulations 1995 Ref: S.I.1763. London: HMSO, 1995b.

Djuretic T, Ryan MJ, Fleming DM, Wall PG Infectious intestinal disease in elderly people. CDR Review 1996; 6 (8): 107–12.

Evans HS, Maguire H Outbreaks of infectious intestinal disease in schools and nurseries in England and Wales 1992 to 1994. CDR Review 1996; 6 (7): 103–8.

Ryan MJ, Wall PG, Adal EK, Evans HS, Cowden JM Outbreaks of infectious intestinal disease in residential institutions in England and Wales, 1992–1994. Journal of Infection 1997; 34: 49-54.

Viral Gastro-enteritis Sub-Committee of the PHLS Virology Committee. Outbreaks of gastro-enteritis associated with SRSVs. PHLS Microbiology Digest 1993; 10 (1): 2–8.

Wall PG, de Louvois J, Gilbert RJ, Rowe B Food poisoning: notifications, laboratory reports, and outbreaks – where do the statistics come from and what do they mean? CDR Review 1996; 6 (7): 93–100.

Wilcox MH Comment – *Clostridium difficile* infection. Surgical Infection 1995; 7 (3): 74–8.

Working Party of the PHLS Salmonella Committee The prevention of human transmissions of gastrointestinal infections, infestations, and bacterial intoxications. A guide for public health physicians and environmental health officers in England and Wales. CDR Review 1995; 5 (1)1: 157–72.

Chapter 15
Bloodborne infections

LESLY FINN

Introduction

Bloodborne infections are those where the blood contains infectious agents that can be transferred into the body of another person giving rise to infection (Advisory Committee on Dangerous Pathogens, 1995). Factors involved in the risk of transmission include: the length of time that the infectious agent remains in the blood, the amount of agent that is present, its virulence (i.e. its ability to cause disease), and the susceptibility of the recipient.

Of particular concern are those diseases where infectious agents may be present in the blood but where the affected individual may be asymptomatic. Within healthcare settings there is a risk of both occupational and patient exposure to these agents. The most significant are human immunodeficiency virus (HIV) and the viruses causing hepatitis B and hepatitis C.

Human immunodeficiency virus (HIV)

Worldwide, the majority of HIV infections are caused by human immunodeficiency virus type 1 (HIV 1). A second virus, HIV 2, is found mainly in West Africa but has been detected in individuals in other areas of sub-Saharan Africa, the USA, India and Europe. A further virus, a sub-type of HIV 1, has recently been recognized and is referred to as HIV 0.

HIV is a retrovirus. Retroviruses contain two strands of RNA and are able to transcribe their RNA into a DNA copy within a host cell by means of an enzyme, reverse transcriptase, contained within the virus particles. The HIV virus binds through fusion of its major envelope glycoprotein, gp120, with a specific cellular receptor, the

CD4 antigen, present on the surface of certain cells. These CD4 receptor cells include helper T-lymphocytes, mononuclear phagocytes, macrophages and glial cells in the brain.

After binding to a cell the HIV virus enters and forms a DNA copy through reverse transcription. This copy is then integrated into the host cell DNA, where it remains in a relatively inactive state.

Several factors are thought to be involved in activation of the virus, which is followed by the production of new virus particles. Over time cell damage occurs, and there is a continuing reduction in the numbers of circulating helper T-cells and other CD4 cells, resulting in an increasingly compromised immune response and, in some individuals, progressive brain damage.

Following initial infection there is a 'window period' before development of antibodies (seroconversion). Seroconversion generally occurs within 3 months, and is often accompanied by a self-limiting illness resembling glandular fever. Progression from initial HIV infection to the severe immune dysfunction known as acquired immuno-deficiency syndrome (AIDS) varies from individual to individual and may take years. Infectious virus is present at all stages of the illness but infectivity is higher at the time of seroconversion and during the later stages (Advisory Committee on Dangerous Pathogens, 1995).

Prevalence of HIV and AIDS in the UK

From the time that reporting began in 1982 to the end of December 1997, a total of 15,074 cases of AIDS (13,401 males and 1,693 females) were reported in the UK, with two of the four Thames regions accounting for over 69% of cases (PHLS, 1998).

The incidence of HIV infection amongst blood donors has been found to be 1:30,400 in new donors and 1:287,000 or less in those who have given blood before (Advisory Committee on Dangerous Pathogens, 1995). Results obtained so far from a major programme of unlinked anonymous serological surveys indicate that London is the focus of the epidemic.

In the period October 1984 to the end of December 1999, 40,372 cases of HIV infection were reported in the UK. Infections were reported from all regions in England, Wales, Northern Ireland and Scotland. The two Thames regions accounted for 66% of the reported cases (PHLS, 2000).

Hepatitis B virus

The hepatitis B virus is a major cause of acute and chronic hepatitis, cirrhosis and hepatocellular carcinoma worldwide. It is a double-stranded DNA hepadnavirus and the whole virus is called the Dane particle.

Acute infection with hepatitis B usually resolves uneventfully, but 5–10% of patients do not clear the infection and become chronic carriers. A small proportion of carriers go on to develop chronic active hepatitis and cirrhosis (Crowe, 1994). Fulminant hepatic necrosis occurs in fewer than 1% of cases of acute hepatitis B infection.

There are multiple markers in the blood comprising both HBV antigens and antibodies for HBV infection. While contributing to the diagnosis and staging of the disease, interpretation of HBV serology is complicated. For example, hepatitis B surface antigen (HBsAg) is a marker for early acute or chronic infection. Diagnosis of acute disease can be made when HBsAg and HB 'e' (envelope) antigen (HBeAg) are present in the blood together with IgM antibody to hepatitis B core antigen (IgM Anti-HBc).

The presence of IgG core antibody (Anti-HBc) is a marker for past infection. A chronic carrier state is indicated when a person remains HBsAg positive, together with 'e' antigen (HBeAg-positive) but has no Anti-HBs, for at least six months. Heightened infectivity is strongly correlated with the presence of the 'e' antigen (HBeAg) and no Anti-HBe (Tilton, 1994).

Prevalence of hepatitis B in the UK

There has been a marked decrease in the number of overt cases of hepatitis B in the UK in recent years although, as with HIV, the true extent of infection within the population is not known with certainty (Advisory Committee on Dangerous Pathogens, 1995). Over the last few years around 500 cases of acute hepatitis infection have been reported annually to the PHLS while 1:1,500 new blood donors is found to be HBsAg positive.

Hepatitis C virus

Worldwide there may be as many as 500 million carriers of the hepatitis C virus (BMA, 1996). It had been recognized since the

1970s that there was a non-A and non-B agent which resulted in chronic liver disease in post-transfusion patients. However, it was not until 1989 that hepatitis C virus (HCV) was cloned and tests developed for blood product screening and diagnosis (Main, 1995).

HCV is a positive stranded RNA virus and at least 28 genotypes have been reported. These genotypes have distinct geographical distributions and may be associated with variations in viral replication, disease-inducing activity and response to the limited treatment currently available (BMA, 1996).

The incubation period is in the range of 1 to 26 weeks and only about 5% of acute HCV infection is associated with signs and symptoms of acute hepatitis (BMA, 1996). There is no test at present for the antigens of HCV in serum and infection is usually diagnosed by serological tests for antibodies to the virus. These are often negative for up to three months after acute illness (Main, 1995).

Up to 80% of those who are anti-HCV positive may continue to carry the virus, which may cause ongoing liver damage, and between 10 and 20% with chronic infection will develop cirrhosis. Chronic effects after acute infection may not appear for between 20 and 40 years (BMA, 1996).

Prevalence of hepatitis C in the UK

The extent of HCV in the UK is unknown at present, although it has been suggested that as many as 615,000 people may be currently infected. Of 2,081 laboratory tests on injecting drug users attending services across the country, 60% were positive for antibodies to HCV – indicating current or past infection.

In North London the incidence of blood donors positive for HCV antibodies was 1:1,400 (BMA, 1996). As with hepatitis B the incidence in the general population is likely to be higher than that found in blood donors due to the self-selection process, i.e. certain groups at high risk of infection are asked not to volunteer for blood donation.

Retrospective analysis of 144 positive HCV antibody tests in a London teaching hospital found that 10 of 38 patients (26%) with chronic liver disease had no history of recognizable potential exposure to blood or blood products (Esfahani et al., 1995), representing 7.5% of the total sample. A further three patients with chronic liver damage, one surgeon, one nurse and one maintenance engineer, had no identifiable potential risk factors other than employment in hospitals (Esfahani et al., 1995).

Sources of infection

One important factor common to bloodborne viruses is that, in addition to blood, other body fluids may also contain significant amounts of virus (UK Health Departments, 1998). These other body fluids are:

- cerebrospinal fluid
- vaginal secretions
- peritoneal fluid
- semen
- pericardial fluid
- amniotic fluid
- pleural fluid
- breast milk
- synovial fluid
- all unfixed tissues and organs

Excreta and secretions i.e. urine, faeces, sputum, tears, sweat and vomit are considered to present little risk from bloodborne infection unless they contain visible blood. However, they may pose a risk of infection for other reasons.

Routes of transmission

For bloodborne infection to occur blood or body fluid containing sufficient virus to cause an infection must enter the body. The possible routes of transmission are:

Percutaneous exposure through:

Major routes

- sharing injecting equipment
- skin puncture by contaminated sharp objects such as needles, instruments or glass
- transfusion of infected blood products (this is now a remote risk in the UK as all blood donations are screened for HBV, HCV, and HIV)

Less common routes

- contamination of open wounds and skin lesions
- human bite (transmission of HBV and HIV have been documented but not quantified) (Jeffries, 1995)

Mucocutaneous exposure through:

Major routes

- sexual intercourse
- childbirth and/or breastfeeding in infected mothers

Less common routes

- contamination of mucous membranes of the eye, nose or mouth (transmission of HBV and HIV following exposure of mucous membranes has been documented but not quantified) (Jeffries, 1995).

The main features of HIV, HBV and HCV are set out in Table 15.1.

Risks to health workers

Risk of occupational transmission occurs whenever there is exposure to blood or body fluids. Both in hospital and community settings it is those who are regularly involved in invasive procedures, i.e. any use of needles, or instruments in penetrating the body, or otherwise in contact with blood or body fluids, who are most at risk. Examples include surgery, obstetrics and gynaecology, dentistry, accident and emergency work, post-mortem, venepuncture and phlebotomy. Ancillary and other staff may also be put at risk through careless disposal of sharps, linen and clinical waste.

Many other occupations involve possible contact with blood, body fluids or tissues, needles and contaminated sharp objects. Examples include custodial services, emergency services, funeral directors, acupuncturists, medical/dental equipment repair, local authority services, environmental health personnel, practitioners in tattooing and body piercing and vehicle recovery services.

HBV is known to pose the greatest risk to healthcare workers, although there is little risk of infection for anyone who has been fully immunized and who has shown an adequate immune response (Jeffries, 1995).

Table 15.1 Main features of hepatitis B, hepatitis C and HIV

	Hepatitis B	Hepatitis C	Human Immunodeficiency Virus (HIV)
ROUTES OF TRANSMISSION	Parenteral: spread by blood, blood products or body fluids (e.g. via transfusion, shared IV needles, contaminated sharps/ equipment, broken skin)	Parenteral: spread by blood, blood products or body fluids (as for hepatitis B)	Parenteral: spread by blood, blood products or body fluids (as for hepatitis B
	Sexual: exposure to vaginal secretions and semen during unprotected sexual intercourse	Sexual: rare	Sexual: body fluids (as for hepatitis B)
	Perinatal: from infected mother to neonate neonate before/during birth or breastfeeding	Perinatal: rare, not thought to occur via breastfeeding	Perinatal: from infected mother to neonate (as for hepatitis B)
INCUBATION	45 to 160 days	7 to 180 days	Weeks to years
INFECTIVITY PERIOD	Before symptoms appear (may remain asymptomatic). May continue for life if chronic carrier	Before onset of symptoms (>90% are asymptomatic) May continue for life if a chronic carrier	For life, once infected
PROGNOSIS	Majority recover Fulminant hepatic necrosis in 1% Chronic carrier state in 5–10% Chronic HBV is associated with cirrhosis and cancer of the liver	Chronic infection in up to 80% Cirrhosis develops in 10–20% of those with chronic infection Unknown number develop liver cancer	Over time continuing CD4 cell depletion leads to increasing immuno- suppression, opportunistic infections and eventual death for the majority
PREVENTIVE MEASURES	Universal precautions Vaccine available	Universal precautions No vaccine	Universal precautions No vaccine

Worldwide the incidence of occupationally acquired HIV infection is small, reflecting its low infectivity outside the main routes of transmission (Shanson, 1991). Up to September 1993 there had been 64 documented cases of seroconversion worldwide of healthcare workers infected with HIV through contact with their patients, four of the cases having occurred in the UK (PHLS, 1993).

Studies in the USA and Europe show that HCV infection is present in healthcare workers although, on current evidence, seroprevalence is low and in some countries no different from that found in blood donors (PHLS Hepatitis Subcommittee, 1993).

Sharps injury is by far the most commonly reported exposure amongst health workers. The risk of contracting HBV following a single percutaneous injury in an unvaccinated individual exposed to HBeAg-positive blood is 30%. Following a single parenteral inoculation of HIV-infected blood the risk is almost 100 times lower at 0.36%. The risk following similar exposure to HCV infected blood remains to be defined but is currently thought to be 3–10% (Jeffries, 1995).

Risk of exposure during surgery and other invasive procedures was illustrated by an outbreak of 4 cases of hepatitis B infection which occurred amongst theatre and ITU staff at a London hospital. The outbreak followed emergency surgery upon a young accident victim who was HBeAg-positive but who was asymptomatic at the time of admission (Shanson, 1986).

A revised scheme for the surveillance of healthcare workers who have been exposed to bloodborne viruses in the course of their work was introduced in July 1997. The scheme aims to monitor the exposure of healthcare workers to patients who are seropositive for HIV, hepatitis B surface antigen or hepatitis C virus. From July to December 1997 CDSC received 66 reports of exposure (46 percutaneous and 18 mucotaneous) to one or more of these viruses (PHLS, 1998).

Risks to patients

There is a greater risk of transmission from patient to healthcare worker than vice versa. However, patients can be put at risk through exposure to contaminated instruments or equipment during invasive procedures or from an infected healthcare worker during an exposure-prone procedure.

Transmission to patients during invasive procedures

A dramatic example of how exposure to even a minute amount of HBV infected blood may result in nosocomial infection occurred in the USA. Twenty-six patients became infected during blood-sugar sampling as a result of a nurse's repeated failure to change the platform on a spring-loaded finger-stick device (Polish et al., 1992).

In the UK four cases of acute hepatitis B occurred in a group of 12 volunteers who had taken part in the same trial in a residential unit for drugs trials. This involved regular blood samples being taken from the volunteers via intravenous cannulae. The outbreak investigation revealed that another member of the group was an HBeAg-positive carrier and that the group had been exposed to a number of hazardous practices:

i)   doctors were reported as not always washing their hands or changing gloves (if worn) between cannula insertions;
ii)   it was not usual practice for staff to wash their hands or change gloves between volunteers when taking blood samples;
iii) kidney dishes used to transport samples and equipment were not decontaminated or discarded between volunteers;
iv)   equipment contaminated with blood was sometimes left on bedside lockers.

It was concluded that transmission of HBV most likely occurred through blood to blood contact between volunteers during cannula sampling (Vickers et al., 1994).

Because of the long incubation period and possible asymptomatic carriage of a bloodborne virus, the fact that a single case is connected with a particular invasive procedure, or that several cases share a common source, may go unrecognized. While there have been no documented cases of hepatitis C virus transmission through contaminated equipment or poor aseptic technique, person to person spread of HIV during minor surgery has occurred in this way. In New South Wales four women and one man who had undergone minor surgery in the same consulting room on the same day were subsequently found to be HIV positive. Investigations determined that only the man had any identifiable risk factors for HIV infection prior to surgery. All the patients, whose ages ranged from early 20s to mid-80s, had undergone minor procedures for removal of skin lesions carried out by an experienced consultant surgeon in his consulting rooms in November 1989. The surgeon alone prepared the operation field, performed the procedures and decontaminated the instruments. It was suspected by the investigating team from the Public Health Department, New South Wales Division, that some failure of infection control practice had occurred resulting in the transmission of HIV from the man to the four women, although the precise mechanism was undetermined. (Chant et al., 1993).

In another outbreak in New South Wales 5 out of 13 patients who had had surgery in the same operating session were subsequently found to be HCV positive. Investigations suggested that transmission may have been associated with contaminated anaesthetic circuitry, in particular laryngeal masks. (Chant et al., 1994).

Transmission to patients from infected healthcare staff

For the majority of procedures in the healthcare setting, the risk of transmission from staff infected with a bloodborne virus is remote. However, there are certain procedures that have been shown to carry an increased risk of exposure and where worker to patient transmission has occurred.

Exposure-prone procedures are defined as:

> Those where there is a risk that injury to the worker may result in the exposure of the patient's open tissues to the blood of the worker. These procedures include those where the worker's gloved hands may be in contact with sharp instruments, needle tips or sharp tissues (spicules of bone or teeth) inside a patient's open body cavity, wound or confined anatomical space where the hands or fingertips may not be visible at all times. (UK Health Departments, 1993 and 1994).

HIV transmission from a healthcare worker to patients has been reported, involving a dentist with AIDS in the USA, although the exact mode of transmission remains uncertain (UK Health Departments, 1994). A further case of HIV transmission from an infected surgeon to a patient in France has also been reported (PHLS, 1997). All retrospective studies undertaken worldwide on patients potentially put at risk of HIV during exposure-prone procedures have failed to identify anyone infected by this route.

However, in order to protect patients, all healthcare professionals who know or suspect that they are HIV-positive must not undertake exposure-prone procedures and must seek expert medical and occupational health advice (UK Health Departments, 1994).

Transmission of hepatitis B from healthcare workers to their patients is known to occur and there is an association between outbreaks and HBeAg positivity. The majority of outbreaks of HBV have involved cardiovascular surgeons, gynaecologists and dentists, with the greatest risk of transmission being to those undergoing major surgery. Healthcare professionals who are HBeAg-positive must not undertake exposure-prone procedures (UK Health Departments, 1993). An addendum to this guidance also states that blood samples taken from healthcare workers to test their immune status must be taken by a member of the local incident investigation team, in order to ensure that the blood is not substituted for someone else's (UK Health Departments, 1996).

An outbreak of hepatitis C in five patients following open-heart surgery by an infected surgeon has been reported. This outbreak followed a previously reported case of hepatitis C infection following cardio-thoracic surgery. Healthcare professionals who are anti-HCV positive are currently allowed to undertake exposure-prone procedures unless they have been shown to have been associated with transmission of the virus (BMA, 1996).

Control measures for prevention of bloodborne viruses

Universal precautions

It is not possible to identify all people who may be infected with bloodborne viruses, therefore guidance to protect healthcare workers against HIV and hepatitis viruses has been issued based on the concept of 'universal precautions' (Advisory Committee on Dangerous Pathogens, 1990 and 1995; UK Health Departments, 1998). Instead of relying on being able to identify 'high-risk' patients, the application of universal precautions requires that ALL blood and body fluids are regarded as potentially infectious and appropriate protective action taken. The primary counter-infection measures applicable at all times and in all settings are set out in Table 15.2.

Table 15.2 Control measures against bloodborne infections

- **wash hands** before and after every patient contact, and immediately after direct contact with blood or body fluids, avoid hand to mouth/eye contact

- **wear gloves** when contact with blood or body fluids, mucous membranes or non-intact skin is anticipated, and wash hands after their removal

- **prevent puncture wounds, cuts and abrasions** in the presence of blood and body fluids

- **protect skin lesions and existing wounds** by means of waterproof dressings and/or gloves

- **avoid use of, or exposure to, sharps** and sharp objects when possible, but where unavoidable take particular care in their handling and disposal

- **avoid contamination of the person** by use of waterproof or water-resistant clothing, plastic apron, etc.

- **wear rubber boots or plastic disposable overshoes** to protect shoes; when the floor is contaminated with blood, wash hands after removing footwear

- **control surface contamination** by blood and body fluids by containment and appropriate decontamination procedures (adapted from ACDP, 1995)

Risk assessment

Application of these precautions, particularly with regard to necessary protective clothing, will vary according to the degree of anticipated contact with blood, body fluids or tissues. The risk of exposure must be assessed for each procedure and the appropriate action taken (Table 15.3).

Adopting safer practices and systems

Invasive procedures

Work by Mast and Geberding suggests that glove materials of any type will reduce the volume of blood inoculated in any needlestick injury by 50% (Royal College of Pathologists, 1992). The use of protective gloves is to be recommended for any invasive procedure involving needles, e.g. undertaking venepuncture, phlebotomy or injections, suturing, tattooing, body piercing.

Table 15.3 Risk assessment and recommended protective measures

RISK ASSESSMENT	EXAMPLES	PROTECTIVE MEASURES
HIGH RISK: contact with blood is probable, potential for uncontrollable bleeding, splashing or spattering with blood is likely	major surgery, gynaecology, obstetric procedures, post mortems, major accident and victim-release work	full range of protective clothing (gloves, water-repellent gown or apron, protective headwear, mask, eye protection, protective footwear)
MEDIUM RISK: contact, splash or spattering with blood is possible	intra-arterial procedures, insertion/removal of intravenous/arterial cannulae, dental procedures, minor surgical procedures	gloves, protective apron/gown, eyewear and mask
LOW RISK: contact with blood is possible	administration of IV, IM or SC injections, phlebotomy, tattooing, acupuncture, body piercing, first aid to cuts/abrasions	gloves to be worn
NO RISK: risk of contact with blood highly unlikely	most non-invasive clinical or patient care, day to day social activity	none necessary

Intra-operative exposures carry the highest risk of exposure and the percutaneous injury rate has been observed to vary according to type of surgery performed. Perforation rates for single gloves during surgical procedures vary from 11–54%, but perforation of the inner glove when two pairs are worn has been reported to be 2% (Jeffries, 1995). The adoption of double-gloving, particularly where the field of manoeuvre is confined and/or visualization of the operation site is restricted, would significantly reduce the risk of injury and possible cross-contamination between surgeon and patient.

Other measures to reduce percutaneous exposure to blood that can be applied to all operative procedures include avoiding manual retraction of tissues, the use of blunt needles for deep suturing, the introduction of hand shielding, e.g. reinforced gloves and thimbles for the non-dominant hand, and ensuring that instruments not in use are removed from the surgical field. Avoiding holding an instrument stationary over an incision while sharp instruments are passed in and out of the wound would also significantly reduce the incidence of sharps injuries during surgery (Royal College of Pathologists, 1992).

Safer systems

Manufacturers are developing safer systems designed to reduce exposure risks to blood and body fluids, e.g. single-use blood glucose monitoring devices with retractable needles. When purchasing equipment or medical devices, priority should be given to safety with regard to risk of exposure to blood or body fluids during use. The safe decontamination of the item must also be considered carefully.

Vaccination

Although there are no vaccines available to protect against hepatitis C or HIV infection, hepatitis B virus is fully preventable. The need for immunization will be determined as part of risk assessment under the COSHH Regulations (Health and Safety Executive, 1994).

All healthcare staff who are exposed to blood, tissues or other body fluids in the course of their work should be immunized against hepatitis B (UK Health Departments, 1993 and 1998). The vaccine is safe and effective and requires the administration of three doses. Individuals who continue to be at risk should receive a booster dose every three to five years unless they have already received a booster following possible exposure.

Antibody response must be checked following the primary course of vaccine as not everyone will produce protective levels of anti-HBs. A fourth dose may be required before they are adequately protected. Around 10% of people fail to respond after four doses and must be informed of their continued susceptibility and advised to have HBV immunoglobulin after contact with HBV-positive blood.

Management of exposure to blood or body fluids

Immediate action following exposure:

- wash off splashes on skin with plenty of soap and water;
- if the skin has been punctured or broken, encourage bleeding but without pressing or sucking the wound;
- splashes to the eye, nose, or mouth should be washed out with copious amounts of water (sterile water for the eye if available);
- record the source of contamination, i.e. name of source (if known), type of fluid, type of injury, and how it occurred;
- report the injury to the supervisor, line manager or other person responsible for health and safety at work, as in local policy;
- medical advice should be sought from the occupational health department or other medical adviser without delay, in accordance with local policy.

Further action

The local plan for management of exposure should consider:

- the source of contamination and the extent of injury/exposure;
- blood sampling and/or serum sample storage;
- vaccination status;
- provision of immediate and follow-up counselling and support;
- the need for post-exposure prophylaxis;
- completion of accident forms;
- surveillance of incidents;
- review of procedures.

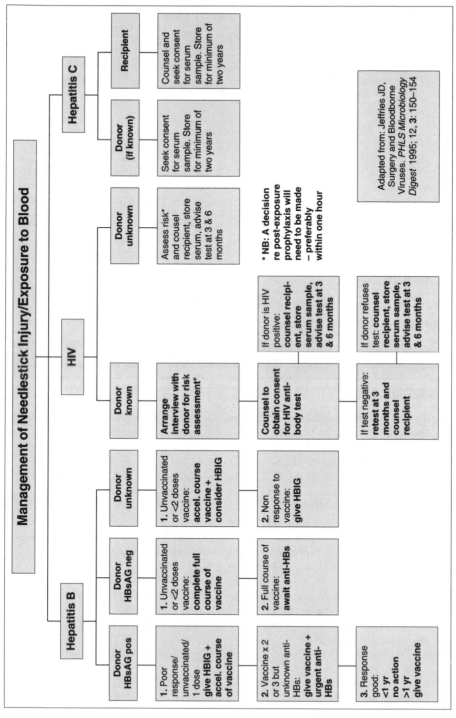

Figure 15.1 Management of needlestick injury/exposure to blood

Guidelines for the management of occupational exposure to hepatitis B virus or HIV are set out in Figure 15.1 (Jeffries, 1995).

> Post-exposure prophylaxis (PEP) should be considered whenever there has been exposure to material known to be, or strongly suspected to be, infected with HIV (UK Health Departments, 1997).

Local PEP policies and procedures need to be agreed and implemented. The Department of Health has issued comprehensive guidelines giving advice on risk assessment following an incident, and including when prophylaxis should be recommended, the choice of antiviral drugs, how to provide a 24 hour PEP advisory service and how to set up local PEP policies and procedures (UK Health Departments, 1997).

Conclusion

In view of the serious nature of bloodborne infections, and the current lack of vaccines or effective post-exposure treatment for hepatitis C and HIV, the prevention of both occupational and patient/client exposure to these viruses is of paramount importance.

References

Advisory Committee on Dangerous Pathogens (ACDP). Protection Against Blood-borne Infections in the Workplace: HIV and hepatitis. London: HMSO, 1995.

BMA. A Guide to Hepatitis C. London: BMA, 1996.

Chant K, Lowe D, Rubin G, Manning W, O'Donoughue R, Lyle D, Levy M, Morey S, Kaldor J, Garcia R, Penny R, Marriott D, Cunningham A, Douglas Tracy G Patient to patient transmission of HIV in private surgical consulting rooms. (Letter) The Lancet 1993; 342: 1548–9.

Chant K, Kociuba K, Prof Munro R, Crone S, Kerridge R, Quin J, Wyland M, Miller G, Turner I, Brown J, Baird L, Prof Locarnini S, Bowden S, Kenrick KG, Maidment C Investigation of possible patient-to-patient transmission of hepatitis C in a hospital. Public Health Bulletin 1994; 5: 47–51.

Crowe HM Forum: A perspective on hepatitis. Asepsis 1994; 16(2): 13–17.

Esfahani RF, Saunders N, Ward KN, Hodgson HJF The spectrum of hepatitis C antibody positive disease in a teaching hospital. Journal of Infection 1995; 30: 115–19.

Health and Safety Executive. Control of Substances Hazardous to Health Regulations. London: HMSO, 1994.

Jeffries DJ Surgery and bloodborne viruses. PHLS Microbiology Digest 1995; 12 (3): 150–54.

Main J Science and clinical practice, hepatitis C: clinical aspects. Journal of Infection 1995; 30: 103–6.

PHLS. Transmission of HIV from an infected surgeon to a patient in France. Communicable Disease Report 1997; 7 (4): 17.

PHLS. AIDS and HIV-1 infection in the United Kingdom: monthly report. Communicable Disease Report 2000; 10(4).

PHLS. Surveillance of healthcare workers with occupational exposure to bloodborne viruses. Communicable Disease Report 1998; 8 (8): 65.

PHLS. Hepatitis Subcommittee Hepatitis C virus: guidance on the risks and current management of occupational exposure. CDR Review 1993; 3 (10): 135–9.

Polish LB, Shapiro CN, Bauer F, Klotz P, Ginier P, Roberto RR, Margolis HS, Alter MJ Nosocomial transmission of hepatitis B virus associated with the use of a spring-loaded finger-stick device. New England Journal of Medicine 1992; 325 (11): 721–5.

Royal College of Pathologists. HIV Infection: Hazards of Transmission to Patients and Health Care Workers during Invasive Procedures. Report of a Working Group of the Royal College of Pathologists: London, 1992.

Shanson D The risks of transmission of the HTLV-111 and hepatitis B virus in the hospital. Infection Control 1986; 7 (2) (suppl.): 128–34.

Shanson D Current surgical controversies over HIV infection. Journal of Hospital Infection 1991; 17: 77–81.

Tilton RC Forum: a perspective on hepatitis. Asepsis 1994; 16 (2): 18–22.

UK Health Departments. Protecting Health Care Workers and Patients from Hepatitis B. HSG (93) 40 and Addendum. London: Department of Health, 1993.

UK Health Departments. AIDS/HIV-infected Health Care Workers: Guidance on the Management of Infected Health Care Workers. London: Department of Health, 1994.

UK Health Departments Executive Letter (96) 77. London: Department of Health, 1996.

UK Health Departments. Chief Medical Officer's Advisory Group on AIDS. Guidelines on Post-exposure Prophylaxis for Health Care Workers Occupationally Exposed to HIV PL/CO (97) 1. London: Department of Health, 1997.

UK Health Departments. Guidance for Clinical Health Care Workers: Protection Against Infection with Blood-borne Viruses. London: Department of Health, 1998.

Vickers J, Painter MJ, Heptonstall J, Yusof JHM, Craske J Hepatitis B outbreak in a drug trials unit: investigations and recommendations. CDR Review 1994; 4 (1): 1–5.

Chapter 16
Catheterization and urinary infection

KATH BANFIELD

Introduction

In a healthy person the urinary tract is usually sterile, except for the distal urethra (Curtis Nickel et al., 1994). And yet, in the National Prevalence Surveys, urinary tract infections accounted for approximately 30% of all hospital-acquired infections, making them the most common infection type found (Meers et al., 1981; Emmerson et al., 1996).

In the wider community, urinary tract infections are also a problem. The annual general practitioner consultation rate of women with cystitis or urinary infection is an estimated 62.5/1000 (RCGP, 1986). In the absence of predisposing factors (Table 16.1), urinary infections are rare in men under the age of 50, but the incidence increases in both sexes with age (Wilkie et al., 1992).

Bacteria can ascend the urinary tract and, if left untreated, serious renal impairment can result, particularly in the presence of abnormalities, pregnancy or diabetes (Hooton and Stam, 1991). In

Table 16.1 Factors predisposing urinary tract infections

- Catheterization
- Surgical instrumentation
- Prostatic disease
- Abnormalities of urinary tract
- Ageing process
- Sexual intercourse
- Diabetes
- Pregnancy
- Altered bladder control
- Urinary calculi
- Functional disability

the case of catheter-associated infection, septicaemia and subsequent death can and does occur (Kunin et al., 1992).

Identification of urinary tract infection

The characteristic symptoms of lower urinary tract infection are dysuria, frequency and suprapubic discomfort (Wilkie et al., 1992; Gray and Malone-Lee, 1995). Elderly patients may present atypically with impairment of continence, falls, immobility, confusion or poor general health (Seyffort, 1991; Nicolle, 1994).

Microbiological examination of urine is often used to confirm the presence of infection. A midstream specimen of urine (MSU) or catheter specimen of urine (CSU) is obtained for this purpose, but interpretation of the results can be confusing. Growth of 10^5 colony-forming units (CFU) of a single type of organism or strain per ml in an uncontaminated MSU is considered significant and indicates that treatment is required (Kass, cited in Gray, 1995; Kass, 1957). However, positive cultures in asymptomatic elderly or catheterized patients are common (Gray and Malone-Lee, 1995; Nicolle, 1994; Ramsay et al., 1989). It has been suggested that asymptomatic bacteriuria is not significant in the development of acute infection and therefore should not be treated unless associated with pregnancy, children under 5 years or instrumentation of the urinary tract (Gray and Malone-Lee, 1995) (see Table 16.2).

Table 16.2 Differentiation of urinary tract infection and asymptomatic bacteriuria

Asymptomatic bacteriuria	Urinary tract infection
Positive growth: Often mixed organisms	Positive growth: $- 10^5$ CFU of one single type of organism/strain per ml $-$ pyuria and/or haematuria
No symptoms or offensive, cloudy, dark urine	Symptomatic: Dysuria: frequency; suprapubic discomfort; pyrexia; raised white cell count
Treatment not indicated unless associated with pregnancy, children <5 years or instrumentation of urinary tract	Treat with appropriate antibiotic

Causative organisms

Urinary tract infections are most commonly caused by Gram-negative bacilli. *Escherichia coli* makes no distinction for age, accounting for the majority of infections in young and old. However, proteus, klebsiella, enterobacter, serratia and pseudomonas are more closely associated with infections in the elderly or catheterized patients (Nicolle et al., 1983; Lye, 1978). Elderly men are more likely to be infected with Gram-positive organisms such as coagulase-negative *Staphylococci* and *Staphylococcus aureus* (Lipsky et al., 1987). However, *Staphylococcus saprophyticus* and occasionally, enterococci, which are both Gram-positive organisms, are associated with infections in sexually active young women. Infection with yeasts may be associated with diabetes, antibiotic therapy, long term catheterization and immunosuppression (Wilkie et al., 1992).

Collection of catheter specimens of urine (CSU)

To avoid unnecessary treatment of asymptomatic bacteriuria it is recommended that routine urine sampling of catheterized patients is not carried out (Falkiner, 1993). The only indications for obtaining a CSU are: if the patient shows signs of infection, e.g. raised white cell count, pyrexia, abdominal pain; and before manipulation or operation on the urinary tract. If a CSU is required it should preferably be obtained before or at catheterization.

A CSU should always be obtained using a sterile needle and/or syringe from the self-sealing sampling port or sleeve on the drainage bag tubing. Occasionally it may be necessary to clamp the drainage tubing below the sampling port for 5 minutes to allow urine to collect before specimen collection. Studies have shown there is a high likelihood of port contamination which can result in misdiagnosis of an infection, a retrograde infection risk and possible cross-infection (Simpson et al., 1995; Wilson and Coates, 1996). To minimize these problems it is recommended that hands are washed and disposable latex or vinyl gloves worn for the procedure. The sampling port should be wiped for 30 seconds with a 70% alcohol wipe and allowed to dry prior to specimen collection. Once obtained, the specimen should be placed in a sterile universal container and sent to the laboratory within 2 hours. If a delay before transport to the laboratory is likely the specimen should be either placed in a refrigerator at 4°C for 24–48 hours or in a universal container with boric acid (Shanson, 1989).

Prevention of non catheter-related UTI

Adequate fluid intake, for example 2–3 litres daily, will promote flushing of the urinary tract and is an essential component of preventing infection. Patients who have had an infection should also be given advice regarding voiding practices. Ensuring complete emptying of the bladder helps to minimize urinary stasis. In women, postcoital voiding and correct hygiene, wiping from the urethra back towards the perianal area, can avoid the problem of ascending bacteria. Maintaining high standards of cleanliness is particularly important if faecal incontinence is present.

Modifications in clothing may help to prevent urinary tract infections, although no research has been found regarding this. Wearing cotton pants and stockings rather than tights should help to maintain normal perineal flora, which protects from infection.

Occasionally, low-dose antibiotic prophylaxis is recommended for prevention of recurrent infections and following acute pyelonephritis in pregnancy. Prophylaxis is also recommended prior to surgical instrumentation of the urinary tract (Wilkie et al., 1992).

Catheter-related UTI

When a patient has an indwelling catheter, bacteriuria (which is the presence of bacteria in the urine) inevitably develops. One study showed that within 72 hours of catheterization, 44% of patients had bacteria in their urine. Within 17 days of catheterization this prevalence had increased to 90% (Crow et al., 1986). However, many cases of bacteriuria are NOT infection. Many patients have what is termed asymptomatic catheter-associated bacteriuria which, as previously mentioned, should not be routinely treated with antibiotics (Gray and Malone-Lee, 1995). Although asymptomatic bacteriuria is a common occurrence, many patients develop symptomatic catheter-related infections which do require treatment.

In the first National Infection Prevalence Survey a total of 545 hospital-acquired urinary infections were reported, and 332 of these were found in catheterized patients (Meers et al., 1981). Despite this significant link between catheters and infections, catheters are a common and essential part of patient care in hospitals, at home and in continuing-care facilities (Table 16.3). Nurses can exert a major influence on the prevention of catheter-related urinary infection, since they are involved in the decision to catheterize, the actual catheterization procedure and subsequent management (Crow et al., 1986; Crow et al., 1988). Guidelines for the management of indwelling urethral catheters were developed by Ward et al (1997). In recognition of the important relationship between catheters, urinary infection and the nurse's role, the remainder of this chapter covers issues which are essential to facilitate evidence-based patient care.

The decision to catheterize

A catheter is a foreign body which bypasses the body's natural defence mechanisms. One author describes a catheterized bladder as a 'continuous culture apparatus' (Falkiner, 1993). Hence, the decision to catheterize requires considerable assessment of the perceived risks and benefits. In order to prevent catheters being used inappropriately, it has been suggested that they should only be used out of medical necessity or irrevocable patient preference (Roe, 1993). However, catheters have become an essential part of patient care and the indications for catheterization are numerous (see Table 16.4).

Table 16.3 Prevalence of catheterized patients

Location	Prevalence of catheterized patients
Hospital	10–12%
Home	4%
Continuing care facilities	16–28%

(Figures taken from Roe, 1993)

Table 16.4 Some indications for catheterization

- Retention of urine
- Care of debilitated patients with incontinence
- Pre-operative drainage to facilitate surgery
- Postoperative drainage
- Paralysis and spinal cord injury
- Bladder irrigation
- Measurement of urinary output
- Urodynamic investigations
- Diagnostic purposes
- Administration of cytotoxic therapy

(Slade and Gillespie, 1985).

Once the decision to catheterize is made, a knowledge of the different types of systems available is essential to give patients an informed choice about their individual care. Catheters may be intermittent or indwelling and enter the body via the urethra or via a suprapubic tract.

Intermittent self-catheterization

Intermittent self-catheterization reduces the risk of urinary tract infections (Wyndaele and Maes, 1990; Hunt et al., 1984; Hunt et al., 1996). It is suitable for patients with high residual volumes of urine due to neuropathic or atonic bladder caused, for example, by paralysis or spinal cord injury (Haynes, 1994). The patient, or carer, passes a catheter via the urethra into the bladder at least 4 times daily and therefore good eyesight, manual dexterity and motivation are essential (Hunt et al., 1996; Haynes, 1994; Moore, 1995).

Various sizes and lengths of intermittent catheters are available to suit males, females and children (Willis, 1995). Most are made of plastic and can be reused over a period of 5–7 days (Department of Health, 1996). These are washed in warm, soapy water, shaken to remove excess moisture and stored in a designated container between uses (Hunt et al., 1984). Single-use self-lubricating catheters are a more recent and popular addition to the range of intermittent catheters. They need to be soaked in water for 30 seconds prior to use, which reduces friction when they are inserted into the urethra (Willis, 1995).

In hospitals, where nursing or medical personnel may pass intermittent catheters, an aseptic technique should be used. However, intermittent self-catheterization is a clinically clean procedure and thus the patient and/or carer must be made aware of the need for good handwashing and general hygiene prior to and following each catheterization (Haynes, 1994). Improper technique or misuse of intermittent catheters can result in urinary tract infections (Wyndaele and Maes, 1990).

Suprapubic catheters

Suprapubic catheters are indwelling catheters that have been inserted into the bladder via the anterior abdominal wall. This is usually a surgical procedure. If used, they avoid some of the problems associated with urethral catheters: the genitalia are catheter-free for sexually active patients; urethral erosion and inflammation are avoided; and wider lumen catheters can be used if blockage is a problem (Hollander and Diokno, 1993).

Suprapubic catheters may be used for patients with a urethral fistula, urethral stricture or other obstruction (Slade and Gillespie, 1985). However, urethral incontinence can occur unless the urethra is oversewn, but this removes the alternative route for drainage should the catheter become blocked (Haynes, 1994).

Studies examining the comparative risk of infection from suprapubic and urinary catheters have been reviewed (Stickler and Zimakoff, 1994). Although the lower density of bacteria on the abdominal skin should reduce the risk, it is suggested that suprapubic catheters merely delay the onset of infection rather than prevent it.

Once a suprapubic catheter is inserted a channel is established within approximately 10 days and the same principles used for care of an indwelling urethral catheter should be applied (Getliffe, 1993a). When changing a suprapubic catheter, it must be re-inserted within 20 minutes to maintain patency of the tract.

Indwelling urethral catheters

Inappropriate choice of urethral catheter can predispose the patient to infection. It results in inflammation of the urethra and bladder mucosa which can become a focus for infection. Also blockage and bypassing can occur which require repeated bladder washouts or premature change of catheter. The range of catheters available is vast. Nurses involved in catheterization need to be aware of the indications for use of each type, to choose a catheter appropriate to the needs of an individual patient and minimize the risk of infection (Falkiner, 1993; Pomfret, 1996). Choice of catheter is based on three criteria:

Duration of catheterization

Catheters are manufactured using a variety of materials. Table 16.5 classifies the different types of catheters by the recommended time they may remain in a patient. These times should be used as an approximate guide only. It is recommended that when long-term catheters are removed the lumen should be examined for encrustation and the optimum time for a catheter established on the basis of these findings (Wilde, 1990).

Table 16.5 Types of catheters available

DURATION	MATERIAL	COMMENTS
Short-term 1–14 days	Plastic/PVC	Rigid; wide lumen facilitates drainage.
	Latex/latex with outer silicone coating	Elastic; relatively cheap; associated with encrustation and trauma if left in situ; absorption of water reduces internal lumen.
Medium-term – up to 28 days	PTFE	Smoother than latex and therefore more resistant to encrustation. Minimal absorption of water.
Long-term – up to 3 months	Silicone	Wider crescent-shaped lumen; prone to encrustation.
	Silicone-coated latex (coating on inner and outer surfaces)	Smoother, therefore more resistant to encrustation; minimal absorption of water.
	Hydrogel-coated latex	Most compatible with human tissue; reduces trauma; least prone to encrustation and bacterial adherence.

(Talja et al., 1990; Roberts et al., 1993).

Dimensions

Catheter diameter – the urethra is not circular in cross section and therefore catheters can distort and distend its normal shape, resulting in tissue damage and bypassing (Pullan et al., 1982). To avoid such complications the general rule is to select a catheter with the smallest possible diameter. A 12–16 Ch catheter is usually appropriate unless debris or blood clots are draining when a catheter >16 Ch should be used (Falkiner, 1993).

Balloon size – a catheterized bladder is in a collapsed state and therefore the weight of large balloons can create irritation and residual urine which can become the focus for infection. Unless postoperative haemostasis is required, a 10 ml balloon should be used in preference to a 30 ml balloon (Falkiner, 1993; Pomfret, 1996).

Catheter length – catheter lengths vary for children, males and females. The male or standard length catheter is the longest. Female catheters are shorter to avoid kinking and are more discreet but are not always suitable for obese patients (Pomfret, 1996).

Catheter design – catheters have either two or three channels. All catheters have one channel for drainage of urine and another to fill the balloon which retains the catheter in place. Some have a third channel to facilitate irrigation or instillation of medication without disconnecting the drainage bag (Getliffe, 1993a). A further feature that requires consideration is the shape and design of the catheter tip. The Tieman tip is slightly curved to negotiate strictures; the Couvalaire or whistle tip has drainage eyes near the tip to allow drainage of debris and blood clots; the Roberts tip has one eye above the balloon and one below to minimize residual urine (see Figure 16.1).

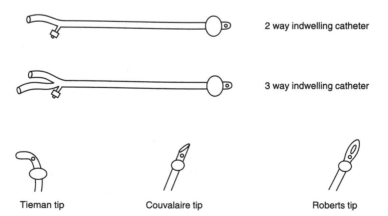

Figure 16.1 Types of catheters

Why catheters predispose to UTI

When a urethral catheter is in place, the organisms that cause either 'asymptomatic bacteriuria' or 'symptomatic infection' can gain access to the urinary tract by two main routes: on the catheter itself, either on insertion or by travelling up between the catheter wall and urethra once in place; and via the lumen of the catheter.

Along each of these routes there are several entry points for infection (see Figure 16.2).

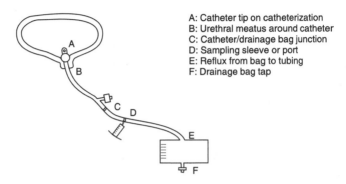

A: Catheter tip on catheterization
B: Urethral meatus around catheter
C: Catheter/drainage bag junction
D: Sampling sleeve or port
E: Reflux from bag to tubing
F: Drainage bag tap

Figure 16.2 Points of entry for infecting organisms

Endogenous catheter-related infections resulting from the patient's own urethral or faecal flora occur in a high percentage of patients and increase with the length of time a catheter is in place (Warren et al., 1982).

Exogenous catheter-related infections result from contamination of the drainage system. This may be due to incorrect handling and maintenance of the drainage system or environmental cross-infection (Platt et al., 1983; Sanderson and Alshafi, 1995; Bukhari et al., 1993).

Retrograde contamination of a catheterized bladder is explained by the phenomenon of bacterial biofilms (Curtis Nickel et al., 1994). Bacteria have been shown to bind to the internal surfaces of the drainage system, forming a creeping biofilm able to travel against the forces of gravity and urinary flow. It is these biofilms that give rise to a colonized catheter or asymptomatic bacteriuria. A catheter-related urinary tract infection can result if these bacteria adhere to the bladder surface.

Prevention of catheter-related UTI

Catheterization

With the exception of intermittent self-catheterization, an aseptic technique should always be used to catheterize a patient. If, in addition to asepsis, every effort is made to eliminate contaminants from the urethra and periurethral skin, then the risk of contaminating the catheter with subsequent introduction of bacteria to the bladder is reduced (Stickler, 1990).

The urethra is made up of delicate tissue and is susceptible to damage on insertion of a catheter, therefore the use of a lubricant is recommended (Courcy-Ireland, 1993). Correct application of a sterile gel preparation actually opens the urethral folds, making the orifice easier to identify, and reduces the risk of a break in the aseptic non-touch technique through misplacement of the catheter.

Once a catheter is inserted either a drainage bag or catheter valve must be attached and every effort made in subsequent management to maintain a 'closed system'. The introduction of the closed drainage system has been described as the most important aspect in prevention of catheter-related urinary tract infection (Stickler, 1990).

Meatal cleansing

Meatal cleansing using antiseptics was once common practice, the aim being to reduce ascending bacteria along the outer walls of the catheter. This is no longer recommended. It is suggested that use of antiseptics removes urethral flora which actually protect the urinary tract from more harmful organisms (Stickler and Chawla, 1987). However, it is desirable to keep the urethral meatus clean and free from debris. For this purpose the use of soap and water once or twice daily, particularly following defecation, is recommended (Falkiner, 1993; Stickler, 1990; Stickler and Chawla, 1987). Carers can introduce infection when handling the catheter, therefore it is preferable for patients to carry out their own meatal cleansing where possible.

Emptying and changing drainage systems

When emptying a catheter drainage bag, there is a high possibility that the nurse's hands will become contaminated (Glenister, 1987).

To avoid this, hands should be washed and either disposable latex or vinyl gloves worn (Slade and Gillespie, 1985). To prevent cross-infection between patients, a new pair of gloves should be used and hands washed following removal of the gloves.

Urine should be drained from the drainage bag using a non-touch technique, either directly into the toilet or into a disposable or heat-disinfected receptacle – one per patient (Falkiner, 1993; Slade and Gillespie, 1985). If possible, patients should be taught to empty their own drainage bags and the need for handwashing before and after the procedure emphasized.

Once the drainage tap is closed, it is not uncommon for a drop of urine to remain suspended from the outlet (Glenister, 1987). Environmental contamination with urine from this source should be prevented by wiping the tap with a tissue after closure. If spillage of urine does occur then the local policy for decontamination of body fluid spillage should be followed.

To reduce the risk of urinary reflux up the drainage tube which may lead to subsequent bacteriuria, bags should not be allowed to overfill and should be correctly positioned (Burke et al., 1986); Mulhall, 1992). Correct positioning of the drainage bag also prevents traction, which can damage the urethral and bladder mucosa (Lowthian, 1989). Hence it is recommended that a suitable hanger is used to position drainage bags below the level of the bladder, without touching the floor (Mulhall et al., 1988). Attaching a link-drainage bag to a leg bag can facilitate correct positioning for bed fast patients (Lowthian, 1988). In hospital it is particularly important that, whether the link-bag is drainable or non-drainable, it must not be re-used. Once it has been disconnected from the drainage systems it must be disposed of as clinical waste. Those considering re-use of such devices should refer to the Medical Devices Agency guidance (MDA, 1994).

In the UK, the Department of Health recommends that drainable catheter bags are changed every 5–7 days to reduce ascending infection without frequent breaks of a 'closed' system (Department of Health, 1996). However, it is interesting to note that routine bag changing is avoided completely in the US Centres for Disease Control recommendations (Wong, 1983). Here, bags are changed only when the catheter is changed, if sediment accumulates, or when the bag becomes odorous or leaks.

One means of alleviating the dilemma of when to change drainage bags is the use of catheter valves. It is also far more discreet. To date there are no published studies examining the relative infection risks, but catheter valves may be a useful alternative to drainage bags in patients who are able to empty their bladders regularly (Roe, 1993; Fader et al., 1997; German et al., 1997). Catheter valves attach directly to the catheter and are replaced when the catheter is changed, or at weekly intervals, depending on the manufacturers' recommendations.

Prevention of encrustation

A common problem for patients with long term indwelling catheters is bypassing or painful retention. This may be due to twisted or kinked drainage tubing, constipation or bladder spasm but is most commonly caused by encrustation (Getliffe, 1993b). Encrustation occludes the lumen of the catheter or forms around the drainage eyes at the tip of the catheter thereby blocking the passage of urine (Getliffe, 1994). Patients have been classified into 'blockers' and 'non-blockers' – blockage being associated with alkaline urine, with high ammonium concentration, female patients and poor mobility (Getliffe, 1994). Figure 16.3 shows relationship between encrustation and bacteriuria.

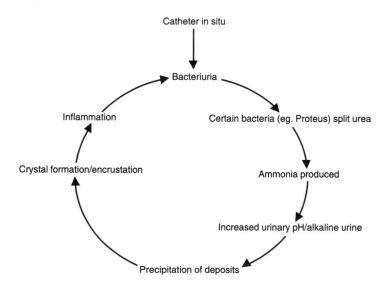

Figure 16.3 Relationship between encrustation and bacteriuria

To prevent encrustation it seems reasonable to break this sequence of events by reducing urinary pH. Possible remedies are increasing fluid intake to 3l daily (Lowthian, 1991); taking oral ascorbic acid or drinking 400 ml cranberry juice daily. Research has provided no conclusive evidence to either support or refute the effectiveness of any of these measures (Kunin, 1987; Getliffe, 1994). However, as no harmful side effects have been reported such interventions may be indicated for patients with repeated episodes of blockage.

Catheter blockage is often treated with a bladder washout. However, unless a three-way catheter is used, carrying out a bladder washout entails breaking the closed drainage system with the risk of subsequent introduction of bacteria (Glenister, 1987). Bladder washout solutions can cause chemical irritation of the bladder mucosa and use of antibacterial washouts predisposes the development of antibiotic resistant urinary pathogens (Warren et al., 1978; Getliffe, 1993b). Furthermore, they are ineffective in the prevention or treatment of catheter-related urinary tract infection (Stickler, 1990; Stickler and Chawla, 1987). Consequently, bladder washouts should be used only when the benefits of removing blockage outweigh the inherent risks of infection and irritation. Indeed, one author suggests it is more effective to remove and replace a blocked catheter rather than attempting a bladder washout (Lowthian, 1991). Alternatively, three-way catheters could be used for persistent 'blockers' to facilitate irrigation without breaking the closed system (Falkiner, 1993; Willis, 1995). If a washout is indicated it is suggested that instillation of 10–20ml of solution should be sufficient to remove a blockage without producing irritation of the bladder mucosa (Getliffe, 1993a). Table 16.6 shows the solutions available and their indications for use.

Assuring quality of care for catheterized patients

Whether patients undergo long or short-term catheterization a commitment to assuring the quality of their care is essential. Patients need to be enabled to live with a catheter whilst avoiding the potential risks and complications associated with it. Quality of care can be enhanced through numerous strategies (Parsley and Corrigan, 1994). Policy formulation and standard setting, education and audit are described here as examples of approaches towards the assurance of quality care.

Table 16.6 Bladder washout solutions

SOLUTION	INDICATION FOR USE	COMMENT
Saline 0.9%	Postoperative bleeding	Continual irrigation
Solution G (citric acid 3.23%)	Remove encrustation	Retain for 15 minutes
Solution R (citric acid 6%)	Remove encrustation	Use prior to catheter removal if crystal formation on catheter tip likely
Mandelic acid	Remove encrustation	Not recommended for routine use due to irritant effect
Chlorhexidine	Decrease bacteriuria	Not routinely recommended due to development of resistant bacteria

Policy formulation and standard setting

Formulation of a policy and standard for discharge of patients from hospital with a catheter has been described in the literature (Pomfret, 1992; Pomfret, 1993). The development of such documents aims to facilitate the consistent implementation of evidence-based care. In the author's place of work the infection control and continence advisory nursing staff, together with a ward sister, carried out an extensive literature review of all aspects of catheter care. The results of this review were merged with existing aspects of good practice to form a draft policy for care of catheterized patients in hospital and the community which incorporated standards for care. Comments upon the content and presentation of this document were elicited from relevant colleagues. These included a urologist, a general practitioner, a microbiologist, and, most importantly, a representative sample of the hospital and community nursing staff who would be putting it into practice.

Education

Formulation of a policy alone is insufficient to improve the quality of patient care. Staff need to be aware of the changes in current practice required to conform to the policy and understand why these changes are necessary. Consequently, several educational sessions were held, and with the support of senior nursing colleagues, a link nurse from each hospital and community ward or team attended an update. Information was then cascaded from these link nurses to their colleagues.

The importance of patient education was emphasized at each training session. Previous studies have identified deficits in the information received by patients regarding catheter care (Roe, 1989; McCullough, 1989). A supply of patient education booklets was provided for each area and staff were encouraged to teach patients and/or carers self-care. This can be achieved by demonstrations of practice followed by supervised practice until the patient and/or carer feels sufficiently confident and competent to carry out unsupervised care.

Audit

As illustrated by the audit cycle featured in Chapter 10, once a protocol or policy is drawn up, practice needs to be monitored, findings reported back to the staff responsible for that practice and the either practice or the protocol updated as necessary (Shaw, 1990).

Audits of catheter-related practice were carried out prior to the implementation of the catheter policy and following education and implementation. Staff in each area were asked to complete audit forms for catheterized patients within a specified time period. Information collected included background information e.g. reason for and estimated duration of catheterization; observable practice e.g. catheter type, length of time since drainage bag change; a review of the patient's records to monitor the extent of documentation; and questions to the patient to estimate his/her level of knowledge. Results of the first audit were fed back to staff at the aforementioned training sessions to highlight areas of good and poor practice. Results of the second audit were publicized at the local Nursing Practice advisory group and Infection Control link nurses group, and written reports were circulated to all areas. Such widespread feedback is essential to close the audit loop or cycle.

These audits were useful in identifying very specific areas of practice that needed addressing. One example was the apparently inappropriate use of catheters with 30 ml balloons. On closer investigation each of these patients identified by the audit had been catheterized in a particular theatre. On visiting this theatre it was found that only catheters with 30 ml balloons were stocked because no one had ever questioned this practice. Once awareness of the problems associated with routine use of large balloons was increased, theatre stocks were modified appropriately.

The latter audit also highlighted areas of the policy which required updating or amendment. One example was a comment that patients were discharged from hospital with a variable quantity of drainage bags and, occasionally, without information about how to obtain further supplies. As a result of this, a recent addition to the policy is a list of the number of drainage bags which should be given to a newly catheterized patient on discharge. A form is also completed listing the Drug Tariff order codes of each patient's drainage bags. This is faxed to the patient's general practitioner and the patient is advised to contact him/her for further supplies.

A further simple example of how the audit helped to improve the policy came from information regarding documentation. The policy states that on catheterization, amongst other information, the 'batch number' of the catheter should be recorded, but the audit showed that this was not happening. On questioning staff, it was found that nowhere on the catheter packaging was the 'batch number' stated. Following discussion with the manufacturers it was found that what the policy referred to as the 'batch number' was printed as the 'lot number'. This minor modification in the policy was easily ratified and publicized.

As previously mentioned, a commitment to provide quality care to catheterized patients is essential. Working through the audit cycle was useful in sustaining a high level of commitment.

References

Bukhari SS, Sanderson PJ, Richardson DM et al. Endemic cross-infection in an acute medical ward. Journal of Hospital Infection 1993; 24: 261–71.

Burke JP, Larsen RA, Stevens LE Nosocomial bacteriuria – estimating the potential for prevention by closed sterile urinary drainage. Infection Control 1986; 7 (suppl 2): 96–9.

Cools HJM, Van der Meer JWM Restriction of long term indwelling catheterisation in the elderly. British Journal of Urology 1986; 58: 683–8.

Courcy-Ireland KD An issue of sensitivity: use of analgesic gel in catheterising women. Professional Nurse 1993; 738–41 August.

Crow RA, Chapman RG, Roe BH, Wilson JA A Study of Patients With an Indwelling Urethral Catheter and Related Nursing Practice. University of Surrey: Nursing Practice Unit 1986.

Crow R, Mulhall A, Chapman R Indwelling catheterisation and related nursing practice. Journal of Advanced Nursing 1988; 13: 489–95.

Curtis Nickel J, Costerton W, McLean RJC, Olson M Bacterial biofilms: influence on the pathogenesis, diagnosis and treatment of urinary tract infections. Journal of Antimicrobial Chemotherapy 1994; 33 (suppl. A): 31–41.

Department of Health Welsh Office. Drug Tariff. London: HMSO, 1996.

Emmerson AM, Enstone JE, Griffin M, Kelsey MC, Smyth ETM The second national prevalence survey of infection in hospitals – overview of results. Journal of Hospital Infection 1996; 32: 175–90.

Fader M, Pettersson L, Brooks R, Dean G, Wells M, Cottenden A, Malone-Lee J, A multi-centre comparative evaluation of catheter valves. British Journal of Nursing 1997; 6(7): 359–69.

Falkiner FR The insertion and management of indwelling urethral catheters – minimising the risk of infection. Journal of Hospital Infection 1993; 25: 79–90.

German K, Rowley P, Stone D, Kamav U, Blackford HN Comparing the use of a catheter valve leg bag in urethrally catheterised male patients. British Journal of Urology 1997; 79(1): 96–8.

Getliffe KA, Mulhall AB The encrustation of indwelling catheters. British Journal of Urology 1991; 67: 337–41.

Getliffe K Care of urinary catheters. Nursing Standard 1993a; 7(44): 31–4.

Getliffe K Informed choices for long-term benefits: The management of catheters in incontinence care. Professional Nurse November 1993b; 122–6.

Getliffe K The characteristics and management of patients with recurrent blockage of long-term urinary catheters. Journal of Advanced Nursing 1994; 20: 140–49.

Glenister H The passage of infection. Nursing Times 1987; 83 (22): 68–73.

Gray RP, Malone-Lee J Review urinary tract infection in elderly people: time to review management? Age and Ageing 1995; 24: 341–5.

Haynes S Intermittent self-catheterisation – the key facts. Professional Nurse 1994; 100–104 November.

Hollander JB, Diokno AC Urinary diversion and reconstruction in the patient with spinal cord injury. Urologic Clinics of North America 1993; 20 (3): 465–74.

Hooton TM, Stamm WE Management of acute uncomplicated UTI in adults. Med Clin North Am 1991; 75: 339–57.

Hunt GM, Whitaker RH, Doyle PT Intermittent self catheterisation in adults. British Medical Journal 1984; 289: 467–8.

Hunt GM, Oakeshott P, Whitaker RH Intermittent catheterisation: Simple, safe, and effective but underused. British Medical Journal 1996; 312: 103–7.

Kass EH Asymptomatic Infections of the Urinary Tract, 1956. Cited in Gray and Malone, 1995.

Kass EH Bacteriuria and the diagnosis of infections of the urinary tract: with observations on the use of methionine as a urinary antiseptic. Arch Intern Med 1957; 100: 709–14.

Kunin CM Detection, Prevention and Management of Urinary Tract Infections, 4th Edition. Philadelphia: Lea and Febiger, 1987.

Kunin CM, Chin QF, Chambers S Indwelling urinary catheters in the elderly. American Journal of Medicine 1987; 32: 405–11.

Kunin CM, Douthitt S, Daning J et al. The association between the use of urinary catheters and morbidity and mortality among elderly patients in nursing homes. American Journal of Epidemiology 1992; 135: 291–301.

Lipsky BA, Ireton RC, Fihn SD et al. Diagnosis of bacteriuria in men: Specimen collection and culture interpretation. Journal of Infectious Disease 1987; 155: 847–54.

Lowthian P Steps to combat infection. Nursing Times 1988; 84 (12): 64–6.

Lowthian P Preventing trauma. Nursing Times 1989; 85 (21): 73–5.

Lowthian P Using bladder syringes sparingly. Nursing Times 1991; 87 (10): 61–3.

Lye M Defining and treating urinary infections. Geriatrics 1978: 71–7.

McCullough J Catheter care at home. Community Outlook March 1989; 4–8.

Medical Devices Agency (MDA). The Re-use of Medical Devices Supplied for Single Use Only. MDA DB 9501. London: MDA, 1995.

Meers PD, Ayliffe GAJ, Emmerson AM et al. Report of the national survey of infection in hospital Journal of Hospital Infection 1981; 2 (suppl): 23–8.

Moore KN Intermittent self-catheterisation: Research-based practice. British Journal of Nursing 1995; 4 (18): 1057–63.

Mulhall A, Chapman R, Crow R The acquisition of bacteriuria. Nursing Times 1988; 84 (4): 61–2.

Mulhall A The bladder model: clinical implications. Nursing Standard 1992; 7 (5): 25–7.

Nicolle LE, Bjornson J, Harding GKM, MacDonell JA Bacteriuria in elderly institutionalised men. New England Journal of Medicine 1983; 309: 1420–5.

Nicolle LE Urinary tract infection in the elderly. Journal of Antimicrobial Chemotherapy 1994; 33 (suppl. A): 99–109.

Parsley K, Corrigan P Quality Improvement in Nursing and Healthcare. London: Chapman and Hall, 1994.

Platt R, Polk BF, Murdock B et al. Reduction of mortality associated with nosocomial urinary tract infection. Lancet 1983; 1: 893–7.

Pomfret IJ Standards for catheter care. Journal of Community Nursing August 1992; 4–8.

Pomfret IJ Standard update for catheters. Journal of Community Nursing August 1993; 8–14.

Pomfret IJ Catheters: design, selection and management. British Journal of Nursing 1996; 5 (4): 245–51.

Pullan BR, Phillips JI, Hickey DS Urethral lumen cross sectional shape: its radiological determination and relationship to function. British Journal of Urology 1982; 54: 399–407.

Ramsay JWA, Garnham AJ, Mulhall AB et al. Biofilms, bacteria and bladder catheters: A clinical study. British Journal of Urology 1989; 64: 395–8.

Roberts JA, Kaack MB, Fussell EN Adherence to urethral catheters by bacteria causing nosocomial infections. Urology 1993; 41(4): 338–42.

Roe B Catheter care revisited. Nursing Standard 1989; 3 (51): 32–4.

Roe BH Catheters in the community. Nursing Times 1989; 85 (36): 43–4.

Roe B Catheter-associated urinary tract infection: a review. Journal of Clinical Nursing 1993; 2: 197–203.

Royal College of General Practitioners, Office of Population Censuses and Surveys, Department of Health and Social Security (RCGP). Morbidity Statistics from General Practice, Third study 1981–82. London: HMSO, 1986.

Sanderson PJ Preventing hospital acquired urinary and respiratory infection. British Medical Journal 1995; 310: 1452–3.

Sanderson PJ, Alshafi KM Environmental contamination by organisms causing urinary tract infection. Journal of Hospital Infection 1995; 29: 301–3.

Seyffort G Drug Dosage in Renal Insufficiency. Kluwer Academic Publishers, 1991.

Shanson DC Microbiology in Clinical Practice , 2nd Edition. London: Wright, 1989.

Shaw CD Criterion based audit. British Medical Journal 1990; 300: 649–51.

Simpson LR, Babb JR, Fraise AP Infection risk and potential contamination of urine specimens associated with sample port design of catheter leg bags. Journal of Hospital Infection 1995; 30: 95–102.

Slade N, Gillespie WA The Urinary Tract and the Catheter. New York: Wiley, 1985.

Stickler DJ, Chawla JC The role of antiseptics in the management of patients with long-term indwelling bladder catheters. Journal of Hospital Infection 1987; 10: 219–28.

Stickler DJ The role of antiseptics in the management of patients undergoing short-term indwelling bladder catheterization. Journal of Hospital Infection 1990; 16: 89–108.

Stickler DJ, Zimakoff J Complications of urinary tract infections associated with devices used for long-term bladder management. Journal of Hospital Infection 1994; 28: 177–94.

Talja M, Korpela A, Jarvi K. Comparison of urethral reaction to full silicone, hydrogel-coated and siliconised latex catheters. British Journal of Urology 1990; 66: 652–7.

Ward V, Wilson J, Taylor L, Cookson B, Glynn A Preventing Hospital-Acquired Infection: Clinical Guidelines. London: PHLS, 1997.

Warren JW, Platt R, Thomas RJ et al. Antibiotic irrigation and catheter-associated urinary tract infections New England Journal of Medicine 1978; 299 (11): 570–73.

Warren JW, Tenney JH, Hoopes JM et al. A prospective microbiologic study of bacteriuria in patients with chronic indwelling urethral catheters. Journal of Infectious Disease 1982; 146: 719–23.

Wilde MH Foley. Catheter management at home. Home Healthcare Nurse 1990; 9 (3): 39–45.

Wilkie ME, Almond MK, Marsh FP Diagnosis and management of urinary tract infection in adults. British Medical Journal 305 1992; (6862): 1137–41.

Willis J Intermittent catheters. Professional Nurse 1995; 10 (8): 523–8.

Willis J Catheters: Urinary tract infections. Nursing Times 1995; 91(35): 48–9.

Wilson M, Coates D Infection control and urine drainage bag design. Professional Nurse 1996; 11(4): 245–52.

Wong ES Guideline for prevention of catheter-associated urinary tract infections. American Journal of Infection Control 1983; 11: 28–33.

Wyndaele JJ, Maes D Clean intermittent self catheterisation: A 12 year follow up. The Journal of Urology 1990; 143: 906–8.

Chapter 17
Cannula-associated infection

CHRISTINE PERRY

Introduction

Invasive cannulae are now commonly used within healthcare settings to facilitate the treatment of patients with a number of conditions. These cannulae range from intravascular catheters to intraperitoneal catheters for dialysis purposes and epidural cannulae for anaesthesia and analgesia. The presence of an invasive cannula breaches one of the body's defence mechanisms to infection, the skin, and therefore creates an access point for micro-organisms and the potential for infection (Ward et al., 1997).

Intravascular cannulae

The use of peripheral cannulae (PCs) and central venous cannulae (CVCs) within acute healthcare settings has become widespread, with their use in outpatient and community settings also increasing. Indications for the use of venous cannulae include: haemodynamic monitoring, infusion of fluids, resuscitation, chemotherapy, parenteral nutrition and haemodialysis. The length of time cannulae remain in situ is dependent on cannula material, usage and ensuing complications.

Short-term cannulae are often made of polytetrafluoroethylene (Teflon) or polyvinylchloride (PVC). Short-term PCs generally have only one lumen and can be ported or unported. They are secured in place by the use of an adhesive dressing. Short-term CVCs vary from single to triple lumen, are generally inserted directly into the vein without skin tunnelling and may be sutured in place for security.

Cannulae designed for long-term use are made of materials associated with low tissue reactions such as silicone. Long-term

CVCs are frequently inserted surgically by tunnelling through the skin. Some long-term lines incorporate a Dacron cuff which is attached to the segment of catheter which lies in the skin tunnel. This causes tissue granulation and fibrosis, helping to secure the catheter and acting as a barrier to migration of micro-organisms along the skin tunnel.

Epidemiology and microbiology

Phlebitis is often a reported complication of peripheral cannulae, which may not always be due to infection but can be due to mechanical factors and chemical reactions. The phlebitis may, however, provide a focus for the adherence of micro-organisms, with subsequent infection. Infection rates for peripheral cannulae are difficult to ascertain as studies often give rates of phlebitis rather than infection. One recent study showed a phlebitis rate of 9.7% following educational and other interventions (Stonehouse & Butcher, 1996). Infection rates for CVCs can be variable, with reported rates being between 3 and 10% (Maki, Ringer and Alvarado, 1991). Some authors report rates as high as 42% (Conly, Grieves and Peters, 1989). This variation between reported infection rates is likely to be due to cannula usage and patient factors such as impaired immune response. In a recent national survey, PCs accounted for 1.9% and CVCs for 2.0% of all hospital-acquired infections (Emmerson et al., 1996). Reports of rates of IV cannula related infection in the community are not as numerous as hospital rates. American studies have shown intravenous cannulae used in the community to have infection rates varying between 1.5% and 4.5% (Markel, 1994; White and Ragland, 1994).

A large number of infections associated with cannulae are due to coagulase negative staphylococci, particularly *Staph. epidermidis*, a skin commensal that may migrate along the cannula from the skin, and has a propensity for attachment to plastic cannula material. *Staph. aureus* and enterococci are also reported as being common causes of infection, as are fungi for immunosupressed persons (HICPAC, 1996).

Factors that increase the risk of infection in peripheral cannulae are:

•   Cannula material and size – the size of the cannula should be the smallest possible lumen for the type of fluid to be infused.

- Site of insertion – flexures should be avoided due to the risk of mechanical damage when limbs are moved.
- Duration of cannulation.
- Insertion technique – prevention of contamination at the point of insertion being important.
- Type of infusate – glucose and the administration of antibiotics are particularly associated with an increased risk.
- (HICPAC, 1996).

Factors that increase the risk of CVC infection are:

- Jugular or femoral insertion sites – femoral insertion sites particularly increase the risk due to the close proximity of the urinary tract and anus, combined with a skin fold which provides ideal conditions for microbial proliferation.
- Dressing type – traditional transparent film dressings may increase the level of moisture, leading to bacterial proliferation.
- Duration of cannulation.
- Number of lumens within the line – triple lumens have been associated with increased infection risk due to additional access points for micro-organisms.

(Elliott, 1993).

Cannula-related infection

Diagnosis of infection

Diagnosis of cannula-related infection can be difficult, but should be suspected in any patient with a cannula who presents with a fever and no indication of other sites of infection. Localized site infection may be characterized by erythema, oedema, tenderness and purulent exudate. With tunnelled cannulae, these signs and symptoms may be present along the tunnel. Systemic infection may be characterized by a low-grade pyrexia and a raised white cell count (Elliot, 1993). Diagnosis can be confirmed microbiologically by the isolation of the same micro-organism from blood cultures taken from both the cannulae and a separate peripheral blood sample. If cannulae are removed due to suspected infection, the cannula tip should be sent to the microbiology laboratory for culture. The most commonly accepted method of culture is for the cannula tip to be rolled across an agar plate which is incubated overnight (Maki et al., 1977). The number of bacterial colonies are then counted, with greater than 15 colony forming units indicative of cannula infection, in association with clinical signs and symptoms. The presence of bacteria in the blood is termed bacteraemia, if this is accompanied by signs and symptoms of infection and illness, this is termed septicaemia.

Routes of infection

The predominant routes of cannula infection are migration of micro-organisms from the insertion site and via the lumen of the cannula from contaminated connections and hubs. Other less common routes are: via the tip of the cannula at the time of insertion; via contaminated infusion fluids or seeding of organisms on the cannula; or via the bloodstream from a distant site in the body (Figure 17.1). Strategies for the prevention of cannula infection are therefore based around these routes of contamination.

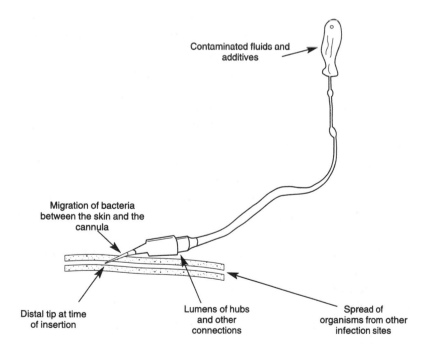

Figure 17.1 Entry sites for micro-organisms

Prevention of infection

Aseptic technique

The key preventative measure underlying cannula care is aseptic technique, with particular emphasis on handwashing before any manipulation of the cannula. In accordance with principles of universal precautions, gloves should be worn to protect the health-care worker if there is a risk of contact with blood. For manipulations of CVCs it is suggested that sterile gloves are worn (Elliott et al., 1994). Whether sterile gloves are required for manipulations of PCs is less clear and no consensus has been reached (HICPAC, 1996). Insertion of CVCs should be carried out with maximum aseptic precautions, wherever possible, including handwashing with an antiseptic followed by an alcohol rub, and the wearing of sterile gloves and gown, theatre-type mask and hat (Elliott et al., 1994).

Skin preparation

Cleansing of the skin prior to insertion of a peripheral or central venous cannula is important to prevent contamination of the cannula at this time. A swab impregnated with 70% alcohol is generally used prior to PC insertion, which is convenient and has good antibacterial properties (Ayliffe et al., 1993). However, time must be allowed for the alcohol to evaporate and care taken not to recontaminate the site after it has been cleansed. Prior to central venous cannula insertion, other antiseptics may be used. Chlorhexidine 2% in an aqueous base has been shown to be effective (Maki et al., 1991), but the use of this is limited as single-use sachets are not currently available commercially in the United Kingdom. For this reason, chlorhexidine in an alcohol base is often used. Chlorhexidine is more effective against Gram-positive organisms, e.g. staphylococci and enterococci, than Gram-negative organisms, e.g. pseudomonas (Ayliffe et al., 1993). Another antiseptic commonly used prior to CVC insertion is povidone-iodine, which has a wide antibacterial spectrum (Ayliffe et al., 1993). Whichever antiseptic is used, a good technique is important and it is necessary to allow adequate drying time.

Dressing

The purpose of a dressing covering an intravenous (IV) line is to: protect the insertion site; secure the cannula to prevent mechanical damage to the vein; and to exclude micro-organisms from the insertion site. The choice of dressing for cannula sites varies according to cannula usage and patient factors. It is recommended that roll tape is not used to secure cannulae because these tapes, which are commonly used for many purposes, can be heavily contaminated with micro-organisms (Oldman, 1991). The properties of an ideal IV line dressing include the following:

- Waterproof
- Impervious to bacteria
- Prevent buildup of moisture and skin maceration
- Securely fix the cannula
- Allow easy visual inspection of the IV site
- Sterile and cut to size
- Easy to apply
- Easy to remove without dislodging the cannula
- Allow minimal dressing changes

(Infection Control Nurses Association, 1991).

Tape and gauze dressings have been used successfully for a number of years, with several studies showing them to be effective (Shivnan et al., 1991). These types of dressing are generally easy to apply, which is an important consideration for patients caring for their own IV lines in the community. Disadvantages of these dressings include: frequent changing may be required, especially if they become wet or dislodged; the exit site is not visible without disturbing the dressing; and frequent dressing changes increase costs and nursing time.

Transparent polyurethane film dressings have become popular as IV line dressings. These dressings have the following advantages: waterproof; easy visual inspection of the site; good cannula security. Concern has been expressed over whether moisture retention is increased under these dressings, leading to an increase in colonization

of micro-organisms around the IV site (Conly et al., 1989). Techno-
logical developments in relation to the moisture vapour permeability
of these dressings have been shown to be effective in reducing infection rates (Wille et al., 1993). Other recent advances in cannula dressings have included the addition of a film 'window' to gauze dressings,
allowing early detection of phlebitis, and the addition of gauze wings
to film dressings, thus enhancing cannula security.

The frequency of dressing changes will be determined by the
type of dressing used (Glynn et al., 1997). It should also be weighed
against the exposure of the IV site to external micro-organisms and
should, where practical, coincide with other manipulations of the
cannulae. The dressing will require changing in any of the following
circumstances: blood or moisture build up beneath the dressing;
strikethrough; lifting of dressing edges; and wet or soiled dressing.

Once cuffed long-term lines are secure, and incisions used for
insertion are healed, the use of a dressing is no longer essential
(Pritchard and Mallet, 1993).

Dressing regimes

At each dressing change the IV site should be inspected for signs of
inflammation, infection and cannula security. As has been previously
noted an aseptic technique should be used. If there is a need to
remove debris or exudate sodium chloride 0.9% (normal saline) or
water may be used, but should be followed by cleansing with an antiseptic such as chlorhexidine or povidone-iodine (Elliot et al., 1994).
Care should be taken to ensure the compatibility of antiseptics with
CVCs, as the integrity of silicone-based cannulae may be damaged
by prolonged contact with alcohol-based antiseptics (Department of
Health, 1993). Acetone and ointments have been suggested in some
dressing regimes; however, their efficacy has not been demonstrated
(Maki and McCormack, 1987; Jarrard and Freeman, 1977) and the
use of antibiotic ointments which are not fungicidal may lead to an
increase in fungal infections. Once long-term cuffed lines are secure,
cleansing techniques as described above are unnecessary and they
can be cleaned as part of general hygiene.

Infusion lines, hubs and connectors

There is good evidence to suggest that IV lines (administration sets
and connections) can safely be left in situ for 48–72 hours (Maki et

al., 1987) and some recommendations consider 72 hours to be the minimum time for line changes (HICPAC, 1996). Any connections, piggy back tubing or stopcocks should be considered as part of the IV line for the purposes of changing. It is important to document the date and time of changing lines to facilitate this regular change. Consideration must also be given to drug and infusate manufacturers' instructions which may specify times for line changes.

Administration sets used for blood should be changed every 12 hours (McClelland, 1996). Administration sets used for lipid-containing total parenteral nutrition should be changed every 24 hours. All equipment used for IV infusions should be checked before use for sterility and date of expiry. A luer lock connector should be included on all IV equipment to help prevent accidental disconnection.

Contamination of stopcocks has been found to be present in 45–50% of IV lines (HICPAC, 1996), with ensuing colonization of the cannula tip and bloodstream infection. Some authors suggest the cleaning of all connections, before manipulation, with an antiseptic providing it is compatible with the device (Elliot et al., 1994). Latex injection ports should be cleaned with an antiseptic and allowed to dry, prior to injecting through the membrane.

Needle-less access devices have recently been introduced with a view to reducing staff needlestick injuries. These devices are based on either a spring-loaded or a slit latex membrane. They have the advantage that bolus injections and administration set connection can be performed without opening the system. The effect of needle-less devices on infection rates is as yet unclear, but evidence is emerging that infection rates may be increased (Russo et al., 1999).

Filters

Filters are available which will filter out particles of above 0.2 microns and are capable of retaining particulate matter, endotoxins and bacteria for up to 96 hours. A reduction in infection rates has not as yet been demonstrated (Spencer, 1990), and as manufacturers are required to filter intravenous fluids to ensure no microbe-size particles remain, their use is still debated. There is no evidence to support the use of micro-aggregate filters for blood transfusions, as a filter is included in the administration set, but it is suggested that leucocyte-depleting filters may be useful in preventing the onset of febrile transfusion reactions in patients requiring regular blood transfusion (McClelland, 1996).

Total parenteral nutrition

Total parenteral nutrition (TPN) is used for patients who are unable to absorb nutrition via the gastric route. Due to the viscosity of TPN and the risk of phlebitis it is administered via IV lines which open into the large central veins. These cannulae can either be inserted centrally or peripherally. It is normal practice to have a line dedicated solely for TPN use, as infection risk is increased due to the nutrient properties of the infusate. It is for this reason that adherence to aseptic technique for any manipulation of the cannula and line is most important. The use of a dedicated team to insert and continue care of these lines has been shown to be effective in reducing infection rates (Hamilton, 1993). If dedicated personnel are not available, staff who are trained and proficient in the care of TPN lines should carry out care.

Infection due to contamination of TPN fluids during manufacture is rare but has been reported (Frean et al., 1994). Strict attention is given to asepsis during compounding of TPN solutions, which generally takes place within laminar flow hoods in pharmacy departments. TPN solutions should be kept refrigerated until use and discarded after 24 hours at room temperature as there is currently insufficient evidence to suggest the safety of infusing them over extended periods. The use of TPN in patients' own homes is increasingly necessitating training and support for patients from dedicated teams to enable safe use in this environment.

Implantable intravascular devices

For patients requiring long-term use of a CVC for chemotherapy, an alternative type of device is a subcutaneous implanted device. These devices consist of a port or reservoir, which is inserted surgically beneath the skin, from which a catheter leads into a central vein (Figure 17.2). To access the system, a 'huber' needle is inserted into the reservoir, through which administration of medication or sampling of blood can take place. These devices were developed in an attempt to reduce the risk of infection, however, no significant reduction in infection rates has been demonstrated (Camp-Sorrell,

1992). Infection of implantable devices is usually manifested by erythema and tenderness over the reservoir or the catheter tract and may lead to the removal of the device. Infection prevention strategies are the same as for conventional central venous catheters and include the cleansing of the skin over the port, with an appropriate antiseptic, prior to accessing with a needle.

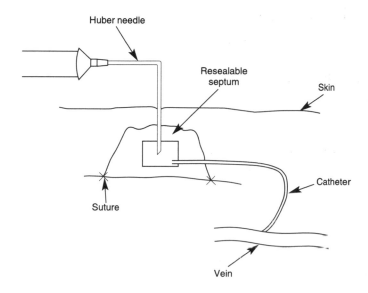

Adapted from Journal of Intravenous Nursing 1992; 5 (15): 264.
Figure 17.2 Design of implantable port

Haemodialysis catheters

Central venous cannulae are useful as temporary access for haemodialysis and for children when surgical construction of an arteriovenous fistula is difficult. A double lumen line is used and should, where possible, be dedicated for dialysis use only. Other uses, for example the administration of drugs, fluid and TPN, should be avoided unless no alternative vascular access is available. Rates of bloodstream infection associated with subclavian dialysis catheters are higher than for other central venous cannulae and dialysis access, and has been attributed to manipulations of the catheter by untrained personnel, duration of catheterization and number of dialysis runs (HICPAC, 1996). The use of an appropriate antiseptic to reduce colonization of skin by bacteria around the dialysis line appears to be important in this group of patients and should therefore be included in any care regime (HICPAC, 1996). It is important to consider that a large proportion of dialysis patients will attend for dialysis as outpatients. Education of patients and their families in the care of these lines will be important in the prevention of infection.

Catheters for CAPD

Continuous ambulatory peritoneal dialysis (CAPD) is a form of renal replacement therapy that involves the infusion and drainage of a dialysis fluid via a catheter inserted through the abdominal wall into the peritoneal space. Patients with CAPD catheters will be at risk of both exit site infection and peritonitis. The organisms which most commonly cause infection are *Staph. aureus*, *Staph. epidermis* and *Pseudomonas* spp. Exit site infections are characterized by redness or induration, or the presence of purulent discharge from the exit site (Twardowski, 1992). Culture of organisms from the exit site is not indicative of infection alone. Tunnel infections are characterized by induration or redness of the area associated with tenderness or pain, with or without abscess formation (Gokal et al., 1993). Peritonitis is indicated by cloudy dialysis fluid, abdominal pain, fever and a raised white cell count in the dialysis fluid (Keane et al., 1993). Rates of infection are often quoted in episodes per patient year. A multicentre study showed a variation in exit site infection rates from 0.27 episodes per patient year to 0.71, depending on the care regimes (Luzar et al., 1990a). The same study showed peritonitis rates to be 0.446–0.574 per patient year.

Pre-insertion prevention

Prevention of infection begins before insertion of the CAPD catheter. An appropriate site of insertion on the abdomen should be selected which will avoid excessive movement of the catheter and excessive pressure. Preparation of the skin should be as for a surgical procedure. If hair removal is necessary this should be performed as near in time to the insertion as possible and using a method that will limit damage to the skin (Gokal et al., 1993). There is some evidence to suggest that nasal carriage of *Staph. aureus*. increases the risk of subsequent infection, and some authors recommend the eradication of this by the use of mupirocin (Luzar et al., 1990b). This approach should be used with caution, due to the risk of developing resistance to mupirocin with prolonged use (Herwaldt, 1993). Antibiotic prophylaxis may be used at the time of insertion with vancomycin or cephalosporins being recommended (Gokal et al., 1993).

Post-insertion prevention

The exit site dressing should be left in situ for several days unless there is a need to change this due to leakage or strikethrough. A non-occlusive dressing is recommended due to the moisture buildup beneath occlusive films (Gokal et al., 1993). Once the exit site has healed the dressing is often dispensed with, unless it is needed for comfort. The catheter should be secured to prevent mechanical damage. Cleansing around the site with soap and water is sufficient once healing is complete; however some regimes suggest cleansing with a skin disinfectant for the first few weeks after insertion (Twardowski, 1992). Scrupulous adherence to aseptic technique during dialysis exchanges, both by healthcare workers and clients, is important for infection prevention.

Treatment of infection

If infection of an exit site or tunnel is suspected, this may be treated by systemic antibiotics and the cauterization of over-granulated tissue around the cannula (Twardowski, 1992). For patients with peritonitis, antibiotics can be given intraperitoneally by addition to the dialysis fluid (Keane et al., 1993). If treatment of infection is unsuccessful, removal of the CAPD catheter may be necessary.

Epidural cannulae

Epidural catheters are now widely used for anaesthesia and analgesia in surgical and maternity patients. Infection may be limited to the exit site or may cause epidural abscess or meningitis. Organisms associated with epidural catheter infection are *Staph. aureus*, *Staph. epidermidis* and *Pseudomonas* spp. Rates of infection have been reported to be 4% (Holt et al., 1995), which is similar to rates for IVs. Infection prevention for epidural cannulae should include disinfection of the skin prior to insertion under aseptic conditions, daily observation of the exit site and cleansing of the exit site with an antiseptic at

Table 17.1 Example of an audit tool

INFECTION CONTROL – CANNULATION AUDIT

HOSPITAL:
WARD: PT No   No OF CANNULAE:

RISK ASSESSMENT CRITERIA	DATE	COMMENTS

Cannula in use?
Cannula *not* in use?
Type of dressing
      occlusive
      non-occlusive
      tape
      other

Condition of dressing
      satisfactory
      unsatisfactory

Infection signs
      oedema
      erythema
      localised skin temp
      tenderness
      exudate

Giving set change
      within 24° of initial visit
        48°
        72°
        >72°

Use of multiple inlet devices
      3-way tap
      traffic light manifold
      Y-line
      other

dressing changes (Holt et al., 1995). Infection may be indicated by fever and back pain, following which exit site and aspirate from the catheter should be cultured. Further neurological examinations, scans and lumbar puncture may also be necessary to detect neurological involvement. Treatment will involve the removal of the cannula and the administration of antibiotics.

Education and audit

With the current usage of invasive cannulae, care of these devices is inevitably a common component of nursing care for patients. All staff with clinical input should be familiar with national recommendations and local policies for cannula care. Education of staff, patients and carers is an important part of infection reduction strategies, however, varying success in reducing infection rates have been reported using education alone in relation to IV therapy (Cohran et al., 1996; Stonehouse and Butcher, 1996).

Audit is useful to establish whether practice reflects current recommended cannula care strategies as opposed to providing infection rates (see Table 17.1). Several studies have demonstrated a lack of good practice in relation to IV care (Lundgren et al., 1993; Nelson et al., 1996; Glynn et al., 1997). Lundgren et al. (1993), Nelson et al. (1996) and Stonehouse and Butcher (1996) provide definitions for audit of peripheral cannulae care, Elliot et al. (1995) provide an audit programme to review patient management and hospital practices for CVC care, and Lawrance (1994) provides documentation used to audit central venous cannulae infection on a bone marrow transplant unit. Wilson et al (1994) audited infection in CAPD to establish whether alterations to management regimes reduced infection rates. These audit programmes are readily adaptable for use within any healthcare setting and could provide a basis for assessing and improving levels of care.

References

Ayliffe GAJ, Coates D, Hoffman PN Chemical Disinfection in Hospitals, 2nd Edition. London: Public Health Laboratory Service, 1993.

Camp-Sorrell D Implantable Ports: Everything you always wanted to know. Journal of Intravenous Nursing. 1992; 15 (5): 262–73.

Cohran J, Larson E, Roach H, Blane C, Pierce P Effect of intravascular surveillance and education program on rates of nosocomial bloodstream infections. Heart & Lung 1996; 25 (2): 161–4.

Conly JM, Grieves K, Peters B A prospective randomised study comparing transparent and dry gauze dressings for central venous catheters. Journal of Infectious Diseases 1989; 159 (2): 310–19.

Department of Health. Degradation of Silicone Tubing by Alcohol-based antiseptics. (Hazard Warning Notice 93:7). London: HMSO, 1993.

Elliott TSJ Line-associated bacteraemias. Communicable Disease Report Review 1993; 3 (7): R91–R96.

Elliott TSJ, Faroqui MH, Armstrong RF, Hanson GC Guidelines for good practice in central venous catherization. Journal of Hospital Infection 1994; 28 (3): 163–76.

Elliott TS, Faroqui MH, Tebbs SE, Armstrong RF, Hanson GC An audit programme for central venous catheter-associated infections. Journal of Hospital Infection 1995; 30 (3): 181–91.

Emmerson AM, Enstone JE, Griffin M, Kelsey MC, Smyth ETM The second national prevalence survey of infection in hospitals – overview of the results. Journal of Hospital Infection 1996; 32 (3): 175–90.

Frean JA, Arntzen L, Rosekilly I, Isaacson M Investigation of contaminated parenteral nutrition fluids associated with an outbreak of Serratia odorifera septicaemia. Journal of Hospital Infection 1994; 27 (4): 263–73.

Glynn A, Ward V, Wilson J, Charlett A, Cookson B, Taylor J, Cole N Hospital-Acquired Infection: Surveillance, Policy and Practice. London: PHLS, 1997.

Gokal R, Ash SR, Helfrich GB, Holmes CJ, Joffe P, Nichols WK, Oreopoulos DG, Riella MC, Slingeyer A, Twardowski ZJ, Vas S Peritoneal catheters and exit-site practices: toward optimum peritoneal access. Peritoneal Dialysis International 1993; 13 (1): 29–39.

Hamilton H Care improves while costs reduce. Professional Nurse 1993; 8 (9): 592–6.

Herwaldt LA Staphylococcus aureus nasal carriage: role in continuous ambulatory peritoneal dialysis associated infections. Peritoneal Dialysis International 1993; 13 (suppl. 2): S301–S305.

Holt HM, Andersen SS, Andersen O, Garhn-Hansen B, Siboni K Infections following epidural catherization. Journal of Hospital Infection 1995; 30 (4): 253–60.

Hospital Infection Control Practice Advisory Committee (HICPAC). Infection Control Hospital Epidemiology 1996; 17 (7): 438–73.

Hospital Infection Control Practices Advisory Committee. Guidelines for prevention of intravascular-device-related infections. Infection Control and Hospital Epidemiology 1996; 17 (7): 438–73.

Infection Control Nurses' Association. Intravenous Line Dressings: Principles of Infection Control. London: Royal College of Nursing, 1991.

Jarrard MM, Freeman JB The effects of antibiotic ointment and antiseptics on the skin flora beneath subclavian catheter dressings during intravenous hyperalimentation. Journal of Surgical Research 1977; 22 (5): 521–26.

Keane WF, Everett ED, Golper TA, Gokal R, Halstenson C, Kawaguchi Y, Riella M, Vas S, Verbrugh HA Peritoneal dialysis-related peritonitis treatment recommendations, 1993 update. Peritoneal Dialysis International 1993; 13 (1): 14–28.

Lawrance T Central venous line audit. Paediatric Nursing 1994; 6 (4): 20–23.

Lundgren A, Jordfeldt L, Ek AC The care and handling of peripheral intravenous cannulae on 60 surgery and internal medicine patients: an observational study. Journal of Advanced Nursing 1993; 18 (6): 963–71.

Luzar MA, Brown CB, Balf D, Hill L, Issad B, Monnier B, Moulart J, Sabatier JC, Wauquier JP, Peluso F Exit-site care and exit-site infection in continuous ambulatory peritoneal dialysis (CAPD): results of a randomised multicenter trial. Peritoneal Dialysis International 1990a; 10 (1): 25–9.

Luzar MA, Coles GA, Faller B, Slingeneyer A, Dah Dah G, Briat C, Wone C, Knefati Y, Kessler M, Peluso F Staphylococcus aureus nasal carriage and infection in patients on continuous ambulatory peritoneal dialysis. New England Journal of Medicine 1990b; 322 (8): 505–9.

Maki DG, McCormack KN Defatting catheter insertion sites in total parenteral nutrition is of no value as an infection control measure. American Journal of Medicine 1987; 83 (5): 833–40.

Maki DG, Botticelli JT, LeRoy ML, Thielke TS Prospective study of replacing administration sets for intravenous therapy at 48- vs 72-hour intervals. Journal of the American Medical Association 1987; 258 (13): 1777–81.

Maki DG, Ringer M, Alvarado CJ Prospective randomised trial of povidone-iodine, alcohol, and chlorhexidine for prevention of infection associated with central venous and arterial catheters. The Lancet 1991; 338 (8763): 339–43.

Maki DG, Weise CR, Sarafin HW A semiquantitative culture method for identifying intravenous catheter-related infection. New England Journal of Medicine 1977; 296 (23): 1305–9.

Markel S PIC/PICC and extended peripheral catheters: five years experience in home care. Journal of Home Healthcare Practice 1994; 7 (1): 35–40.

McClelland B (ed.) Handbook of Transfusion Medicine, 2nd Edition. London: HMSO, 1996.

Nelson RRS, Tebbs SE, Richards N, Elliott TSJ An audit of peripheral catheter care in a teaching hospital. Journal of Hospital Infection 1996; 32 (1): 65–9.

Oldman PA A microbiological study of a piece of tape used to secure IV cannulae. Professional Nurse 1991; 6 (5): 265–9.

Pritchard AP, Mallet J Royal Marsden Manual of Clinical Nursing Procedures, 3rd Edition. Oxford: Blackwell, 1993.

Russo PL, Harrington GA, Spelman DW Needleless intravenous systems: A review. American Journal of Infection Control 1999; 27(5): 431–4.

Shivnan JC, Macguire D, Freedman S et al. A comparison of transparent adherent and dry sterile gauze dressings for long-term catheters in patients undergoing bone marrow transplant. Oncology Nurses Forum 1991; 18 (8): 1349–56.

Spencer RC Use of in-line filters for intravenous infusions. Journal of Hospital Infection 1990; 16 (3): 281.

Stonehouse J, Butcher J Phlebitis associated with peripheral cannulae. Professional Nurse 1996; 12 (1): 51–4.

Twardowski ZJ Peritoneal dialysis catheter exit site infections: prevention, diagnosis, treatment and future directions. Seminars in Dialysis 1992; 5 (4): 305–15.

Ward V, Wilson J, Taylor L, Cookson B, Glynn A Preventing Hospital-Acquired Infection: Clinical Guidelines. London: PHLS, 1997

White MC, Ragland KE Surveillance of intravenous catheter related infection among home care clients. American Journal of Infection Control 1994; 22 (4): 231–5.

Wille JC, Blusse van OudAlblas A, Thewessen EAPM A comparison of two transparent film-type dressings in central venous therapy. Journal of Hospital Infection 1993; 23 (2): 113–21.

Wilson APR, Scott GM, Lewis C, Nield G, Rudge C Audit of infection in continuous ambulatory peritoneal dialysis. Journal of Hospital Infection 1994; 28 (4): 265–71.

Chapter 18
Wound infection

ANDREW KINGSLEY

Introduction

Wound infection has been a problem throughout history. It was written about in the 2nd century AD by Galen, who discussed his theory of 'laudable pus' (Cooper and Lawrence, 1996), and Semmelweiss battled with it in the 19th century, but it has only been in the last 50 years, during the age of the antibiotic, that its shadow has been lifted. Wound infection remains a problem today although it is usually easily treated. However, the development of antibiotic-resistant micro-organisms has made the treatment of infection more problematic, requiring more toxic, more expensive antibiotics and often leading to less satisfactory health outcomes for patients. This must shake us out of our complacency. In addition, we are still regularly troubled by the routine pathogens that have always been with us. We may still gain the upper hand in these episodes most of the time but that does not mean to say that they have not caused suffering and consumed valuable health resources along the way.

Healthcare professionals of all disciplines must make every effort to adopt the appropriate measures to prevent the development of wound infection. Such measures will broadly fall into two categories: those aimed at reducing the risk from endogenous reservoirs of micro-organisms, i.e. from the individual's own micro-flora; and those concerned with preventing the transmission of pathogens from exogenous sources, i.e. other people and the environment. Infection prevention and control measures taken should be supported by research considered robust in the light of information available at the time, or based on sound principles which are the logical extension of knowledge of such things as microbial growth patterns and requirements, pathogenesis of infection and transmission of organisms, applied to the practical situation. Equally, those measures that have been discredited, either because they are harmful or because they provide no advantage, should be removed from current use.

There have been two national surveys of infections in UK hospitals, the first in 1980 (Meers et al., 1981) and the second in 1994 (Emmerson et al., 1996). The figures from the first have been widely quoted, so it is interesting to see the latest results as a comparison. Hospital acquired infections had a prevalence of 9.2% in 1980 and 9.0% in 1994. Expressed as a percentage of these figures, surgical wound infection fell from 18.9% to 10.7%. Skin infections, which would have included non-surgical wounds healing by secondary intention, also fell, from 13.5% to 9.6%, which is perhaps some cause for encouragement that progress in preventing wound infection is occurring. However, 413 surgical wound and 370 skin infections were identified by the 1994 prevalence survey, which means that on a typical day in a UK hospital, it is not uncommon to find cases of wound infection.

The costs of wound infection arise in three main areas: actual expenditure on treatment, expenditure associated with lost opportunity or extra bed days consumed, and, most importantly, the unquantifiable but significant social costs of associated morbidity and mortality. The cost of extra bed occupancy caused by infected surgical wounds was estimated to £22.3 million per annum in 1973 (Gilmore and Sanderson, 1975). In an earlier study, 5% of bed strength was lost to the treatment of surgical sepsis (Loewenthal, 1962).

Wound healing

The wound healing process is delayed by the presence of infection. In fact it may not only delay progress but may also increase the size of a wound by necrosing tissue. The mere presence of micro-organisms in a wound or, indeed, the colonization of chronic open wounds often with large numbers of various bacteria will not inevitably lead to wound infection. Amongst these colonies will be found the normal commensal flora and also micro-organisms that are considered pathogenic (see Table 18.1). It might seem a mystery why on some occasions such organisms cause infection and sometimes not, and the answer in each case will lie in the complex balance of the strength or

Table 18.1 Commensal and transient skin flora

Commensal flora	Transient flora
Staphylococcus epidermidis	*Staphyloccus aureus*
Micrococci	(Carriage: 10–30% in general population,
Coryneforms	20–60% in hospital staff)
Small numbers of the following	Enterobacteria, e.g. *E. coli*
may also be present:	*Klebsiella* spp.
Anaerobic cocci, e.g. peptostreptococci	
Anaerobic bacilli, e.g. propionibacteria	

resistance factors of the host against the quantity and virulence of the potential pathogens. The balance between competing microbes may also be important in reducing each other's space and the available nutrients to grow to sufficient inocula to produce infection. The state of the wound is also critical in determining outcome.

Necrotic tissue and excess exudate will support microbial proliferation and a dry wound environment will hinder the activity of the host's tissue repair and infection control cells, both of which have evolved to function and survive in a fluid medium. Healing will also be affected by reduced blood flow, which can be caused in trauma situations, thrombosis and in peripheral vascular disease. This is because blood brings nutrients and oxygen to support the healing process as well as healing cells.

There is debate over whether the presence of bacteria actually delays healing. Prophylactic treatment with topical antiseptics and antibiotics is in most cases not considered appropriate because of the attendant risks of sensitivity reactions and the possible harmful effects to infection control, tissue repair and new tissue cells. In addition such treatments may lead to resistance to the antibiotic used.

Wound healing may be by *primary* or *secondary intention* (see Figure 18.1).

Primary intention: wounds that heal in this way have very little loss of tissue and are closed by sutures, clips or similar methods. Healing is rapid.

Secondary intention: wounds where tissue has been lost and must be filled with granulation tissue and covered by epithelium. These wounds cannot be closed and the healing process takes much longer (University of Dundee, 1993).

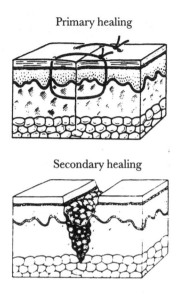

Primary healing

Secondary healing

Figure 18.1 Healing by primary and secondary intention

The wound healing process can be described as a healing cascade where each response initiates another until full repair is effected (Turner, 1993).

For convenience, the healing process can be divided into four stages, but progression across the whole wound is rarely linear; it is rather more common to see different parts of a wound at different stages of the healing route.

Phase 1: acute inflammatory stage

The main elements of this are:

- bleeding with clot formation to control haemorrhage
- inflammation to initiate host defences and tissue repair process
- vasoconstriction to further control bleeding
- vasodilatation to allow leucocytes to enter wound area

Phase 2: destructive stage

The main elements of this are:
- removal of bacteria by neutrophils, polymorphonuclear leuco-cytes and macrophages
- removal of necrotic tissue by macrophages
- attraction of fibroblasts by macrophages to initiate new cell deposition

Phase 3: reconstructive stage

The main elements of this are:

- fibroplasia by fibroblasts laying down collagen network and granulation tissue
- angiogenesis to bring blood supply to new tissue
- epithelialization
- wound contraction (occurs through all phases)

Phase 4: maturation stage

The main element of this is:

- remodelling new tissue to achieve maximum tensile strength

Definition of wound infection

Even with modern methods of prevention, some wounds will at times become infected. When such situations arise, healthcare professionals must be trained and ready to observe and interpret the signs and symptoms and be prepared to act at the earliest opportunity. Swift recognition and prompt treatment will ensure the best outcome, which means the least harm for the patient, minimum additional expense and bed days lost, and least opportunity for the transmission of infection between patients.

It is important to consistently use a clear and simple definition of wound infection in order to ensure early recognition and treatment. Essentially, this will be based on clinical signs and symptoms and not rely on microbiological analysis, which will have the effect of delay-ing therapy whilst results are awaited. A definition of wound infec-tion should include the four cardinal signs: swelling (including lymphadenitis); pain; heat; redness (including lymphangitis) in the tissue surrounding the wound (peripheral cellulitis).

The local indications of redness, swelling, heat and pain are signs of inflammation which would be expected at the site of tissue injury. However, the degrees to which they are present may increase with infection. Pain in the surrounding tissues is likely to be the main symptom that highlights the possibility of wound infection.

Additional signs may be present such as pus, increased level of exudate and offensive odour, all of which could be considered corroborative. Some authors consider the presence of pus to be the only defining diagnostic criterion. Systemic signs are pyrexia and elevated neutrophil count.

The following definition and criteria were used to diagnose infection in one study (Glenister et al., 1992). A wound was defined as 'a break in the epithelial surface (skin or mucous membrane) and the underlying tissue made by some positive act such as an accident or surgical incision'. Burns, leg ulcers and pressure sores were excluded from the definition. All wounds had to have purulent discharge in or exuding from them to be classified as infected. Criteria for surgical wound infection were infection at the incision site (including drains) within 30 days of operation or within one year if an implant was placed.

Due to the ever-diminishing length of patient stay in hospital, postoperative wound infection is likely to show first following discharge. Patients who develop a major infection will probably visit their GP or surgeon for treatment, but minor infection, for example suture abscess, may resolve spontaneously and remain unreported, thereby falsely lowering the incidence of surgical wound infection assuming surveillance is being carried out.

The same study classified an accidental wound as infected if the infection occurred at the wound site. Burns were considered to be infected if either discharge of purulent material or graft rejection occurred, together with clinical signs of infection. Chronic wounds were diagnosed as infected by the clinical signs and symptoms, with or without microbiological evidence.

Using pus as the only diagnostic criterion has been reported to considerably lower the infection rate (Ayliffe et al., 1977). Other criteria to assist in the identification of infection in granulating wounds have been suggested but not validated, in addition to the more traditional criteria of abscess, cellulitis and discharge (Cutting and Harding, 1994).

These are:

- delayed healing
- discoloration
- friable granulation tissue which bleeds easily
- unexpected pain or tenderness
- pocketing or bridging at base of wound
- abnormal smell
- wound breakdown

Whatever the definition, two major factors determine whether a wound will become infected (Kingsley, 1992):

- micro-organic contamination of the wound
- the patient's resistance to that contamination

An equation of these factors was described by Allemeier and Culbertson (1965):

$$\text{Risk of infection} = \frac{\text{Dose of bacterial contamination} \times \text{Virulence}}{\text{Resistance of the host}}$$

The microflora present in a wound relate to the type of wound, the environmental circumstances in which the injury occurred and the site of the wound on the body. Having stated that, *Staphylococcus aureus* is possibly the most commonly found organism (Lawrence, 1993) and the most common cause of wound sepsis. Acute wounds, which are those produced by surgery or trauma in healthy individuals, that heal in a normal time scale have been said to contain micro-organisms similar to that of intact skin. These include aerobic species such as staphylococci, coryneforms (formerly known as diphtheroids), and micrococci, and propionibacterium species (Mertz and Ovington, 1993), which is an anaerobic coryneform. Foreign matter impacted into the wound at the time of the injury results in bacterial contamination. *Clostridium tetani* are rarely isolated from wounds but their possible presence in dirty wounds must be taken into account.

The nature and degree of contamination during a surgical procedure will influence the microbial species present. In particular if the gut is opened or has perforated, it would be expected that intestinal flora such as *Escherischia coli*, *Pseudomonas aeruginosa*, *Klebsiella* species and other coliforms would be present. Bacteroides, another species of Gram-negative bacilli, are strict anaerobes that live in the lower part of the gut, and are the commonest cause of anaerobic infection in man (Thomas, 1988).

Burn wounds are often initially sterile but quickly become colonized with micro-organisms, including potential pathogens such as *Staphylococcus aureus*, beta haemolytic streptococcus Lancefield group A (*Streptococcus pyogenes*), *Pseudomonas aeruginosa* and *Acinetobacter* species. Fungi and yeasts are present about 10% of the time but rarely cause problems (Frame et al., 1992).

The microflora of chronic wounds changes with the stages of healing and they may be colonized by more than 27 separate bacterial species including Gram-positive, Gram-negative, aerobic and anaerobic species (Mertz and Ovington, 1993).

Factors increasing wound infection risks

Factors increasing wound infection risks fall into two categories – those that increase risk for the individual and those that add to the risk of the transmission of infection to others.

Risks to the individual

There are many factors that increase the risks of wound infection for the individual, and additional factors which increase risks for those undergoing surgical procedures (see Table 18.2).

Table 18.2 Factors increasing risks of surgical wound infection

Time on the table – the rate of clean wound infection roughly doubles with every hour. Operations lasting more than 2 hours have an increased risk (Cruse and Foord, 1980).
Abdominal operations
Contaminated and dirty/infected operations
Having three or more diagnoses at time of operation.

General risk factors include

Nature of injury – wounds in which microbial contamination is introduced at occurrence, such as puncture wounds with contaminated items like rusty nails or garden implements; bite wounds where oral flora are introduced; road trauma where dirt and grit are introduced.

Skin flora at time of injury – traumatic wounds can have pathogenic bacteria introduced from what is on the skin at the time, even by sterile objects such as hypodermic needles.

Reduced blood supply – reduced perfusion of the local area around the wound, either through damage to blood vessels at the time of traumatic injury, thrombosis formation, embolism, atherosclerotic changes or surgical technique.

Necrotic tissue – being dead this is avascular and therefore is not perfused with normal defence cells. This decaying medium which may produce anaerobic conditions is good for supporting the growth of pathogens.

Foreign bodies – if left in wounds these act as foci for infection. This includes fibres shed from wound dressings. Implants could be considered here as they reduce the inoculum required to initiate infection.

State of health – if the individual's overall state of health is poor, the risk of infection is increased. The malnourished and the immunocompromised are particularly at risk.

Underlying disease – certain diseases increase the risk of wound infection, including diabetes mellitus and immunosuppressive conditions such as AIDS.

Endogenous carriage of pathogens – between 30% and 50% of the population carry *Staphylococcus aureus*, and 5% to 10% carry beta haemolytic streptococcus group A (Thomas, 1988), providing reservoirs of pathogens in close proximity to wounds in these people.

Drugs – steroids reduce the inflammatory response which is the protective mechanism for the immune system. Equally, immunosuppressive drugs used to treat cancers increase the risk of wound infection.

Age – though this is clearly an irreversible risk factor, the very young have immature immune systems and the old have ageing immune systems, both of which may lead to inadequate responses to the threat of infection.

Taking all the risks listed in Table 18.2 into account, one study calculated that 90% of surgical wound infections occur in patients who fall into these groups and amount to approximately 50% of all surgical patients (Haley et al., 1985).

Infection risks to others

A number of factors will increase the risks of transfer of potentially pathogenic micro-organisms from one individual's wound to another. These include:

Poor hand hygiene – transfer of pathogens from one wound to another by contact route. This will usually be the hands of nurses or doctors, but patients must also be taught to wash their hands after touching their own dressing.

Contaminated equipment and instruments – if equipment and instruments are not decontaminated between patients, transfer of pathogens can occur through this indirect contact route. For example, a footstool used by a patient with a heavily exuding wound may be a source of cross-infection if it is not decontaminated before use by another patient.

Poor dressing technique – can introduce organisms from one wound to another, especially if they are both sited on the same patient.

Removal of dressings – this applies particularly to dry, gauze-type dressings which release many organisms to the air, from where they can find their way into other wounds either directly, or indirectly via contaminated equipment or surfaces.

Prevention of wound infection

A wound, by definition, is a break in the skin and as such represents the breach of the body's primary physical defence mechanism. Therefore all wounds are a potential portal of entry for infecting microbes; it is just the degree to which they are vulnerable to this attack that differs. Prevention of infection of all wounds should be one of the principal tenets of wound care. Any measures taken should have proven benefits in this direction which outweigh any attendant risks to the patient. Prevention strategies centre on the principles of asepsis, antisepsis, prophylaxis, removal of infection foci (foreign bodies, necrotic tissue, excess exudate), occlusion of the wound by dressings, prevention of harm to the body's own infection control and tissue repair cells. The application of these principles may vary for each wound, dependent on individual circumstances. Wounds can be divided into two main groups: those healing by *primary* and by *secondary* intention, or further into four groups: surgical, trauma, thermal and chronic wounds (Miller and Dyson, 1996). These will now be considered in turn.

Surgical wounds

Surgical wounds can be subdivided into planned and emergency groups. It would be reasonable to suppose that emergency surgery carries a higher risk of wound infection because fewer of the infection-influencing factors can be addressed than for planned cases (Kingsley, 1992). Typically the surgical process is divided into three time periods in which prevention activities can be undertaken: pre-, peri- and postoperative.

Pre-operative phase

In this phase, prevention activities centre on maximizing the individual's level of health and reducing the risk of colonization by controlling underlying diseases such as diabetes and concurrent infection that might predispose to wound infection (Ayliffe et al., 1992), reversing malnutrition, and keeping hospital stay as short as possible. Other possible strategies include skin preparation with antiseptic soaps, modified hair removal and antibiotic prophylaxis.

Nutrition: rapid weight loss of more than 10% due to illness is associated with a deterioration in resistance to infection (Sizer, 1996). Estimates of malnourishment among surgical patients have been as high as 20% (Powell-Tuck, 1993), so ensuring that patients are well nourished beforehand may stand them in good stead later.

Hospital stay: pre-operative inpatient stays should be as short as possible, though long enough to ensure adequate preparation of the patient. Shorter stays are associated with lower infection rates

(Cruse and Foord, 1980); this is thought to be due to the reduction in colonization of patients with virulent hospital pathogens. Shorter stays are becoming a reality with the increase in day surgery and pre-operative assessment clinics.

Skin preparation: the benefit of pre-operative bathing with or without antiseptic soaps to reduce skin flora remains unclear. Studies have produced evidence of both benefit (Cruse and Foord, 1980) and no benefit (Rotter et al., 1988). Repeated pre-operative bathing with chlorhexidine has been shown to have a cumulative antibacterial action (Ayliffe et al., 1983). A review of literature by Jepsen and Brut-tomesso (1993) confirmed this view, concluding that showering was more effective than bathing; chlorhexidine was highly effective and two showers were necessary pre-operatively to reduce skin flora. The removal of ingrained dirt is sensible prior to skin disinfection in theatre because, along with skin scales and exudate, it interferes with the action of antiseptics (Mackenzie, 1988).

Hair removal: removal of hair is only necessary if it interferes with surgery. Razor shaving appears to be associated with the great-est risk of infection compared with unshaven sites (Cruse and Foord, 1980), or removal by depilatory cream (Seropian and Reynolds, 1971). The length of time shaving is carried out prior to surgery is also important – the longer the time in advance, the higher the risk. If hair removal is required and a razor is the chosen method, then it should be done as close to the time of surgery as possible, i.e. within one hour.

Bowel preparation: in order to remove as much faecal material as possible and reduce intra-abdominal contamination it is generally advised that bowel preparation is carried out pre-operatively. Regimes vary and care should be taken to ensure low residue diets used in preparation do not cause malnutrition.

Antibiotic prophylaxis: the administration of chemo-prophy-laxis should be restricted to those patients whose risk of infection is high (Thomas, 1988) and when the consequence of infection would be serious (Ayliffe et al., 1992). This is because the use of antibiotics is accompanied by risks of side effects for the patient and the produc-tion of antibiotic-resistant organisms for institutions. Prophylaxis usually consists of one dose of antibiotic given on induction of anaes-thesia.

Peri-operative phase

In this phase, the thrust of prevention is concerned with stopping or minimizing the seeding of the wound site with exogenous flora from the surgical team and the wider environment, and avoiding the transplantation of endogenous organisms, residents and transients, from the skin surface. Efforts are also directed at removing pus and infection foci such as necrotic tissue and preventing them from occurring through drainage of fluid collections. Activities can be divided into four groups: environment, instruments, personnel and patient preparation.

Environment

Operating room cleanliness: surfaces in the operating room should be intact and washable to allow effective cleaning to take place. Surfaces should be maintained ready for use in a clean (that is without visible soiling), dry and dust-free state. Routine cleaning is effected by use of detergent and water. Between cases, decontamination of surfaces soiled with body fluids, contaminated irrigation fluid or solid tissues should involve cleaning and disinfection. Operating rooms maintained in this state are unlikely to contribute to cross-contamination.

Ventilation: ventilation of the operating room using forced, filtered air reduces particulate airborne contamination arising from the patient and personnel. These particles, mostly skin squames, carry viable bacteria, thus reducing their number through ventilation reduces the risk of infection for the patient (Humphreys et al., 1995). There are various levels of filtration and types of ventilation systems that can be achieved and used. The UK norm is plenum ventilation which changes the room air typically 20 times per hour, in combination with incoming air filtration down to 5 microns diameter. Air can be filtered to sub micron level using HEPA (high efficiency particulate air) filters and can be delivered into the room directly above the operative site by laminar (uni-directional) airflow. Allander ventilation or zonal ventilation falls into this category and delivers air changes up to 80 per hour (Hambraes and Laurell, 1980). Air changes in some laminar flow systems can be taken up to several hundred per hour to produce ultra-clean air, which is air carrying

<10 bacteria-laden particles per cubic metre (Lidwell et al., 1982). Ultra-clean air, which can also be produced through use of total body exhaust suits, is considered to be of value in orthopaedic implant surgery, but is unlikely to be of benefit in routine general surgical situations.

Instruments

All instruments entering sterile body cavities must be sterile at the time of use and it is of course standard practice to prevent contamination of the wound from exogenous sources. Where possible the Central Sterile Supplies Department should process the instruments and the use of chemicals such as glutaraldehyde should be avoided in order to eliminate health risks to staff and improve quality controls.

Personnel

Hand hygiene: the objective of handwashing prior to the surgical process is twofold: firstly to remove transient organisms and secondly to reduce the numbers of resident bacteria. The first objective is achieved through use of soap and water to remove physical contamination and loose skin squames on the surface. As for the second, an antiseptic is required – preferably one that has a residual activity on the skin and will maintain that lowered count for a longer period. Antiseptic surgical preparations containing chlorhexidine or povidone iodine are perhaps the most commonly used on hands and forearms, for two minutes (Griffiths-Jones and Ward, 1995). Following the first scrub of the list, alcohol rubs containing chlorhexidine can be used between cases if hands are visibly clean. Two applications of 5 ml on the hands and forearms until evaporated to dryness is advised (Ayliffe et al., 1992). The use of sterile latex gloves is considered standard practice to further reduce risk of transmission of resident skin flora into the wound. However gloves may become punctured during procedures, often without the wearer realizing. Cruse and Foord (1980) recorded that 11.6% were holed by the end of operation, but no wound infections were noted against that series. More recently Lane et al. (1993), in a glove puncture study in orthopaedic operations, found that 29 of 148 gloves were holed at the end of the operation, only 23 of which had been noticed by surgeons during the operation. Hartley et al.(1996) studied the difference to glove puncture rates when using blunt-tipped versus cutting needles during abdominal closure. As might be expected, rates fell dramatically when blunt tips were used, though punctures were not entirely eliminated. It is important to change gloves if punctures occur, and when gloves become wet with alcohol based products which can lead to penetration of the latex (Mellstrom et al., 1992).

Clothing: sterile operating gowns prevent the transmission of microbes in two ways. Firstly, by being changed between patients, they block transmission from one wound to another on the outer surface of the material. Secondly, they prevent the transmission of commensals from the skin of the scrub team. However, to achieve this the material must be tightly woven to prevent this passage and also waterproof to prevent wicking which would otherwise facilitate the transport of microbes through the fabric in either direction. The pores of woven linen are typically about 50 microns square while skin particles on average are smaller at 15 microns square, so penetration is possible (Clark, 1989). Disposable gowns have been shown to reduce wound infection over traditional cotton clothing (Moylan and Kennedy, 1980; Moylan et al., 1987). New-generation re-usable fabric gowns which are waterproof yet vapour-permeable may yet prove to show equal benefit. Charnley total body exhaust suits are the ultimate in patient protection. In effect they seal off the operating personnel completely from the patient. Surgical face masks, on the other hand, do not reduce airborne contamination and do not reduce wound infection in general surgery (Tunevall, 1991). Research to determine the benefit of mask-wearing in specialized fields of surgery, such as orthopaedic joint replacement where the infecting inoculum is smaller (Whyte, 1988), needs to be done (Leyland and McCloy, 1993).

Covering the head is intended to prevent hair falling from the scrub team into the wound. The wearing of surgical hats has little effect on reducing airborne counts of bacteria (Humphreys et al., 1991). However, whether fall out can be prevented and if head cover is valuable in reducing infection has yet to be established, although an outbreak was attributed to hair carriage of *Staphylococcus aureus* in an operating unit (Dineen and Drusin, 1973). It therefore remains reasonable for scrub teams to continue the practice.

Patient preparation

Skin drapes: like gowns, the drapes are considered to provide a barrier to the transmission of organisms. In this case the transmission source is endogenous, from the patient's commensals on surrounding skin. The drape prevents contamination of the surgeon's instruments and hands. Again, this is only likely to occur if the drape remains dry or is waterproof and not compromised by sharp towel clips. The same studies that demonstrated reduced infection rates with disposable instead of cotton gowns were conducted using the same materials for drapes (Moylan and Kennedy, 1980; Moylan et al., 1987). Again it may be argued that there may be benefits to be gained from the use of new generation waterproof/vapour permeable fabric re-usable drapes. Incisional drapes have not been shown to reduce levels of wound contamination from skin organisms or wound infections (Raahave, 1976). Investigations into the effectiveness of wound-edge drapes, which are placed inside the wound, have not clearly established this one way or the other (Whyte, 1988).

Skin antisepsis: the use of antiseptics is advised to reduce skin flora over the wound site (Griffiths-Jones and Ward, 1995), and has been shown to reduce the clean wound infection rate (Cruse and Foord, 1980). Alcoholic chlorhexidine 0.5% or 10% alcoholic povidone iodine is generally recommended (Ayliffe et al., 1992; AORN Recommended Practices Co-ordinating Committee, 1992). The length of application has been questioned, with one review of relevant literature concluding that one-minute applications of 70% isopropyl alcohol followed by application of an antimicrobial adhesive drape to be as effective, or more effective, than longer preps (Jepsen and Bruttomesso, 1993). Alcoholic preparations must be allowed to dry and must not pool in the umbilicus in order to prevent burn injuries from the diathermy.

Normothermia: recently it has been shown that hypothermia may delay healing and predispose patients to wound infections. In a study of 200 patients undergoing colorectal surgery, a normothermic group had a 6% infection rate against a hypothermic group (2°C lower temperature) with a 19% infection rate (Kurz et al., 1996).

Wound closure and dressing: wounds requiring drainage appear to have lower infection rates if drains are brought out through stab wounds rather than the stitch line (Cruse and Foord, 1980). Suction drains help to reduce haematoma formation, which otherwise would be a risk factor for infection.

Microbial contamination leading to wound infection is more likely to be acquired peri- rather than post-operatively, and it is also more likely that these organisms will be of endogenous origin (Ayliffe et al., 1990). According to Hulten (1994) surgically closed wounds usually heal rapidly and re-epithelialization may occur after 24–48 hours. The role of the wound dressing in preventing surgical wound infection is therefore unclear. Non-leaking wounds can be left undressed after 48 hours (Wilson, 1995). Getting stitches wet during personal hygiene activities appears not to be detrimental (Noe and Keller, 1987).

Post-operative phase

In this phase, the prevention activities centre on the speedy rehabilitation of the patient to full health, though perhaps only nutrition, timely removal of wound drains and prevention of wound contamination from exogenous sources have any direct influence over preventing wound infection.

Nutrition

An early resumption of diet or the use of parenteral feeding if this is not possible should build on pre-operative nutritional support to help improve the rate of healing and strength of wounds (Ruberg, 1984) and reduce the risk of infectious complications arising from nutritional deficits (Rhoads, 1980).

Removal of wound drains

Wound drains are used to prevent the type of accumulations of fluids that might occur when infection is present, in presence of fistulae, or when there is leakage of blood, lymph or serum into the wound (Ayliffe et al., 1992). Fluid collections present a risk of infection and need to be drained away. However, any invasive line represents a risk by connecting the outside of the body to the inside. To overcome this risk it is equally logical to remove the drain at the earliest opportunity, i.e. when fluid has stopped collecting. This view is supported by the results of a study suggesting that the likelihood of colonization increases while drainage decreases over time (Drinkwater and Neil, 1995). Attempts must be made to reduce environmental contamination of drains; practices include minimal handling of the drainage equipment, using an aseptic technique and securing them off the floor.

Prevention of contamination

It seems reasonable to prevent additional contamination as so much effort has been devoted to preventing contamination in the perioperative phase of the wound. It has been reported that in a series of colorectal procedures no correlation between faecal contamination of the wound following dressing dislodgement and infection was found (Hulten, 1994). It is not clear what the effects on post-operative wound infection rates are from other types of microbial contamination. In an effort to prevent exogenous contamination patients are often advised not to wet suture lines, and consequently bathing and showering is restricted. However, limited evidence suggests that such avoidance is unnecessary, though it is probably best to wait 24 hours to allow the network of fibrin and the process of epithelialization to establish itself (Noe and Keller, 1987).

Trauma wounds

Trauma wounds are those that have been caused by mechanical damage such as abrasions and lacerations (Miller and Dyson, 1996), penetrating and crushing injuries. Clearly, pre-planned prevention of infection activities is impossible in this group. Efforts to prevent a septic outcome take place after the injurious event. These include debridement of devitalized tissue, and removal of foreign bodies and dirt. If the injured patient requires resuscitation, prompt medical management can reduce the incidence of infection by preventing cellular hypoxia (Wijetunge, 1994). Prompt resuscitation also facilitates the mobilization of host defence mechanisms (Wijetunge, 1994). Trauma wounds will inevitably be contaminated by microorganisms relevant to the nature of the injury and the environment in which it occurred, but most minor trauma will heal without infection occurring. However the need for tetanus immunization should always be assessed and antibiotic prophylaxis considered for puncture wounds caused by bites (Boriskin, 1994).

Thermal wounds

Commonly termed burns, thermal wounds are caused by heat. Dry heat injuries from fire or sun are burns and moist heat injuries from hot liquids are scalds. Conversely excessive cold (frostbite) can also cause tissue damage. Burns as a group also include damage caused by chemicals, friction, radiation and electricity.

Burns are often categorized according to depth of tissue damage, most simplistically as either partial or full thickness. The deeper the damage, the more necrotic tissue is likely to be present, the longer the healing time, and the greater the risk of infection. In major burns, following the initial shock phase, wound infection with its complications of septicaemia and delayed healing is seen as the second major problem faced by the patient (Parker and Copley, 1993). Most burns are sterile at the time of injury but readily acquire bacteria because dead tissue bathed in exudate at 37°C is an excellent growth medium. Colonized wounds put the patient at risk of infection which may not be obvious until septicaemia occurs (Lawrence, 1989). In order to reduce this risk it is common practice to engage in early burn surgery to remove necrotic material and therefore limit the source of nutrition for bacteria (Frame et al., 1992) and to use topical antiseptics. Along with early excision of necrotic tissue the application of various forms of skin graft can also be used to reduce the risk of infection. However, the majority of burns are partial thickness and small to moderate in size, where the risk of systemic sepsis is low (Smith et al., 1994). In these circumstances the value of using topical antimicrobials that may have a delaying effect on healing (Smith et al., 1994) needs to be questioned, as most chronic wounds heal uneventfully in the presence of colonizing bacteria.

In the UK, *Staphylococcus aureus* is the most common pathogen isolated in burns. It has been reported that 74% of burns were colonized with a mean acquisition time of six days. Beta haemolytic streptococcus group A is also found, but much less frequently than *Staphylococcus aureus*. *Pseudomonas aeruginosa*-associated morbidity has apparently declined since the introduction of silver nitrate and silver sulfadiazine in 1970, but antimicrobial-resistant strains of

Pseudomonas aeruginosa, *Staphylococcus aureus* and *Acinetobacter* species have emerged. Fungi are present in as many as 10% of cases but are rarely reported to cause problems (Frame et al., 1992).

The purpose of a burn dressing is to absorb exudate and as far as possible prevent colonization of the wound by pathogenic micro-organisms (Settle, 1986). In large burns, fluid loss can be copious in the early days, so dressings require frequent change to prevent the strike-through of exudate onto the outer dressing surface which would otherwise enhance the rate of colonization by no longer acting as a barrier.

The use of purpose-built environments with ventilation systems to reduce the risk of colonizing wounds at change of dressings and to prevent the transmission of organisms to other wounds has been suggested (Wilson, 1995), but data comparing types of facility indicates that wound colonization is not influenced by this (Frame et al., 1992; Adeniran et al., 1995). As burn wounds inevitably become colonized, strategies to prevent invasion of local tissues and the bloodstream include antibiotic therapy; active and passive immunization; and general supportive measures such as the treatment of diabetes and anaemia. Antibiotic therapy should be aimed at treating pathogens identified through regular culturing of wound swabs, in particular beta haemolytic streptococcus group A and *Pseudomonas aeruginosa*, but only when there is evidence of clinical sepsis (Ayliffe et al., 1992). The use of tetanus prophylaxis should be considered, as with all trauma wounds. Vaccine against *Pseudomonas* spp. has been found useful (Ayliffe et al., 1992) but demonstrations of benefit have not been consistent (Frame et al., 1992).

Chronic wounds

This group includes leg ulcers and malignant wounds and others that develop as a result of adverse underlying pathology. Pressure sores are usually grouped here, though they are mainly caused by the traumatic forces of pressure and shear (Miller and Dyson, 1996).

Chronic wounds heal by secondary intention, and because they are open during this process they will inevitably become colonized with micro-organisms. Colonization is therefore the norm and most open wounds heal uneventfully with its presence. It is interesting to note, though, that one study suggests there is a greater chance of failure to heal if four or more bacterial groups are present rather than any specific type of bacteria (Trengove et al., 1996). Whatever the case, with the presence and quantity of bacteria not being definitive (Thomson and Smith, 1994; Miller, 1996), infection diagnosis must again rely on clinical signs, extensive erythema, oedema, pus, elevated body temperature, raised neutrophil count, pain, change in colour of exudate or uncharacteristic odour (Mertz and Ovington, 1993). The question is therefore: are there any steps worth taking to reduce the risk of infection in chronic wounds? Clearly the best way to prevent infection is to facilitate the fastest healing of the wound. This is best achieved in a moist environment, with causal factors, such as pressure in pressure sores, removed, underlying pathology reversed, e.g. by reducing venous hypertension in venous leg ulcer management or improving blood flow in arterial leg ulcer management, and negating exacerbating factors, such as incontinence and skin sensitivities.

Occlusive dressings have been associated with a wound infection rate of 2.6% compared with 7.1% for non-occlusive dressings (Hutchinson and McGuckin, 1990). The mechanism for this is due to a combination of factors optimizing the micro-environment of the wound and reducing contamination from exogenous sources. The optimal conditions under a dressing are maintenance at body temperature and moisture balance. In an occlusive environment, the host's own infection control system is able to operate (Field and Kerstein, 1994).

Debridement of necrotic tissue by surgical, enzymatic and hydration methods removes a focus for infection. Biochemical evidence demonstrates that nutrition plays an important part in the wound healing process (Ruberg, 1984), but it has been shown that many hospital patients do not consume sufficient levels of nutrients and in some cases are not given adequate quantities on their plates (Sitton-Kent and Gilchrist, 1993). Ensuring adequate intake of all nutrients by whatever route or combination of routes is likely to assist the patient to resist infection.

Wound care can pose iatrogenic risks for wound infection which should be prevented, in particular deposition of non-degradable fibres or dressing detritus into the wound.

Conclusion

Despite advances in prevention strategies, wound infection remains an important cause of morbidity, mortality and additional costs. It is the duty of all professionals involved to take all reasonable precautions every day to prevent the occurrence of wound infection and to keep abreast of advances in the field; for managers of healthcare organizations to support professionals in their efforts; and for the government to fund research into the prevention and treatment of wound infection ensuring the widest dissemination of the findings.

References

Adeniran A, Shakespeare P, Patrick S, Fletcher AJ, Rossi LA Influence of a changed care environment on bacterial colonisation of burn wounds. Burns 1995; 21 (7): 521–5.

Allemeier WA, Culbertson WR Surgical infection. In Moyer, C et al (eds). Surgery, Principles and Practice, 3rd Edition. Philadelphia: Lippincott, 1965.

AORN Recommended Practices Co-ordinating Committee. Recommended Practices: skin preparation of patients. American Operating Room Nurses Journal 1992; 56 (5): 937–41.

Ayliffe GAJ, Brightwell KM, Collins BJ, Newbury EJL, Boonatilake PCL, Etheridge RA Surveys of hospital infection in the Birmingham Region: effect of age, sex, length of stay and antibiotic use on normal carriage of tetracycline-resistant Staphylococcus aureus and on postoperative wound infection. Journal of Hygiene (Camb.) 1977; 79: 299.

Ayliffe GAJ, Noy MR, Babb JR, Davies JG, Jackson J A comparison of pre-operative bathing with chlorhexidine detergent and non-medicated soap in the prevention of wound infection. Journal of Hospital Infection 1983; 4: 237–84.

Ayliffe GAJ, Collins BJ, Taylor LJ Hospital Acquired Infection: Principles and Prevention, 2nd Edition. Oxford: Butterworth-Heinemann Ltd, 1990.

Ayliffe GAJ, Newbury RJL, Geddes AM, Williams JD Control of Hospital Infection: A Practical Handbook, 3rd Edition. London: Chapman and Hall Medical, 1992.

Boriskin MI Primary care management of wounds: suturing and infection control. Nurse Practitioner 1994; 19 (11): 38–58.

Clarke C Re-usable or disposable theatre linen: which is best? Professional Nurse January 1989; 183–5.

Cooper R, Lawrence JC Micro-organisms and wounds. Journal of Wound Care 1996; 5 (5): 233–6.

Cooper R, Lawrence JC The prevalence of bacteria and implications for infection control. Journal of Wound Care 1996; 5 (6): 291–5.

Cruse PJE, Foord R The epidemiology of wound infection: a 10 year prospective study of 62,939 wounds. Surgical Clinics of North America 1980; 60 (1): 27–40.

Cutting KF, Harding KG Criteria for identifying wound infections. Journal of Wound Care 1994; 3 (4): 198–201.

Dineen P, Drusin L Epidemics of post-operative wound infections associated with hair carriers. Lancet 1973; 2: 1157–9.

Drinkwater CJ, Neil MJ Optimal timing of wound drain removal following total joint arthroscopy. The Journal of Arthroplasty 1995; 10 (2): 185–9.

Emmerson AM, Enstone JE, Griffin MC et al. The second national prevalence survey of infection in hospitals: overview of the results. Journal of Hospital Infection 1996; 32: 175–90.

Field CK, Kerstein MD Overview of wound healing in a moist environment. The American Journal of Surgery 1994; 167 (1A) suppl.: 25–65.

Frame JD, Kangesu L, Malik WM Managing flora in burns and trauma units: experience in the United Kingdom. Journal of Burn Care and Rehabilitation 1992; 13 (2): 281–6.

Gilmore OJA, Sanderson PJ Prophylactic intraparietal povidone-iodine in abdominal surgery. British Journal of Surgery 1975; 62: 792–9.

Glenister HM, Taylor LT, Cooke EH, Bartlett CLR A Study of Surveillance Methods for Detecting Hospital Infection. London: PHLS, 1992.

Griffiths-Jones A, Ward K (eds) Principles of Infection Control in Practice. London: Scutari Press, 1995.

Haley RW, Culver DH, Morgan WH, White JW, Emori TG, Hooton TH Identifying patients at high risk of surgical wound infection. American Journal of Epidemiology 1985; 21 (2): 206–15.

Hambraes A, Laurell G Protection of the patient in the operating suite. Journal of Hospital Infection 1980; 1: 15–30.

Hartley JE, Ahmed S, Milkins R, Naylor G Monson JRT, Lee PWR Randomised trial of blunt-tipped versus cutting needles to reduce glove puncture during mass closure of the abdomen. British Journal of Surgery 1996; 83: 1156–7.

Hulten L Dressings for surgical wounds. The American Journal of Surgery 1994; 167 (1A) suppl.: 425–55.

Humphreys H, Russell AJ, Marshall RT, Ricketts VE Reeves DS The effect of surgical theatre head-gear on air bacterial counts. Journal of Hospital Infection 1991; 19: 175–80.

Humphreys H, Stacey AR, Taylor EW Survey of operating theatres in Great Britain and Ireland. Journal of Hospital Infection 1995; 30: 245–52.

Hutchinson JJ, McGuckin M Occlusive dressings: a microbiological and clinical review. American Journal of Infection Control 1990; 18 (4): 257–68.

Jepsen OB, Bruttomesso KA The effectiveness of pre-operative skin preparations: an integrative review of the literature. AORN Journal 1993; 58 (3): 477–84.

Kingsley A Assessment allows action on risk factors: infection control and surgical wounds. Professional Nurse 1992; 7 (10): 644–8.

Kurz A, Sessler D, Lenhardt R Peri-operative normothermia to reduce the incidence of surgical wound infection and shorten hospitalisation. The New England Journal of Medicine 1996; 334 (19): 1209–15.

Lane TV, Shaw M, Newsom SWB Punctures in surgical gloves (letter). The Lancet 1993; 342: 984–5.

Lawrence JC Dressings for burns. The Dressings Times 1989; 2 (3): 1–3.

Lawrence JC Reducing the spread of bacteria. Journal of Wound Care 1993; 2 (1): 48–52.

Leyland M, McCloy R Surgical face masks: protection of staff or patient? Annals of the Royal College of Surgeons 1993; 75: 1–3.

Lidwell OM, Lowbury EJL, Whyte W, Blowers R, Stanley SJ, Lowe D Effect of ultra clean air in operating rooms on deep sepsis in the joint after total hip or knee replacement: a randomised study. British Medical Journal 1982; 285: 10–14.

Loewenthal J Sources and sequelae of surgical sepsis. British Medical Journal 1962; 1: 1437–40.

Mackenzie I Pre-operative skin preparation and surgical outcome. Journal of Hospital Infection 1988; 11 (suppl. B): 27–32.

Meers PD, Ayliffe GAJ, Emmerson AM, et al. Report on the national survey of infection in hospitals, 1980. Journal of Hospital Infection 1981; 2 (suppl.): 1–51.

Mellstrom GA, Lindbury M, Boman A Permeation and destructive effects of disinfectants on protective gloves. Contact Dermatitis 1992; 26: 163–70.

Mertz PM, Ovington LG Wound healing microbiology. Dermatologic Clinics 1993; 11 (4): 739–46.

Miller M The role of infection in wound healing. Nurse Prescriber/Community Nurse August 1996; 33–5.

Miller M, Dyson M Principles of Wound Care. London: MacMillan Magazines Ltd, 1996.

Moylan JA, Fitzpatrick KT, Davenport KE Reducing wound infections: improved gown and drape barrier performance. Archives of Surgery 1987; 122: 152–7.

Moylan JA, Kennedy BV The importance of gown and drape barriers in the prevention of wound infection. Surgery, Gynaecology and Obstetrics 1980; 151 (4): 465–70.

Noe JM, Keller M Can stitches get wet? Plastic and Reconstructive Surgery 1987; 81: 82–4.

Parker JA, Copley JE Burns: Educational Leaflet no. 14 Part 1. Wound Care Society, 1993.

Powell-Tuck J Parenteral Nutrition. Paper presented to the Annual Symposium of the Infection Control Nurses Association, 1983.

Raahave D Effect of plastic skin and wound drapes on the density of bacteria in operation wounds. The British Journal of Surgery 1976; 63: 421–6.

Rhoads JE The impact of nutrition on infection. Surgical Clinics of North America 1980; 60 (1): 41–7.

Rotter ML, et al. A comparison of the effects of pre-operative whole body bathing with detergent alone and with detergent containing chlorhexidine gluconate on the frequency of wound infections after clean surgery. Journal of Hospital Infection 1988; 11: 310–20.

Ruberg RL Role of nutrition in wound healing. Surgical Clinics of North America 1984; 64 (4): 705–14.

Seropian R, Reynolds B Wound infection after pre-operative depilatory versus razor preparation. American Journal of Surgery 1971; 121 (3): 251–4.

Settle JAD Burns: The First Five Days. Romford: Smith and Nephew Pharmaceuticals Ltd, 1986.

Sitton-Kent L, Gilchrist B The intake of nutrients by hospitalised pensioners with chronic wounds. Journal of Advanced Nursing 1993; 18: 1962–7.

Sizer T (ed.) A Report by the Working Party of the British Association for Parenteral and Enteral Nutrition, 1996.

Smith DT, Thomson PD, Garner WL, Rodrequez JL Burn wounds: infection and healing. The American Journal of Surgery 1994; 167 (1A) suppl.: 465–85.

Thomas CGA Medical Microbiology (6th Edition). London: Balliere Tindall, 1988.

Thomson PD, Smith DJ What is infection? The American Journal of Surgery 1994; 167 (1A) suppl.: 75–115.

Trengrove NJ, Stacey MC, McGechie DF, Stingemore NF, Mata S Qualitative bacteriology and leg ulcer healing. Journal of Wound Care 1996; 5 (6): 277–80.

Tunevall TG Post-operative wound infections and surgical face masks: a controlled study. World Journal of Surgery 1991; 15: 383–8.

Turner T The healing process. The Pharmaceutical Journal 1993; 735–7 May 29.

University of Dundee. The Wound Handbook. Dundee: University of Dundee, 1993.

Wijetunge DB Management of acute and traumatic wounds: main aspects of care in adults and children. The American Journal of Surgery 1994; 167 (1A) suppl.: 565–605.

Wilson J Infection Control in Clinical Practice. London: Ballière Tindall, 1985.

Whyte W The role of clothing and drapes in the operating room. Journal of Hospital Infection 11 1988; suppl. C: 2–17.

Chapter 19
Respiratory infection

JANET McCULLOCH

Introduction

Pulmonary infection is a significant cause of morbidity and mortality amongst children and adults in both hospitals and the community. Infection of the upper respiratory tract includes: tonsillitis, mumps, the common cold, diphtheria, pharyngitis, epiglottitis, influenza and whooping cough. Lower respiratory tract infections include bacterial pneumonia caused by: *Streptococcus pneumoniae*, *Staphylococcus aureus*, *Mycoplasma pneumoniae*, *Chlamydia psittacosis*, etc. It also includes pulmonary tuberculosis, respiratory syncytial virus (RSV) and bronchiolitis (Finch and Ball, 1991). These lists are by no means exhaustive.

Chest infection is also one of the most common forms of hospital-acquired infection (Emmerson et al., 1996) and is one of the most expensive to manage. Wenzel (1995) found that hospital-acquired pneumonia accounted for 10% of those deaths attributable to HAI. Some community-acquired infections can also have a serious impact on the hospital workload.

Community-acquired infections

Many community-acquired respiratory infections can be prevented by compliance with the national immunization programme, i.e. diphtheria, mumps, pertussis, pneumococcus and tuberculosis. For others, early recognition, treatment and the introduction of measures to prevent person-to-person transmission are important.

Childhood infections

Some respiratory infections particularly affect infants and children. They include croup, epiglottitis, bronchiolitis and RSV. Bronchiolitis

affects infants, often secondary to infection with RSV or parain-
fluenza viruses. Signs and symptoms are fever, nasal congestion,
cough, wheeze, dyspnoea and conjunctivitis. It tends to occur in the
winter months (Finch and Ball, 1991).

Respiratory syncytial virus is a common viral infection amongst
children, affecting 69% by the age of 1 year and 83% by the age of
two. Although it can be severe in neonates and babies with underlying
disease, in general mortality is low at <1%. Most cases are improved
within 10 days with only symptomatic therapy. It is a common cause of
bronchiolitis, pneumonia and bronchitis in children.

The infection is acquired by inoculation of the virus on to the
nasal or conjunctival mucosa, the virus spreading from cell to cell via
intracytoplasmic bridges called syncytia. Inflammation, oedema and
necrosis of the submucosa develop, leading to occlusion of the small
airways and bronchioles. Air may become trapped, resulting in hyper-
inflation and lung collapse. Regular suctioning, oxygen and fluids are
required. The virus can survive for up to 7 hours outside the body,
therefore transmission may be by direct or indirect contact with secretions (Purssell and Gould, 1997). The infection can spread quickly in
children's wards, therefore single-room isolation or the cohorting of
known or suspected cases is recommended (Doherty et al., 1998).

Children rarely develop a bacterial infection superimposed on a
viral infection; therefore antibiotics are of no use (Davies et al.,
1996).

Influenza

An outbreak of influenza can lead to many additional hospital
admissions and can also affect large numbers of hospital staff, resulting in the curtailment of normal activity. In addition, associated
deaths can be numerous. For this reason the Public Health Laboratory Service in the UK monitors influenza activity nationally by
analysing reports from general practitioners, laboratories, mortality
records, CDSC, boarding schools and the London Emergency Bed
Service. Using this data, the PHLS is able to identify the prevalent
virus and match it with the appropriate vaccine.

Concerns about an influenza pandemic were highlighted when
in 1998 there was an outbreak of avian flu ($H_5 N_1$) in Hong Kong

which led to 18 cases and 6 deaths. Although no person-to-person transmission was identified there was a cull of poultry in Hong Kong and an international alert to raise awareness of cases linked with the country (Dedman et al., 1998; PHLS, 1998). Prior to the annual influenza season, people known to be at particular risk of acquiring influenza are advised to be vaccinated. This includes: people with chronic respiratory disease, chronic cardiac disease, chronic renal failure, diabetes mellitus, the immunosuppressed, and those living in nursing and residential homes. Key healthcare workers such as doctors and nurses may be offered Amantadine hydrochloride during an epidemic, to prevent infection and subsequent service disruption (Department of Health, 1996).

Pneumococcal pneumonia

Streptococcus pneumoniae is a normal commensal in 60% of infants and 30–40% of adults and is the most the common cause of community acquired pneumonia, especially in the elderly and those with under-lying health problems such as cardio-pulmonary disease or alcoholism (Department of Health, 1996). Resistance in the organism to antimicrobials is increasing.

Infection results in the production of rusty, purulent sputum, fever, rigors and consolidation of the lungs. The mortality rate is around 10%. Penicillin is the antibiotic of choice (Finch and Ball, 1991). Vaccination is recommended for individuals at high risk of acquiring severe infection (Department of Health, 1996). Practice nurses can take a proactive role in identifying individuals at risk and promoting uptake of this vaccine (Baird, 1998).

Pneumocystis carinii pneumonia

This is an opportunistic infection associated with immunosuppression, particularly in recipients of donated organs, premature infants and people with AIDS. It is caused by the inhalation of a protozoal parasite, which is thought to be widespread in the environment, or perhaps re-activation of latent infection. Symptoms are mild fever, myalgia, progressive dyspneoa, tachypnoea, cyanosis and unproductive cough. The mortality rate is 30%. The infection is treated with aerosolized pentamidine (Finch and Ball, 1991; Benenson, 1995).

Diphtheria

Diphtheria is caused by the bacterium *Corynebacterium diphtheriae*. Respiratory infection may affect the nose, tonsils or pharynx; and cutaneous infection may affect the skin, conjunctiva or genitals. Respiratory infection is often associated with the development of a white membrane, which is composed of bacteria, macrophages and dead cells extending from the uvular to the soft palate. The toxins can lead to cardiac, adrenal and neurological complications.

Transmission is by droplets and sometimes by contact with contaminated items. The disease is preventable by vaccine and is rare in the UK (see Table 19.1). In the former Soviet Union there has been an epidemic in recent years, causing 52,000 cases and 1,700 deaths in 1995 (Department of Health, 1996). For this reason travellers to these countries may be advised to receive a booster (Benenson, 1995; MacQueen, 1997; Cooper, 1998). Treatment is with antitoxin and erythromycin or penicillin.

Table 19.1 Cases of diphtheria in the UK

Year	Cases	Deaths
1940	46,281	2,480
1957	37	6

(Department of Health, 1996).

Legionnaires' disease

Legionella pneumophila was identified in 1976 following an outbreak of infection amongst those attending a convention in the United States of America. The mortality rate was 16%. The organism survives in stagnant water and is transmitted by inhalation of droplets, which are disseminated by showers, air conditioning plant and spa baths. It mainly affects middle-aged men with an underlying respiratory condition (Finch and Ball, 1991). There have been no cases of person-to-person spread.

In the UK in 1997, there were 226 cases, 80% of which were isolated cases. Over half the cases were associated with overseas travel and the mortality rate was 12% (Joseph et al., 1998). Legionnaires' disease on a cruise ship affected two holiday-makers on separate cruises. The organism was isolated in cabin water supplies and a decommissioned spa pool. The water system had to be re-plumbed, pasteurized and super-chlorinated, and a system introduced to provide continuous dosing for the potable supplies (PHLS, 1998). Outbreaks have also occurred in hospitals in the UK; regulations now exist which specify measures to prevent legionellae in water systems (DHSS, 1986; NHS Estates, 1994).

Psittacosis

Psittacosis infection can result in sub-clinical infection or atypical pneumonia, which may be severe in the elderly. Rarely, complications may include encephalitis, myocarditis and thrombophlebitis. It is caused by exposure to a natural parasite of birds, *Chlamydia psittaci*, and the inhalation of desiccated secretions, droppings and feathers from infected birds. Even transient exposure can lead to acquisition of the infection. Symptoms include pyrexia, rigors, myalgia, malaise, a dry unproductive cough, headache, delirium and sometimes sore throat or laryngitis. If the cough is productive it is muco-purulent. Person to person spread may also be associated exposure to paroxysmal coughing during the acute illness. Care should also be taken to avoid contact with specimens (Finch and Ball, 1991; Benenson, 1995).

Environmental health officers will investigate cases and advise on hygiene, vets should be involved in the management of infected birds.

Tuberculosis

Tuberculosis is a notifiable infection, which may affect the lungs, bones, kidneys, meninges or joints. Primary pulmonary infection is usually symptomless and self-limiting; a lesion (tubercle) develops in the lung then heals and calcifies. Alternatively, the lesion can enlarge and caseate, resulting in what is described as a 'cold abscess', which slowly inflames and results in the formation of scar tissue. The bacilli may get into the bloodstream and lead to generalized infection and septicaemia (miliary TB). Symptoms of TB are cough, haemoptysis, chest pain and expectoration of sputum. Those with miliary TB also experience malaise, weight loss, night sweats and intermittent pyrexia. Re-activation of primary lesions, or re-infection, can occur (Cook, 1996).

In the UK 5,000 new cases are reported annually, and prevalence varies from 4.7:100,000 of the indigenous population, to 101:100,000 amongst the Pakistani and Bangladeshi community and 135:100,000 of Indian origin (Cook, 1996). National guidelines recommend that children aged 10–13 and others at high risk of acquiring infection should be vaccinated. High-risk individuals include:

- healthcare workers
- veterinary workers and farmers
- staff working in prisons, refugee hostels and with the homeless
- immigrants from countries where there is a high prevalence of TB infection and their children
- people who travel abroad regularly
- individuals who have been in contact with cases of active pulmonary TB

(Department of Health, 1996).

TB is transmitted by the inhalation of airborne droplet nuclei, which the infected case expels during talking, coughing and singing. The infection is not highly communicable, but can be spread particularly amongst those who have prolonged close contact with a case, e.g. sharing the same household, or confined workplace. People with HIV infection are also at higher risk. New cases of tuberculosis will be followed up by specialist nurses and are asked to identify possible close contacts. Those with pulmonary tuberculosis are infectious until they have received about 2 weeks of anti-TB therapy. Poor compliance can lead to the development of resistance to the anti-TB drugs. The increase in multi-drug resistance (MDR-TB) is of concern in relation to effective treatment of affected individuals and controlling the spread of resistant strains to contacts. Nurses may be involved in monitoring compliance with therapy and, if necessary, the taking of the medication may need to be directly observed to combat poor compliance (Jamieson, 1997). In the US, this has resulted in a 21% reduction in cases of multi-drug resistance (Morse, 1996; Department of Health, 1998).

Hospital-acquired infection

Hospital-acquired chest infection accounts for about 20% of all HAIs (Emmerson et al., 1996). It is one of the most expensive to treat and the most likely to cause death (Inglis, 1990). Risk factors include:

- infants and young children
- >65 years of age
- underlying disease
- immunosuppression
- cardiopulmonary disease
- thoraco-abdominal surgery
- mechanical ventilation

(CDC, 1997)

Infection may be: **endogenous**, i.e. caused by the aspiration of micro-organisms which colonize the gut and oro-pharynx (e.g. *Klebsiella* spp., *Acinetobacter* spp. and *Pseudomonas* spp.); or **exogenous**, transmitted via contaminated hands, equipment and fluids.

(CDC, 1997; Inglis, 1990)

Mechanical ventilation

Haley et al. (1985) claimed that mechanical ventilation significantly increases the risk of nosocomial infection and causes 17% of all hospital-acquired pneumonias. Increased risk arises from bypassing the first line of natural defences by intubation and ventilation, altered gastric pH and impaired clearance of the respiratory secretions (Inglis, 1990). Glynn et al. (1997) found that hospital-acquired pneumonia was the most common HAI in ITU (see Table 19.2). They identified mechanical ventilation, intubation and the presence of a nasogastric tube to be risk factors for pneumonia, and reported a mortality rate of 22% in this group of patients.

The use of heat-moisture exchange filters can be effective in reducing contamination of ventilator circuits and can eliminate the need for water humidifiers and fluid traps. Boots et al. (1997) found that there was less contamination of ventilator circuits when a heat-moisture exchange filter was used compared to a hot water humidi-

Table 19.2 Hospital-acquired infection in ITU

Hospital-acquired infection	Infection rate in ITU
Pneumonia	45%
Bloodstream infection	22%
Surgical wound infection	9%
Urinary tract infection	5%
Others	19%

(Glynn et al., 1997)

fier. It is also important to ensure that fluids are not allowed to drain back into the tubing or humidifier, etc. (Sproat and Inglis, 1992).

Cadwallader et al. (1990) found that there was confusion amongst ITU staff regarding the optimal frequency of changing ventilator circuits. They found that contamination of circuits was more common when circuits were used on adults than on neonates, and recommended changing circuits every 48 hours for adults and weekly or between cases for neonates, if water humidification was used. If a HME is used the tubing should be changed between cases (Cadwallader et al., 1990). Madeo (1996) identified a need to balance the risk between a) removing the reservoirs of microbes and b) the handling and circuit breaking involved in changing the tubing, and recommended changing the tubing weekly. Stamm (1998) and Gastmeier et al. (1997) carried out a review of literature and came to the conclusion that ventilator tubing should be changed every 7 days.

Contaminated equipment/environment

Humphreys et al. (1991) identified an outbreak of aspergillosis in an intensive care unit. This was related to environmental contamination with *Aspergillus fumigatus* and *A. flavis*, which had been dispersed by building works in previous weeks. It was suggested that patients may have inhaled these organisms when they were disconnected from the ventilator for hand-bagging and suctioning.

Equipment such as endotracheal tubes, laryngoscopes, ventilator circuitry and fluid traps can become colonized and act as a reservoir for bacteria. For example, contaminated laryngoscopes were implicated in an outbreak of *Bacillus cereus* in a neonatal intensive care (Neal et al., 1995). Humidifiers can also act as a reservoir for pseudomonads (Madeo, 1996). Procedures must be in place to ensure they are decontaminated adequately, changed at appropriate intervals and an aseptic technique used when handling equipment.

CDC (1997) classified many items of respiratory equipment as semi-critical (or medium-risk), i.e. it comes into direct or indirect contact with the respiratory tract mucous membranes. These items are required to be single-use only, or sterilized after use. Items identified as such included:

- anaesthetic equipment
- breathing circuits
- bronchoscopes
- endotracheal tubes
- laryngoscope blades
- mouthpieces
- airways
- resuscitation bags
- suction catheters

They did not identify the risk related to pulmonary function test equipment, but suggested that these items be protected with a filter.

Handwashing

Hands will inevitably become contaminated whenever handling tubing, water traps, filters, suction tubing, etc. and may cause cross-contamination. Therefore it is important to decontaminate the hands after handling these items, before handling clean equipment and between patient contacts. Disposable gloves may be worn, but must be changed when contaminated and hands washed.

Suction equipment

Tracheal suctioning can play an important part in preventing respiratory infection, by removing accumulations of secretions from the respiratory tract. The equipment used in suctioning can act as a reservoir for micro-organisms. In addition, suctioning can involve opening the endotracheal tube to the air and generating aerosols, which can contaminate the environment up to one metre away from the patient. Therefore a closed suction system is recommended (Cobley et al., 1991).

Care must be taken during suctioning to avoid introducing micro-organisms into the airways. This is achieved by handwashing prior to the procedure and using a sterile suction catheter only once before discarding it. Secretions are cleared from the tubing using sterile water from a sterile container, which is changed at least daily (Creamer and Smyth, 1996). Tap water contains numerous potential pathogens and if used inappropriately can contribute to chest infection. Gloves are worn during suctioning to prevent contact with respiratory secretions, but may be non-sterile if contained in a box and kept away from possible contamination (Sproat and Inglis, 1992). Creamer and Smyth (1996) recommend changing suction containers daily. Disposable suction liners can be used to reduce this frequency. By eliminating the need to empty out and clean the bottles, disposable liners also protect the handler from exposure to body fluids.

The packaging of sterile endotracheal tubes and suction tubes must be kept intact until the moment of use. If packs are opened in advance of use, the sterility of the equipment cannot be guaranteed. Information regarding size, expiry date and batch numbers will have been removed and exposure to dust, air and humidity may affect the effectiveness of the product.

Suction machines must be kept clean, dry and dust-free. In areas where they are used infrequently, the cleaning of these machines should be part of a regular cleaning schedule, otherwise they may be missed. Disinfectant solutions should not be put into the suction containers, because they do not add to the hygiene quality and will become contaminated in a short period of time. Filters must be in place to protect the machinery from contamination. They must be replaced when wet or discoloured, or as part of a planned preventive maintenance programme.

Nebulizers

Nebulizers are used for the administration of nebulized medication. The fluid reservoirs can quickly become contaminated with Gram-negative organisms and increase the risk of chest infection if they are not managed effectively. Some nebulizer reservoirs (acorns) are single-use only and should be discarded after each use. Others may be re-used on the same patient but must be cleaned and dried between uses to prevent the accumulation of contaminated fluids.

Audit can help to identify practice related to the management of nebulizers and other equipment. Ronchetti (1998) found that only 11% of nebulizers in use were cleaned and stored correctly. Critchley and Roulsten (1993) found that nurses' knowledge of these procedures was poor and only 33% ever cleaned a nebulizer after use. Feedback of results, together with clear guidelines, can help to improve standards.

According to guidelines from the Medical Devices Agency, single-use items may only be re-used if a written risk assessment is carried out and decontamination procedures are identified and documented each time they are carried out. Reprocessing can adversely affect the product; for example the product material may be incompatible with the cleaning fluid or disinfectant (Medical Devices Agency, 1995).

This also applies to respiratory and suction equipment used in the patient's own home. Due to the cost, waste disposable problems and limited storage space there is often pressure in these circumstances to disinfect and re-use the equipment. A risk assessment must be carried out and fully documented when making decisions of this kind.

Conclusion

Respiratory infection is costly in terms of morbidity and mortality, and in relation to the costs of treatment. Some infections may be prevented by immunization; following good infection control practice may prevent others. Identifying individuals at risk of acquiring infection and instituting precautions, or by giving appropriate vaccinations at the earliest opportunity can also help to avoid unnecessary infection.

References

Baird A Pneumococcal vaccine in general practice. Nursing Standard 1998; 12 (44): 38–40.

Benenson AS Control of Communicable Diseases Manual, 16th Edition. Washington: American Public Health Association, 1995.

Boots RJ, Howe S, George N, Harris FM Clinical utility of hygroscopic heat and moisture exchangers in intensive care patients. Critical Care Medicine 1997; 25 (10): 1707–12.

Cadwallader HL, Bradley CR, Ayliffe GAJ Bacterial contamination and frequency of changing ventilator circuitry. Journal of Hospital Infection 1990; 15: 65–72.

Christie P, Abraham W Legionella infections in Scotland: 1997. Communicable Disease and Public Health 1998; 1 (4): 258.

Cobley M, Atkins M, Jones PL Environmental contamination during tracheal suction. Anaesthesia 1991; 46: 957–61.

Communicable Disease Centre (CDC). Guidelines for prevention of nosocomial pneumonia. Morbidity and Mortality Weekly Review 1997; 46 (RR-1): 1–79.

Cook R Tuberculosis. Nursing Standard 1996; 10 (48): 49–52.

Cooper T Deadly souvenir. Nursing Times 1998; 94 (37): 78.

Creamer E Decontamination quality. Nursing Times 199389 (36): 65–8.

Creamer E, Smyth EG Suction: reducing infection risks. Journal of Hospital Infection 1996; 34 (1): 1–9.

Critchley D, Roulsten J Nurses' knowledge of nebulised therapy. Nursing Standard 1993; 24 (8): 37–9.

Davies EG, Elliman DAC, Hart CA, Nicoll A, Rudd PT Manual of Childhood Infections. London: WB Saunders Co Ltd, 1996.

Dedman DJ, Zambon M, Van Buynder P, Ferning DN, Watson JM, Joseph CA Influenza surveillance in England and Wales: October 1997–June 1998. Communicable Disease and Public Health 1998; 1 (4): 244–51.

Department of Health (Welsh Office, Scottish DH, DHSS) (NI). Immunisation against Infectious Disease. London: HMSO, 1996.

Department of Health, Scottish Office, Welsh Office. The Report of the Interdepartmental Working Group on Tuberculosis: The Prevention and Control of TB in the UK. UK Guidance on the Prevention and Control of Transmission of HIV-related TB and Drug Resistance including Multi-drug-resistant TB. London: HMSO, 1998.

Department of Health and Social Security (DHSS). The First Report of the Committee of Enquiry into the Outbreak of Legionnaires' Disease in Stafford in April 1985. London: HMSO, 1986.

Doherty JA, Brookfield DSK, Gray J, McEwan RA Cohorting of infants with respiratory syncytial virus. Journal of Hospital Infection 1998; 38: 203–6.

Emmerson AM, Enstone JE, Griffin M, Kelsey MC, Smyth ETM Second national prevalence study of infections in hospital – overview of results. Journal of Hospital Infection 1996; 32: 175–90.

Finch RG, Ball P Infection. London: Blackwell Scientific Publications, 1991.

Gastmeier P, Wendt C, Ruden H Breathing circuit exchange in intensive care. Once daily once weekly? Anaesthetist 1997; 46 (11): 943–8.

Glynn A, Ward V, Wilson J, Charlett A, Cookson B, Taylor L, Cole N Hospital Acquired Infection: Surveillance, Policies and Practice. London: PHLS, 1997.

Haley RW, Morgan WM, Culver DH, White JW, Emori TG, Mosser J, Hughes JM Update from the SENIC Project. Hospital infection control: recent progress and opportunities under prospective payment. American Journal of Infection Control 1985; 13 (3): 97–108.

Humphreys H, Johnson EM, Warnock DW, Willatts SM, Winter RJ, Speller DCE An outbreak of aspergillosis in a general ITU Journal of Hospital Infection 1991; 18: 167–77.

Inglis TJJ Pulmonary infection in intensive care units British Journal of Anaesthesia 1990; 65: 94–106.

Jamieson S The fight against TB. Nursing Standard 1997; 11 (28): 16.

Joseph CA, Harrison TG, Ilijic-Car D, Bartlett CLR Legionnaires' disease in residents in England and Wales: 1997. Communicable Disease and Public Health 1998; 1 (4): 252–8.

MacQueen S Diphtheria: a changing pattern. Nursing Times 1997; 93 (19): 57–62.

Madeo M Ventilator tubing change times and the Infection Control Nurse. Nursing Standard 1996; 11(6): 44–7.

Medical Devices Agency. The Reuse of Medical Devices Supplied for Single Use Only. MDA DB 9501, 1995.

Morse DI Directly observed therapy for tuberculosis. British Medical Journal 1996; 312: 719–20.

Neal TJ, Hughes CR, Rothburn MM, Shaw NJ The neonatal laryngoscope as a potential source of cross infection. Journal of Hospital Infection 1995; 30: 315–21.

NHS Estates. Control of Legionellae in Healthcare Premises: A Code of Practice HTM 2040. London: HMSO, 1994.

Public Health Laboratory Service (PHLS). Influenza A virus subtype $H_5 N_1$ infection in Hong Kong update. Communicable Disease Review 9 January 1998; 8 (2).

Public Health Laboratory Service (PHLS). Legionella on board a cruise ship. Communicable Disease Review 3 July 1998; 8 (27).

Purssell E, Gould D A common ailment. Nursing Times 1997; 93 (3): 53–8.

Ronchetti T Cleaning up our practice. Nursing Times 1998; 94 (28): 68–71.

Stamm AM Ventilator-associated pneumonia and frequency of circuit changes. American Journal of Infection Control 1998; 26 (1): 71–3.

Sproat LJ, Inglis TJJ Preventing infection in the intensive care unit. British Journal of Intensive Care September 1992; 275–85.

Wenzel RP The economics of nosocomial infections. Journal of Hospital Infection 1995; 31: 79–87.

Chapter 20
Management of known infections

JANET McCULLOCH AND LESLY FINN
and the late **BETTY BOWELL**

Introduction

Those working in healthcare will inevitably have to care for people with known or suspected infection and infectious diseases. This can be alarming if they are not equipped with the knowledge and skills necessary to understand how these infections may be transmitted to others, and their own role in preventing the spread of infection.

For some people the practice of infection control is shrouded in ritual and mystique which can hide the underlying principles. The traditional terms of 'barrier' or 'isolation' nursing can reinforce the concept that the infected patient must be isolated from all contact with others. Neither term helps the practitioner to understand how infection is spread. This can lead to fear and confusion and can also promote the idea that infection control precautions are only required for patients with a known infectious disease. There is less emphasis on the need for everyday infection control practices such as handwashing and the use of protective clothing, which can be described as standard or universal precautions.

Use of isolation

Patients who are nursed in isolation can suffer as a consequence for many reasons. For example, sometimes staff are reluctant to enter the isolation room for fear that they may become infected themselves, or take the infection home to their families. The inconvenience of donning protective clothing may reduce the frequency of contact with others, and they may lack the usual comradeship with other patients and the caring team. In extreme circumstances patients in isolation may even experience a lack of food, if the staff

316

forget to serve those in single rooms! For similar reasons the isolation room may not be cleaned often enough, although its hygiene should be a priority for housekeepers. Patients who require periods of isolation may also experience stress as a result of loneliness; the stigma attached to infection; lack of control; and mental stimulation (MacKenzie and Edwards, 1997; Gammon, 1998; Oldman, 1998). In particular, the elderly may decline physically through lack of exercise, or develop confusion through lack of mental stimulation.

As the isolation of patients with infections may not always be beneficial to them or to others, single-room isolation should be used with great care and the need for isolation re-assessed frequently. The national guidelines for the management of MRSA in hospitals (Department of Health Interdepartmental Working Group, 1998) no longer recommend the isolation of *all* patients colonized or infected with MRSA. Rather the need for isolation should be assessed on the basis of the risk of infection to others who may be exposed to the organism if the patient is not isolated. Sanderson and Richardson (1997) found that the incidence of infection with *Clostridium difficile* did not increase when infected cases were nursed in the main ward instead of in single rooms.

However in many instances single-room isolation of patients with a communicable disease is important for the prevention of spread to others. This may be in order to:

- reduce environmental contamination with the organism (for example if a patient has uncontrollable diarrhoea)
- reduce exposure of those in the vicinity to airborne organisms (for example *Mycobacterium tuberculosis*)
- act as a reminder to carers of the need to carry out specific infection control precautions with an individual patient.

At times it may be impossible to isolate an infectious patient, for example because:

a) there are no single rooms, or isolation ward available
b) many patients have been affected during an outbreak
c) the individual patient requiring isolation is too ill to be nursed in a single room or in a special unit.

In these cases it is particularly important that carers understand the process of infection, so that they know how they can help prevent the transmission of infection. The process of infection is often termed 'the chain of infection'.

Chain of infection

The chain of infection is composed of a number of links that represent the chain of events leading to the transmission of infection. To break the chain requires the removal of just one link. However, in healthcare it is common to remove more than one link. The links in the chain of infection include:

1. an *infectious agent* (bacteria, viruses, fungi, etc.)
2. a *reservoir* for the organism (people, animals, food, water, equipment, etc.)
3. a *portal of exit* for the organism (droplets, excreta, secretions, skin, etc.)
4. a *means of transmission* (contact, inhalation of airborne organisms, injection, ingestion)
5. a *portal of entry* into the body (genito-urinary tract, broken skin, respiratory tract, etc.)
6. a *person at risk* of acquiring the infection (host susceptibility).

One example of how the chain of infection can be applied to practice concerns smallpox. This infection has been eradicated globally so the *infectious agent* will no longer be encountered, except in a limited number of laboratories. As result, healthcare workers are no longer vaccinated against the infection. Previously when smallpox was likely to be encountered, staff had to be vaccinated so that they were not at risk.

When considering healthcare it is often impossible to ensure that one link has been completely removed, so one has to target more than one link in the chain. It is particularly difficult to eradicate the reservoirs of infection and the people at risk, so infection control practice usually focuses on eliminating the means of transmission or 'vehicles' and preventing infectious agents from gaining entry via portals of entry.

Infectious agents

These are many and varied, ranging from the pathogens we face continually on a day-to-day basis to more exotic organisms which we are unlikely to face unless we travel abroad or have contact with a patient infected abroad. It is important to remember that some infections require high numbers of organisms for infection to develop whilst others need only a few micro-organisms. For example, only 100 organisms are sufficient to cause shigella dysentery, but salmonella infection may require 100,000. Host factors also play a part in determining whether clinical infection will develop after exposure to a pathogen and the degree of severity of infection experienced. This may be expressed by the following formula:

$$\text{Risk of infection} = \frac{\text{dose} + \text{time} + \text{virulence of organism}}{\text{host susceptibility}}$$

(Horton and Parker, 1997)

Reservoirs of infection

Reservoirs of infectious agents include humans, animals, the environment, food and water and contaminated items such as the equipment used in patient care, or for cleaning.

Human reservoirs of infection

These may include anyone who is infected by or colonized with an organism that may cause infection in susceptible human beings. One example of this is *Staphylococcus aureus*, which colonizes the skin of approximately 30% of the general population (Shanson, 1989). This organism can reside on the skin, hair and anterior nares of individuals without causing infection or other ill effects. However, should the organism gain entry into a wound or catheter infection may develop. Human beings constantly shed skin scales into the immediate environment and adhering to these shed scales are the micro-organisms which colonize the skin. Many skin commensals will not survive away from the body, but some organisms, such as *Staphylococcus aureus*, can survive in dry environments such as dust. Micro-organisms in dust are unable to cause infection until carried to a susceptible site via another link in the chain: a *means of transmission*.

Staff are important human reservoirs of infection in healthcare, because of their numerous and often intimate contacts with patients, such as when carrying out surgery, intravenous therapy, wound care, catheter care and feeding etc. Their knowledge of infection control should ensure that they practise safely in such a way as to minimize the risk. If they have a communicable infection themselves, such as diarrhoea or chickenpox, they may have to stay away from work or be redeployed to another area until no longer infectious. Unfortunately some infections, such as childhood illnesses, are communicable before the onset of symptoms, and susceptible patients and staff may be exposed to the infection unknowingly.

Environmental reservoirs of infectious agents

In general it is considered that environmental reservoirs are less of a problem than they were once thought to be. Floors, walls, toilets and drains appear to contribute little to the transmission of infection. To some extent the use of disinfectants for the environment is now considered to be money poured down the drain; it produces the typical 'hospital smell' but does not contribute to the control of infection.

The most important environmental reservoirs are:

- dust
- liquid residues
- spillages of body fluids

Dust is composed of skin scales and other debris and can contain a wide variety of micro-organisms, some of which are pathogenic such as *Staphylococcus aureus*, *Streptococcus* and *Clostridium difficile* spores. Although some micro-organisms survive in dust they cannot grow or multiply in this environment. To reduce the risks associated with dust it is important to keep dust levels to a minimum by dusting at an appropriate frequency. The frequency will vary from place to place. A busy ward may need dust removal several times a week because of the number of people present and the intensity of activity. Less busy areas, such as a care home or even a health centre, may need to be dusted less frequently. The method of cleaning is important so that the dust is completely removed and is not simply transported to another area. For example, dusters and feather dusters may simply move the dust around. A more effective method is to damp-dust using disposables such as paper roll. An alternative is to use a product that attracts dust, such as a static mop.

Liquid residues (or dregs of fluid) can be important reservoirs, even in clean containers such as jugs and washbowls. Some organisms do not merely survive in residues of liquid, they can thrive and multiply to a potentially infectious dose. The pathogenic organisms that may be present in these damp items include *Pseudomonas aeruginosa*; *Eschericia coli* and other coliforms.

There have been many instances in which liquid residues have been implicated in cross-infection. Poor disinfection of breast pumps was the cause of an outbreak of *Serratia marcescens* in a neonatal care unit (Gransden et al., 1986); condensate from ventilator water traps was implicated in an outbreak of *Klebsiella pneumoniae* (Gorman et al., 1993) and flasks of hexetidine used for mouthwashes were found to be contaminated with *Serratia marcescens* (Bosi et al., 1996). Even holy water has been identified as a risk factor (Rees and Allen, 1996). Removal of liquid residues is simple – it entails either physically drying articles with a cloth/paper or turning hollow items upside down to allow the dregs to drain away. The organisms that thrive in these damp conditions cannot stand to be dried out and will quickly die.

Spillages of body fluids inevitably contain micro-organisms, some of which will be pathogenic. For example, diarrhoea may contain *Salmonella* spp. or *Clostridium difficile*, blood spillages could be infected with HIV or hepatitis. Spillages of body fluid pose a direct risk of infection to the person who is clearing the spillage away, and an indirect risk to other susceptible individuals who may come into contact with the contaminated environment later, if the cleaning method has not been effective. Protective clothing is essential when dealing with spillages. The body fluid should be removed using paper roll and the surface cleaned thoroughly and dried. Consideration should be given to the need for disinfection of the surface, although often cleaning will suffice. It should be remembered that disinfectants are less effective in the presence of organic material.

None of the reservoirs listed above can transmit infection by themselves; they all require a means of transmission, or vehicle, to carry the organisms from the reservoir to a person at risk of acquiring the infection.

Means of transmission of infection

Means of transmission include direct and indirect contact with a reservoir of the infectious agent (this includes sexual contact), inhalation, ingestion, and injection of the organisms. Except for direct contact, a vehicle is required to convey pathogenic micro-organisms from the reservoirs to those individuals at risk of acquiring the infection. Vehicles of transmission of infection, like the reservoirs, can be human, environmental or related to equipment (see Figure 20.1). There is often little that can be done to eliminate the infectious agents or their reservoirs and it is impossible to develop immunity to all infections, therefore eliminating the means of transmission is a key link in the chain to target.

Direct contact

Contact is the most common method of transmitting infection, and most direct contact occurs via human hands. Hands are easily contaminated by their contact via reservoirs of infection and may directly cause infection in the host or may act as a vehicle and carry pathogenic organisms to others who may be susceptible. Contaminated hands are the vehicles that have been most frequently implicated in the transmission of infection, consequently it is well documented that handwashing is the most important infection control activity. However it has often been observed that it is a practice that is frequently neglected or poorly practiced (Bowell, 1992a; Gould et al., 1996; Perry and Gore, 1997).

Handwashing

Taylor (1978a and b) demonstrated that nurses routinely missed some areas of the hands when hand washing. The areas omitted included the tips of the fingers, the thumbs, between the fingers, backs of the hands, and the wrists. The Infection Control Nurses' Association has produced a comprehensive guide to handwashing (ICNA, 1997).

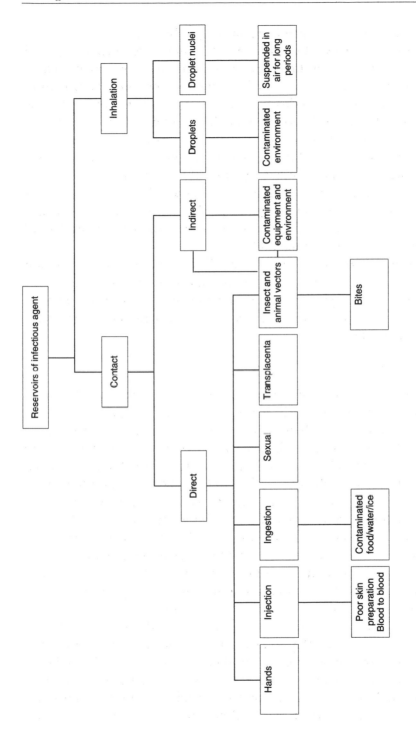

Figure 20.1 Methods of transmission of infection

There are three main handwashing techniques:

Social handwashing removes transient organisms acquired through carrying out direct care, and from the environment. These may be pathogens, commensals or environmental organisms from the contacts. Social handwashing is carried out after contact with the patient, after using the toilet and before eating or preparing meals. etc. Soap and water is adequate for this purpose.

Aseptic handwashing disinfects the hands by removing transient organisms and eliminating much of the commensal flora from the outer surfaces of the skin. It is carried out prior to invasive procedures, or after direct care for patients with infectious diseases. Washing with soap and water, followed by an application of alcohol handrub, is a common method.

Surgical scrub involves the application of an antiseptic lotion which is applied to the hands, wrists and forearms. It takes longer and eliminates a greater volume of commensal flora. It is used prior to surgery or prior to the insertion of long-term invasive devices such as Hickman lines.

Method of handwashing

The basic handwashing method is similar whether applied as a social, aseptic or surgical technique. After thoroughly wetting the hands, a measure of handwashing agent is applied and the hands rubbed together so that all parts are covered, without adding more water. Care must be taken to include the tips of the fingers, between the fingers, the nailbeds, thumbs, backs of the hands and the wrists. Rubbing need not take more than 20 seconds. For a surgical scrub, the hands should be lathered for 2 minutes and a disposable brush may be used before the first case (Ayliffe et al., 1992). Brushing should not be overdone, as this could damage the skin and increase the bacterial count on the hands. After washing the lather should be completely rinsed away under running water (see Figure 20.2).

Drying the hands is an important sequel to handwashing. In clinical areas paper towels are recommended and cotton towels should not be used. Paper towels may be harsh on the hands and some are not very absorbent, but they are completely disposable. It must be remembered that the towel holders need to be kept clean inside and out. After carrying out a surgical scrub the hands are dried using sterile paper towels. Cotton towels are quickly contaminated and can act as a reservoir.

1.   2.   3.

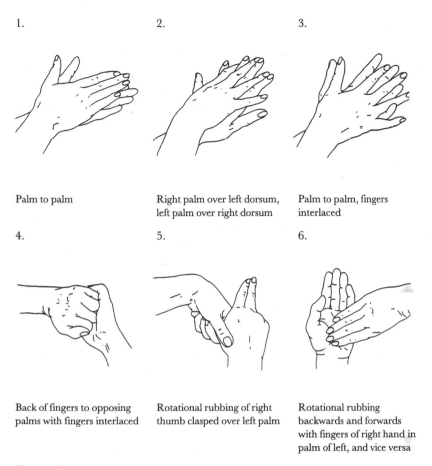

Palm to palm   Right palm over left dorsum,   Palm to palm, fingers
                          left palm over right dorsum   interlaced

4.   5.   6.

Back of fingers to opposing   Rotational rubbing of right   Rotational rubbing
palms with fingers interlaced thumb clasped over left palm backwards and forwards
                                                            with fingers of right hand in
                                                            palm of left, and vice versa

Figure 20.2 6-step hand hygiene technique

Hot air driers are effective if used correctly (Matthews and Newsom, 1987). However, they have a number of features that mean that they must be used with care. For example, they take several seconds to work so there is a temptation to stop before the hands are dry. They are also rather noisy for use in patient care areas and require a constant electricity supply. It has also been reported that bacteria or viruses which are suspended in the air are conveyed by the drier directly on to the hands or on to the mucous surfaces of the nasal passages. Electric driers are commonly found in public toilets, as they do away with the need for constant re-supplying of paper towels, and they keep the toilets tidier, but hot air driers are not recommended for use in clinical areas or where food is being prepared.

Handwashing agents

The type of solution used to wash hands is less important than the handwashing technique used. The most expensive bactericidal agent is of little use if it does not have contact with the fingers and the thumbs. Some handwashing agents can themselves pose an infection risk. For example, bar soap is a convenient agent, but left wet in a soap dish it becomes an ideal medium for the growth of micro-organisms which can then recontaminate the hands. For this reason, in clinical settings, liquid soap dispensers should be provided. These should be designed so that the soap canisters are completely discarded when empty rather than being topped up with soap, which could become contaminated over time.

Other handwashing agents include chlorhexidine, povidone iodine and alcohol handrub. Chlorhexidine and povidone are often used for surgical scrubbing. These agents are also sometimes employed for routine handwashing during outbreaks of infection.

Alcohol handrubs are useful agents for disinfecting the hands prior to invasive procedures. Organic matter on the hands should be removed by cleaning before applying alcohol handrub which destroys commensal flora living near the surface of the skin. The alcohol must be rubbed into all surfaces of the hands until it has evaporated.

Alcohol can be used to ensure effective skin decontamination, following a social hand wash, after giving care to patients with infectious diseases. It can also be applied to hands between contacts with patients as an aid to preventing the transmission of micro-organisms, if the hands are visibly clean. This is particularly useful in that the user can be decontaminating his/her hands while moving on to the next task without having to go to the sink.

Sexual contact

Certain infections are directly transmissible via sexual contact and this subject is comprehensively discussed in Chapter 13.

Ingestion

Ingestion of pathogens may occur directly by eating contaminated food, water, ice, or indirectly by transferring organisms in the environment to the mouth via hands or contaminated equipment such as cutlery or feeding tubes. Prevention of transmission via this means is covered in Chapter 8.

Injection/inoculation

Pathogenic organisms may be injected into the body directly or indirectly. Direct injection can occur if the skin is not thoroughly cleaned prior to administering injected medication or setting up an intravenous infusion. In this example the patient may become infected with his or her own skin organisms. It can also occur if the practitioner does not handwash before giving the injection and transfers their own bacteria into the patient. Direct injection/inoculation can also occur if there is direct transfer of blood from one person to another, for example if a surgeon is cut during an operation and bleeds into the patient's open wound.

Indirect injection can occur where equipment has become contaminated with blood and is used to inject others. Examples of this include inoculation injury sustained during re-sheathing or the handling of used needles; sharing used needles; not replacing the platforms or lancets of blood letting devices used for glucose monitoring (Department of Health, 1990). Prevention of infection via injection requires safe disposal of sharps, adequate skin preparation prior to invasive procedures and good practice during surgery.

Insect and animal vectors

Certain vectors, such as the mosquito, louse and tick, may directly transmit infection usually by biting. Others, such as the fly, rat and mouse, may be the indirect cause of infection, by contaminating the environment or in particular food. Food preparation areas must have pest control systems in place. In clinical areas vectors must be discouraged by, for example, not allowing clinical waste to accumulate, repairing holes in walls, etc. Some vectors are seasonal and should be dealt with swiftly should they appear.

Transplacental

Some micro-organisms can cross the placenta to infect the foetus in utero, sometimes with devastating effects. Examples include rubella, chickenpox, shingles, cytomegalovirus, hepatitis and HIV. This issue is dealt with more thoroughly in relevant sections.

Indirect contact

Role of the environment

Although the environment is less significant in the spread of infection, outbreaks of gastroenteritis have been attributed to environmental contamination. It is also known that MRSA, hepatitis B, tuberculosis and *Clostridium difficile* survive for long periods in the environment (Hoffman, 1993). Therefore, care should be taken to ensure that the environment is kept clean.

Certain conditions are more likely to result in environmental contamination than others; these include MRSA, diarrhoea and exuding cellulitis. These patients should be nursed in a single room until they are assessed as no longer posing a risk to others. This practice helps to prevent others coming into contact with the contaminated environment and developing infection themselves.

Unfortunately environmental hygiene in hospitals has not had a high profile in recent years and the standards of cleanliness may have suffered where there have been reductions in the hours of cleaning services available. Effective cleaning is more complicated than many imagine (see Table 20.1). It requires appropriate:

- methods
- products
- equipment (vacuums, high dusters etc.)
- frequencies
- storage of equipment
- training
- standards
- audit

Incorrect cleaning methods can contribute to the spread of infection and be injurious to health. COSHH assessments must be carried out and protective clothing used. In some healthcare settings responsibility for cleaning which had been removed from the remit of nurses, allowing them to concentrate on clinical care, is now being returned to the management of nurses. Often this is done to ensure that the housekeeper is part of the caring team and improve communication and supervision. However, nurses may not have the time to supervise and do not have the specialist knowledge of cleaning methods, products and equipment. Should the day-to-day supervision of housekeepers

Table 20.1 Example of a hygiene audit tool

Standard: Clinical areas (wards)
The environment and furniture will be clean, dry and dust free. There will be no evidence of smears or scuff marks and there will be an even appearance. Equipment used for handwashing or general cleaning will also be kept replenished and bins lined with the correct colour bag. Stocks of perishable goods are used in rotation and discarded or used before expiry date.

Clinical areas	Y/N	Comments
Beds Bed tables Lockers Chairs Over-bed light and panel Curtains Hand washbasin Liquid soap, paper towels Pedal bin High dusting Low dusting		
SCORE		
Bathroom/toilet Bath/shower Toilet Bidet Hand washbasin Liquid soap, paper towels, toilet roll		
SCORE		
Utility rooms High dusting Low dusting Macerator/washer Sinks Liquid soap, paper towels Cleaning roll, detergent Pedal bins		
SCORE		
Kitchen High dusting Low dusting Fridge/ice maker Microwave oven		

(contd)

Table 20.1 (contd)

Clinical areas	Y/N	Comments
Trolleys Dishwasher Cupboards Food stocks Hand washbasin Liquid soap, paper towels Paper roll, detergent Floor		
SCORE		
Action plan		

be devolved to the ward manager it is important that an expert housekeeping manager is retained (or is accessible) to ensure that safety standards continue to be met across the organization (Thompson and Hempshall, 1998). The Infection Control Nurses Association in conjunction with the Association of Domestic Managers (1999) developed standards for hygiene in hospitals which have been adopted as national standards by the Department of Health.

Role of equipment

Contaminated equipment has frequently been implicated in the indirect transmission of infection. Examples include wooden tongue depressors used as splints on neonates (PHLS, 1996); endoscopes (McGrath, 1998); neonatal laryngoscopes (Neal et al., 1995); lancets for blood glucose monitoring (Department of Health, 1990); vaginal speculae (Department of Health, 1994); mattresses (Loomes, 1988); blood-gas analyzer (Garland et al., 1996) and many more examples.

Equipment must be safe for its purpose and decontaminated adequately after use and whenever contaminated (King, 1998). This includes clinical items such as drip stands and syringe drivers, commodes, suction machines, ECG machines, ultrasounds, etc. These items are usually not cleaned by housekeepers and can be neglected by nursing staff. Chapter 9 discusses this topic in more detail.

Inhalation

Some infections may be contracted through inhalation of the pathogens and transmission may be via *droplets* or *airborne droplet nuclei*

(Hospital Infection Control Practices Advisory Committee, 1996).

Respiratory droplets are generated and expelled during coughing, sneezing, talking, suctioning and bronchoscopy. The droplets are large and quickly fall to the ground. In order to inhale droplets one has to be very close to the infected person. However the organisms contained in the droplets may survive for some time in the environment and may be picked up unintentionally on the hands and subsequently inoculated on to the mucous membranes of the eyes or mouth. Chickenpox, the common cold and influenza are transmitted in this manner and it is thought that viral gastroenteritis may also be spread this way.

Droplet nuclei are expelled in the same manner. They are very small, no more than 5 micrometers in size, and they can remain suspended in the air for long periods. Pulmonary tuberculosis is transmitted by droplet nuclei. It is recommended that people with TB who need to be admitted to hospital and whose sputum is smear positive should be nursed in a single room with the door closed, or preferably in a single room with negative air pressure (Department of Health Interdepartmental Working Group, 1997 and 1998).

Portals of entry

Portals of entry are the routes by which pathogens gain entry to the body, and they may be natural or artificial. Natural portals of entry include the eyes, mouth, rectum, vagina, urethra, breaches in the skin, etc. Artificial portals of entry breach the natural defences of the body and are more common in patients receiving medical treatment. They include: intravenous cannulae, PEG tubes, tracheostomies, Hickman lines, urinary catheters, surgical drains, stomas, epidural catheters, etc.

Patient-related portals of entry

Glynn et al. (1997) found that invasive devices increase a patient's risk of infection sevenfold. This risk must be related to the fact that invasive devices are portals of entry. In contemporary healthcare, medical treatment often requires the employment of invasive devices. It must be recognised by all involved in their management that devices such as these, while assisting in the treatment of clinical conditions, can also contribute to morbidity. Invasive sites may become infected by the patient's own organisms (particularly staphylococci or coliforms), or by other pathogens. Invasive devices must be used with care, avoided where possible and removed as soon as possible if infection is to be prevented. Following the work of Glynn et al. (1997), Ward, Wilson, Taylor, Cookson and Glynn (1997) produced clinical guidelines for a number of invasive procedures. The principles of care are outlined in Table 20.2.

Table 20.2 Principles of care with invasive devices

* aseptic handwashing before and after contact with invasive devices
* change lines at appropriate intervals
* keep tubes and drainage bags off the floor
* apply appropriate dressings
* change dressings at appropriate intervals and when contaminated
* keep the skin clean and dry
* remove when no longer required

Staff-related portals of entry

Healthcare workers are generally fit and healthy and their portals of entry are protected by the body's normal non-specific defence system (see Chapter 1). The nature of their work is such that they may be exposed to particularly hazardous substances and therefore extra care is needed to protect them from infection.

In order to prevent pathogens gaining entry into their own bodies, healthcare workers need to practice safely at all times. This will include:

* protecting any open wounds or cuts on parts of the body which come into contact with body fluids (e.g. the hands) with a good quality dressing such as a waterproof island plaster;
* handwashing after handling any body fluid or after removing protective clothing;
* wearing appropriate personal protective clothing. Protective clothing must be worn whenever contact with a body fluid is anticipated, regardless of the patient's known condition. A risk assessment chart is provided in Table 20.3.

It is important to remove protective clothing once the procedure for which it was worn has finished, otherwise the clothing itself can transmit organisms into the environment or equipment.

Table 20.3 Risk assessment chart

Risk	Action	Aim
Body fluid in contact with hands	Wear disposable gloves Remove when procedure is completed Wash hands	Prevent direct contact Avoid indirect spread of infection via gloves Avoid indirect spread via the hands
Body fluid contact with clothing	Wear disposable apron If high volume, wear a fluid repellent disposable gown Remove when procedure completed Wash hands	Prevent direct contact Avoid spread of infection via apron Avoid indirect spread via the hands
Body fluid contact with mouth	Wear fluid repellent face mask Use a barrier for mouth-to-mouth contact Remove after procedure completed Wash hands	Prevent direct contact Avoid indirect spread via the hands
Body fluid contact with eyes	Wear eye protection (face mask with integral visor, goggles, full head visor, safety spectacles) Remove after procedure completed. Discard or disinfect as appropriate Wash hands	Prevent direct contact Avoid indirect spread via the hands
Patient's sputum is smear positive to *M. tuberculosis*	Wear high-efficiency particulate filter mask during: • long periods of contact • cough induction • bronchoscopy until the patient has received anti-TB therapy for 2 weeks and responded	Prevent inhalation of *M. tuberculosis*

People at risk

Everyone is at risk of acquiring infection, although for some infections immunity can be acquired naturally or artificially (see Chapter 1). Bowell (1992a and b) devised a risk assessment tool to help practitioners identify patients with specific risk factors. Factors included individual factors such as extremes of age, malnourishment, immobility etc.; local factors which affect blood supply such as ischaemia; invasive factors such as IV therapy, surgery, implants, etc.; drugs such as antibiotics, steroids and cytotoxics; underlying disease such as diabetes, HIV and AIDS.

Some people are at particular risk of infection due to their lowered immunity (patients with an immunosuppressive illness such as AIDS, or receiving cytotoxic drugs) or because they are more likely to be exposed (healthcare workers or intravenous drug users). Patients with lowered immunity will require extra care, particularly when hospitalized. This may simply mean additional handwashing or even the use of positive air pressure single rooms. Where possible healthcare workers should be protected by vaccination, in particular against hepatitis B, tetanus and BCG. Those working in areas of higher risk may receive other vaccinations. During outbreaks of infection, such as influenza, key carers may also be given specific vaccination to prevent infection and ensure staffing levels can be maintained during the crisis.

Applying the chain of infection to practice

The concept of a 'chain of infection' can be used to help understand the rationale underpinning the precautions taken for a particular infection. The Royal College of Nursing used the model to illustrate the chain of events of hepatitis infection (Royal College of Nursing, 1998). Examples are presented in Figure 20.3.

Planning care

The prevention and control of infection must be an integral part of any care plan and just like every other aspect of care the first stage is an assessment of the risks. Each patient must be assessed with regard to:

a) their own risk of acquiring infection (immune status, general condition, invasive devices, etc.)

b) whether they pose risks to others (known or suspected underlying infection, loss of body fluids, e.g. bleeding, diarrhoea, expectoration, etc.)

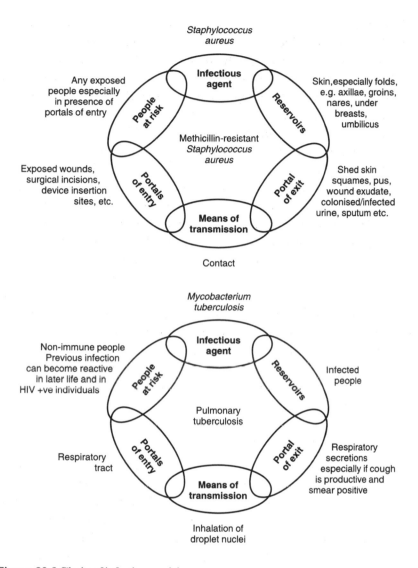

Figure 20.3 Chain of infection model

Having assessed the risks a care plan can be written which aims to prevent or control infection either by protecting vulnerable portals of entry, by providing appropriate accommodation, or by rendering safe any potential vehicles of spread (Bowell, 1992a and b). Patients who have the same infectious disease may need quite different care plans because of individual factors which influence the infection risks. For example, a person with salmonella who has the mental and physical ability to get themselves to the toilet and wash their own hands, will need a different care plan to someone who is confused and frail and who cannot even get themselves out of bed. Likewise a person with a communicable infection will need their care plan revised if their physical or mental state changes. For example the risks associated with a person with hepatitis B infection undergoing dental extraction will be different before, during and after surgery. Figure 20.4 (pp. 338–9) gives an example of risk assessment and planning guide.

When devising plans of care, reference must be made to the local infection control policy, procedures which incorporate infection control principles and to current regulations and national guidance. For example, there is guidance available relating to the management of people with tuberculosis (Department of Health – Interdepartmental Working Group on Tuberculosis, 1996 and 1998); MRSA (Report of Working Party 1998); transmissible Spongiform encephalopathy agents (Advisory Committee on Dangerous Pathogens/Spongiform Encephalopathy Advisory Committee 1998); viral haemorrhagic fever (Advisory Committee on Dangerous Pathogens 1998); antimicrobial resistance (Department of Health, Standing Medical Advisory Committee 1998); bloodborne viruses (UK Health Departments– Expert Advisory Group on AIDS and the Advisory Group on Hepatitis 1998).

Implementing the care plan

Care plans are important as means of communicating a care programme, providing a record of care given, ensuring continuity of care and assisting in the evaluation of interventions. Accurate documentation is required by employers, the United Kingdom Central Council for Nursing, Midwifery and Health Visiting and the Courts (UKCC, 1998). Producing comprehensive documentation may appear to be time-consuming to practitioners and low on their list of priorities. Research has shown that nurses' documentation of infection control precautions is inadequate, even when they are provided with a core care plan (Finn, 1997). Efforts should be made to ensure that actions taken to prevent infection and its transmission are incorporated into assessment documents, care pathways, care plans etc. An example of a core care plan is shown in Figure 20.5 (p. 340).

A care plan cannot be implemented without the necessary resources, so managers have a duty to ensure that these are assessed periodically and a supply maintained. Resources include: an adequate supply of single rooms; availability of handwash basins complete with soap and towels; protective clothing; linen bags and waste containers; sharps boxes; supplies of clean linen and cleaning materials, etc.

Relevant aspects of the care plan must also be communicated to those who need to know and who are involved in the patient's care. This may include: the patient and his/her visitors; other professionals; housekeepers; porters; radiographers; other clinical staff to whom the patient is being transferred e.g. District Nurses and Nursing Home managers. The need for confidentiality should also be considered. Gammon (1999) demonstrated that when patients in isolation were given information and assisted with developing coping strategies, their stress was reduced and self-esteem increased.

Managing specific infections

Certain infections can cause a great deal of concern for the affected patients affected, their visitors and the staff who are part of the caring team in both hospital and community situations. This may be because the infections are particularly life-threatening, because they involve the tracing of contacts or because they can elicit an emotive response from elements of the media. Examples of three such infections are outlined below.

Meningococcal disease

Meningococcal disease is comparatively rare with around 2,000 cases per year being confirmed by culture. Transmission of *Neisseria meningitidis* is by droplets and the organism quickly dies outside the human host (PHLS, 1995). Around 10% of the population normally carry meningococci in their upper respiratory tract and there is a carriage rate of up to 25% in young adults in 'closed or semi-closed' communities, such as schools, colleges and military barracks. It is not yet understood why exposure to the organism leads to invasive disease in certain individuals.

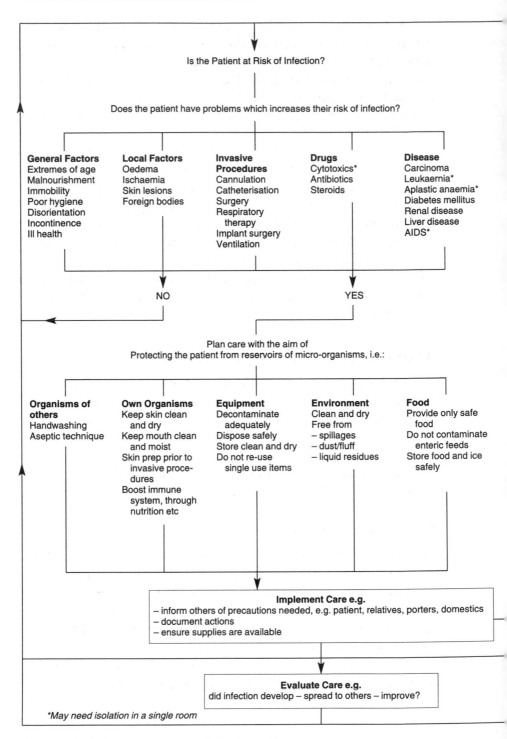

Is the Patient at Risk of Infection?

Does the patient have problems which increases their risk of infection?

General Factors	**Local Factors**	**Invasive Procedures**	**Drugs**	**Disease**
Extremes of age	Oedema	Cannulation	Cytotoxics*	Carcinoma
Malnourishment	Ischaemia	Catheterisation	Antibiotics	Leukaernia*
Immobility	Skin lesions	Surgery	Steroids	Aplastic anaemia*
Poor hygiene	Foreign bodies	Respiratory		Diabetes mellitus
Disorientation		therapy		Renal disease
Incontinence		Implant surgery		Liver disease
Ill health		Ventilation		AIDS*

NO   YES

Plan care with the aim of
Protecting the patient from reservoirs of micro-organisms, i.e.:

Organisms of others	**Own Organisms**	**Equipment**	**Environment**	**Food**
Handwashing	Keep skin clean	Decontaminate	Clean and dry	Provide only safe
Aseptic technique	and dry	adequately	Free from	food
	Keep mouth clean	Dispose safely	– spillages	Do not contaminate
	and moist	Store clean and dry	– dust/fluff	enteric feeds
	Skin prep prior to	Do not re-use	– liquid residues	Store food and ice
	invasive proce-	single use items		safely
	dures			
	Boost immune			
	system, through			
	nutrition etc			

Implement Care e.g.
– inform others of precautions needed, e.g. patient, relatives, porters, domestics
– document actions
– ensure supplies are available

Evaluate Care e.g.
did infection develop – spread to others – improve?

*May need isolation in a single room

Figure 20.4 Infection assessment and planning guide

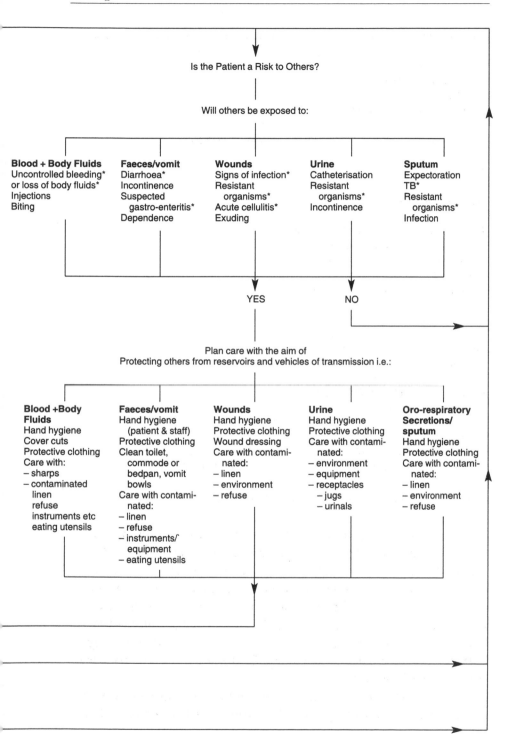

Is the Patient a Risk to Others?

Will others be exposed to:

Blood + Body Fluids
Uncontrolled bleeding*
or loss of body fluids*
Injections
Biting

Faeces/vomit
Diarrhoea*
Incontinence
Suspected
    gastro-enteritis*
Dependence

Wounds
Signs of infection*
Resistant
    organisms*
Acute cellulitis*
Exuding

Urine
Catheterisation
Resistant
    organisms*
Incontinence

Sputum
Expectoration
TB*
Resistant
    organisms*
Infection

YES   NO

Plan care with the aim of
Protecting others from reservoirs and vehicles of transmission i.e.:

Blood +Body Fluids
Hand hygiene
Cover cuts
Protective clothing
Care with:
– sharps
– contaminated
    linen
    refuse
    instruments etc
    eating utensils

Faeces/vomit
Hand hygiene
    (patient & staff)
Protective clothing
Clean toilet,
    commode or
    bedpan, vomit
    bowls
Care with contami-
    nated:
– linen
– refuse
– instruments/
    equipment
– eating utensils

Wounds
Hand hygiene
Protective clothing
Wound dressing
Care with contami-
    nated:
– linen
– environment
– refuse

Urine
Hand hygiene
Protective clothing
Care with contami-
    nated:
– environment
– equipment
– receptacles
    – jugs
    – urinals

Oro-respiratory Secretions/ sputum
Hand hygiene
Protective clothing
Care with contami-
    nated:
– linen
– environment
– refuse

Assess potential problems	List current problems	Signature	Date
1. Diarrhoea* 2. Incontinent of faeces* 3. Dependence for use of toilet 4. Dependence for hygiene			

Problems marked * indicate a high risk of transmission to others

Nursing interventions	Signature	Date + time

If high risk of spread, single room with en-suite toilet
If low risk allocate own toilet/commode
Gloves for handling contaminated items
Apron for contact with contaminated items
Hand wash:
    -After removing protective clothing
    -Before leaving the room
    -After using the toilet
    -Before eating
Dispose of faecally soiled waste in yellow bag
Place faecally soiled linen in red alginate bag
Provide patient with Fact Sheet
Clean room/equipment daily and on discharge or transfer into main ward		

Notes:
- Inform infection control if two or more cases
- There is no need to obtain faecal samples if the symptoms resolve

Figure 20.5 Example of a core care plan (*Clostridium difficile*)

Cases of meningococcal disease occur throughout the year and there is a higher incidence in the winter months. Types B and C are the most commonly occurring strains causing invasive meningococcal disease in the UK and account for around 60–65% and 35–40% of isolates respectively. The disease can affect any age group, but the young are the most vulnerable with the highest number of cases being seen in the under 4s and the next highest in those aged between 15 and 19 years. Group C disease is relatively more common in older cases.

The disease may present as meningitis, meningococcal septicaemia or, most commonly, a combination of the two. The case fatality rate varies from around 5% for meningitis alone to 20% for septicaemia alone. Rapid diagnosis and treatment is the key factor in a favourable prognosis and Benzylpenicillin should be given prior to admission to hospital in all suspected cases (Department of Health, 1999).

The signs and symptoms of meningococcal disease can include fever, stiff neck, severe headache, photophobia, vomiting and drowsiness. In cases of septicaemia, and in many cases of meningitis, there is also a rash that does not blanch under pressure.

Close contacts of a confirmed or probable case are likely to be carrying the causative organism and are offered chemoprophylaxis in order to eradicate it.

A close contact is usually defined as someone having close prolonged contact, such as living in the same household or having intimate relations with the index case, during the week prior to the onset of symptoms. Prophylaxis is given to reduce the risk of exposure to other susceptible persons within that particular social group but will not prevent the illness in someone who is already incubating the disease. Guidance on the management of clusters is available (Stuart et al., 1997).

Chemoprophylaxis can do harm as well as good by eliminating protective commensal organisms and encouraging the development of antibiotic-resistant strains of meningococci; it may also have harmful side effects. Public health authorities arrange for contact tracing in cases of meningococcal disease and advice should always be sought from the Consultant for Communicable Disease Control before prophylaxis is given to people who are concerned that they may be contacts.

There is now a vaccine against serogroup C meningococcal disease which has become part of the national immunization schedule and offers long-term immunity.

Tuberculosis

Tuberculosis (TB) is caused by the bacterium *Mycobacterium tuberculosis*. It is usually an infection of the lungs, although other body parts can be affected. In general TB is remarkably difficult to catch. People can have natural resistance to many infections, including TB. The general rise in living standards over the past 100 years has helped to raise the level of this natural resistance.

Tuberculosis of the lung (pulmonary TB) can give symptoms of cough with phlegm (sometimes with blood in it), breathlessness, fever, loss of weight and poor appetite. People can be completely cured with modern anti-TB treatment.

TB can only be passed on by someone who is ill with an active TB infection in the lungs. Just being in the same room as someone who has TB is not enough to catch the disease. It depends on being in close contact with an infected person who has a productive cough. Someone who has pulmonary TB but who does not have a cough is not infectious to others. Close contact means that the contact has to be frequent or prolonged. This would normally be people living in the same household or who are very close friends of the person with TB.

When infectious TB is suspected or diagnosed, it is recommended that all close contacts of that patient should be screened. Contacts are usually tested a few weeks later by using a simple skin (Heaf) test which is examined a week later. A negative skin reaction to the Heaf test would indicate that the person may have no immunity to the disease and the test may be repeated in a couple of months. If there is still no reaction, immunization against TB (BCG vaccine) may be carried out.

A positive Heaf test would confirm a previous BCG vaccination, or that at some time the person being tested has been in contact with TB and has developed a natural immunity. At this stage it would be necessary to check that anyone with natural immunity has no infection present and a chest X-ray would be carried out. The chest X-ray would be not taken until 2 to 3 months after the contact with TB infection occurred, as the disease develops very slowly and it would not be possible to see any infection on X-ray sooner than this.

All necessary screening is organized by the TB services. The contact does not need to see anyone else or change anything they do whilst waiting for this to take place, but should see their GP if they become unwell.

Healthcare staff caring for someone with active pulmonary TB are not routinely screened. It is recommended that only those giving close and regular/repeated prolonged care involving sputum-productive procedures should be screened with the Heaf test or chest X-ray as described above.

Isolation requirements for cases of *Mycobacterium tuberculosis*

Patients, regardless of HIV status, with potentially infectious tuberculosis (i.e. sputum negative, but culture positive or culture results unknown) need not be isolated in a single room unless there are significantly immunocompromised patients within the ward or area.

All patients with suspected or confirmed infectious tuberculosis, regardless of HIV status, should be nursed in a single room until three consecutive good quality sputum samples are smear negative or the diagnosis is excluded. Where the room is in or near a ward or area in which significantly immunocompromised patients are located, the isolation room should be at negative air pressure which is continuously and automatically monitored.

HIV-related tuberculosis

Although probably no more likely to acquire infection following exposure to *M. tuberculosis* HIV-infected individuals are at significantly increased risk of progressing to active tuberculous disease once infected. In the UK, the overlap between HIV and tuberculosis is still quite small. There is no evidence that HIV-infected individuals with tuberculosis cough up greater quantities of infective bacteria but, because they progress faster to active disease following primary exposure, the pool of infection that others may be exposed to may be greater.

Multiple-drug resistant tuberculosis (MDRTB)

Drug-resistant TB is still relatively rare in the UK. There is no evidence that drug-resistant tuberculosis, including MDRTB, is more infectious than drug-sensitive TB, patients with MDRTB are likely to remain infectious for a longer period of time because the available treatment regimes are less effective. Because of these differences necessary isolation precautions, treatment regimes and contact tracing will differ from those described above in the case of HIV-related or multiple-drug resistant tuberculosis (Department of Health Interdepartmental Working Group on Tuberculosis, 1998).

However, early identification and treatment of tuberculosis is the single most important means of control. Tuberculosis should be suspected in any patient, regardless of HIV status, with a persistent cough lasting more than three weeks with or without weight loss, loss of appetite, fever, night sweats or the coughing up of blood.

Methicillin-resistant *Staphylcoccus aureus* (MRSA)

Staphylcoccus aureus may colonize the skin, particularly the anterior nares, skin folds, hair lines, umbilicus, etc., in up to 30% of the healthy population. Only if the organism invades the skin or deeper tissues and multiplies, causing a localized or systemic response, e.g. inflammation, is the patient said to be clinically 'infected'.

Outbreaks of infection with antibiotic-sensitive strains of *Staphylcoccus aureus* are well documented, but strains of *Staphylcoccus aureus* resistant to penicillin were first isolated soon after the antibiotic was introduced. This is due to the production of a penicillinase or beta-lactamase enzyme produced by *Staphylcoccus aureus*. New penicillins became available in the 1960s, which were not easily destroyed by this enzyme; for example methicillin, the forerunner of flucloxacillin. Although methicillin is no longer used as an antibiotic to treat patients 'methicillin resistance' is interpreted as meaning 'flucloxacillin resistance', as flucloxacillin remains a commonly used antibiotic.

In recent decades the organism has demonstrated its ability to develop resistance to a range of antibiotics, but different strains vary in their sensitivity to antibiotics. Some strains of MRSA also have a greater propensity to spread and are known as 'epidemic' strains (termed EMRSA). Sixteen epidemic strains of MRSA have so far been identified in the UK and in recent years the most common strains to affect healthcare have been EMRSA-15 and EMRSA-16.

MRSA in general is no more or less pathogenic than sensitive strains. However, should infection develop, the range of effective antibiotics will be more limited and these may be more costly and potentially more toxic. Consequently it is considered prudent to continue to take infection control precautions to prevent transmission of the organism, especially in those patient groups that are more susceptible to infection.

Individuals may acquire MRSA as a natural consequence of long-term exposure to antibiotics, particularly if the courses have not been completed or the dosage has been inadequate. Acquisition of MRSA often occurs as a result of exposure to the organism in a clinical environment, for example during an outbreak in hospital.

MRSA is transmitted in the same ways as sensitive strains of staphylococcus i.e. it may be:

Endogenous – the bacteria may be transferred from one part of a colonized person's body to another site (e.g., nose to wound).

Exogenous – transmitted from person to person by direct contact with the skin or contaminated environment or equipment. Skin scales may be disseminated by natural desquamation and become airborne by movement. This can be a particular problem if the patient has a skin condition such as psoriasis or is heavily colonized. Airborne skin scales may contaminate other people or the environment some distance away and staphylococci can survive for long periods in dust which acts as a reservoir.

Prevention of transmission of MRSA is essentially the same as for other organisms which are transmitted by the contact route, but there may be additional specific practices for MRSA specified in local policies:

Universal precautions

Hand hygiene:

- after each patient contact
- after handling body fluids and items contaminated with body fluids
- after removing protective clothing
- before handling invasive devices

Cleanliness of:

- general environment – horizontal surfaces, sinks, baths, etc.
- patient-related equipment (beds, furniture, monitors, IV counters, etc.)
- soft furnishings (curtains, bedding, etc.)
- wearing disposable gloves, aprons when handling body fluids
- safe disposal of waste

- maintaining safe staff: patient ratio
- avoiding overcrowding patients
- avoiding unnecessary transfers of patients between wards

Additional precautions

- isolation of patients with a known or suspected infection
- an isolation unit/ward/side room may be required
- affected patients may require systemic antibiotics or topical treatment
- keeping the door to isolation room closed as much as possible (especially during bedmaking, wound care, suctioning or moving and handling the affected patient)
- screening of other patients (contacts, admissions, discharges, transfers)
- screening of staff lesions/skin sites
- careful deployment of agency/bank nurses

The combined Working Party of the British Society for Antimicrobial Chemotherapy, the Hospital Infection Society and the Infection Control Nurses Association (1998) has revised the guidelines for the management of MRSA in hospitals. The Working Party identified factors which increase the risk of infection with MRSA, i.e. the presence of patients with intravenous devices, surgical wounds, pressure sores and those in intensive care units (see Table 20.4). It recommended that in those areas where particularly vulnerable patients are nursed, every precaution should continue to be taken to prevent the spread of MRSA. However, in situations where the risks of developing infection are low, efforts should be concentrated on providing routine infection control practice to a high standard.

This risk assessment is consistent with previous guidelines issued by the Department of Health related to the management of people with MRSA in nursing and residential homes (Department of Health, 1996). People in the general community who acquire MRSA are unlikely to develop serious MRSA infection because they do not have high risk factors such as invasive devices, deep tissue wounds and severely depressed immunity. Therefore the guidance from the Department of Health stresses the importance of standard infection control procedures as identified above. It also recommends

Table 20.4 MRSA risk assessment chart

Risk category			
High	Moderate	Low	Minimal
Intensive care	General surgery	Elderly (acute)	Elderly (long stay)
Special care baby unit	Urology	General medical	Psychiatric
Burns unit	Neonatal	Children (not neonate)	Psycho-geriatric
Transplant unit	Gynaecology		
Cardiothoracic	Obstetric		
Orthopaedic	Dermatology		
Trauma			
Vascular			
Regional, national, International centres			

that MRSA-positive patients in residential and nursing homes should not be isolated, but permitted to socialize as normal, although they should not share a room if they or their room mate has a chronic open wound or catheter.

In the patient's own home the risks are even lower and there should be no restrictions to a normal life. People with MRSA are able to work, socialize and go to the pub, hairdresser, etc., as usual and do not need to restrict contact with friends, children or the elderly.

Community healthcare workers should practise standard precautions as normal, such as an aseptic technique for wound care. They should be sure to decontaminate their hands after giving care, either using soap and water or alcohol handrub. In clinics and surgeries, it is also important to maintain a clean working environment, avoiding the buildup of dust. Patients with MRSA do not stay long in waiting rooms or treatment rooms, therefore the risk of spread is low.

Should patients who have previously been MRSA-positive be re-admitted to hospital, the admitting ward should be informed so that they can take appropriate actions according to local policy. This may involve screening the patient's carriage sites, applying topical treatment or even providing single room accommodation, depending upon the assessment of risk.

The presence of MRSA can sometimes cause concern amongst staff, patients and visitors. This is often based on a lack of knowledge about the organism and misconceptions about the risks of infection and procedures to prevent transmission. Communication is essential in relieving anxiety, and this can take the form of information leaflets for patients, visitors and staff; the provision of notices which describe succinctly the necessary precautions or organizing training or special team meetings during outbreaks to include support staff and others involved in giving care. The patient needs to know how their care may be affected by MRSA, why they may be in a single room and how long the precautions will be required. It is also important to ensure that other staff understand the actions they need to take, for example that cleaners need to keep the isolation room especially clean, or the community nurse may need to continue care at home.

Conclusion

The control and prevention of infection must form part of every patient's care. It does not only become important when a patient is known to have an infection, or when an outbreak occurs. Good infection control will prevent infection developing and prevent outbreaks. It is not easy to measure what has been avoided, and consequently infection control may have a low priority for care staff. Unfortunately, it is also not always possible to clearly demonstrate cause and effect so that, for example, if a patient develops an urinary tract infection no one may recognize that it was caused by the poor handwashing technique of the person inserting the catheter.

It is the small things that can make all the difference – the care taken when hand washing, keeping the catheter off the floor, keeping the patient's mouth and skin clean, keeping patient equipment clean. It is not only part of 'basic nursing' care, it is everyone's basic care, from the doctor to the porter. We all have our part to play. No one will ever say 'well done, you've prevented another infection', but if we all practice conscientiously we will all know that we have contributed to a reduction in infection.

References

Advisory Committee on Dangerous Pathogens. Management and Control of Viral Haemorrhagic Fevers. London: UK Health Departments, 1998.
Advisory Committee on Dangerous Pathogens – Spongiform Encephalopathy Advisory Committee (1998). Transmissible Spongiform Encephalopathy Agents: Safe Working and the Prevention of Infection London: HMSO, 1998.

Ayliffe GAJ, Lowbury EJL, Geddes AM, Williams JD Control of Hospital Infection: A Practical Handbook, 3rd Edition. London: Chapman and Hall Medical, 1992.

Benenson AS (ed.) Control of Communicable Diseases Manual (16th Edition). Washington: American Public Health Association, 1995.

Bosi C, Davin-Regli A, Charrel R, Rocca B, Monnet D, Bollet *Serratia marcescens* nosocomial outbreak due to contamination of hexetidine solution. Journal of Hospital Infection 1996; 33: 217–24.

Bowell B Hands up for cleanliness. Nursing Standard 1992a; 6: 24–5.

Bowell B Protecting the patient at risk. Nursing Times 1992b; 88 (3): 32–5.

Bowell B A risk to others. Nursing Times 1992c; 88 (4): 38–40.

Department of Health. Safety Action Bulletin (SAB(90)78): Lancing devices for multi-patient capillary-blood sampling: avoidance of cross infection by correct selection and use. London: Department of Health, 1990.

Department of Health. Safety Action Bulletin 108-SAB(94)22. Instruments and Appliances Used in the Vagina and Cervix: Recommended Methods for Decontamination. London: DoH, 1994.

Department of Health – Interdepartmental Working Group on Tuberculosis. The Prevention and Control of Tuberculosis in the United Kingdom: Recommendations for the Prevention and Control of Tuberculosis at a Local Level. Department of Health and the Welsh Office. London: HMSO, 1996.

Department of Health – Interdepartmental Working Group on Tuberculosis. The Prevention and Control of Tuberculosis in the United Kingdom: UK Guidance on the Prevention and Control of 1. HIV-related Tuberculosis. 2. Drug-resistant, Including Multiple Drug-resistant, Tuberculosis Department of Health, Scottish Office and Welsh Office. London: HMSO, 1998.

Department of Health. Meningococcal Infection PL/CMO/99/1. London: Department of Health, 1999.

Finn L Nurses' documentation of infection control precautions: 2. British Journal of Nursing 1997; 6 (12): 678–84.

Department of Health. MRSA: What Nursing and Residential Homes Need To Know. London: Department of Health, 1996.

Department of Health – Standing Medical Advisory Committee. The Path of Least Resistance. London: HMSO, 1998.

Elliot T, Hastings M, Desselberger U Lecture Notes on Medical Microbiology, 3rd Edition. London: Blackwell Science Ltd, 1997.

Gammon J Isolated instances. Nursing Times 1999; 95 (2): 57–66.

Gammon J Analysis of the stressful effects of hospitalisation and source isolation on coping and psychological constructs. International Journal of Nursing Practice 1998; 4 (2): 84–96.

Garland SM, Mackay S, Tabrizi S, Jacobs S *Pseudomonas aeruginosa* outbreak associated with a contaminated blood-gas analyzer in a neonatal intensive care unit Journal of Hospital Infection 1996; 33 (2): 145–51.

Glynn AA, Ward V, Wilson J, Charlett A, Cookson B, Taylor L, Cole N Hospital Acquired Infection: Surveillance, Policies and Practice. London: Public Health Laboratory Service, 1997.

Gorman LJ, Sanai L, Notman AW, Grant IS, Masterton RG Cross infection in an intensive care unit by *Klebsiella pneumoniae* from ventilator condensate. Journal of Hospital Infection 1993; 23: 27–34.

Gould D Nurses' hands as vectors of hospital acquired infection: a review. Journal of Advanced Nursing 1991; 16: 1216–25.

Gould D, Wilson-Barnett J, Ream E Nurses' infection control practice: hand decontamination, the use of gloves and sharp instruments. International Journal of Nursing Studies 1996; 33 (2): 143–60.

Gransden WR, Webster M, French GL, Phillips An outbreak of Serratia marcescens transmitted by contaminated breast pumps in a special care baby unit. Journal of Hospital Infection 1986; 7: 149–54.

Hoffman P *Clostridium difficile* and the hospital environment. PHLS Microbiology Digest 1993; 10 (3): 91–2.

Horton R, Parker L Informed Infection Control Practice. London: Churchill Livingstone, 1997.

Hospital Infection Control Practices Advisory Committee. Guideline for isolation precautions in hospitals: Part 2 recommendations for isolation precautions in hospitals. American Journal of Infection Control 1996; 24 (1): 32–52.

Infection Control Nurses Association. Guidelines for Hand Hygiene, 1997.

Infection Control Nurses Association/Association of Domestic Managers. Standards for Environmental Cleanliness in Hospitals. Northumberland: ADM/ICNA, 1999.

King S Decontamination of equipment and the environment. Nursing Times 1998; 12 (52): 57–64.

Loomes S Is it safe to lie down? Nursing Times 1988; 84: 63–5.

MacKenzie D, Edwards A MRSA: the psychological effects. Nursing Standard 1997; 12 (11): 49–53.

Matthews JA, Newsom SWB Hot air electric hand driers compared with paper towels for the potential spread of airborne bacteria. Journal of Hospital Infection 1987; 9: 85–8.

McGrath S Cleaning up the act. Nursing Times 1998; 94 (19): 59, 60, 63.

Neal TJ, Hughes CR, Rothburn MM, Shaw NJ The neonatal laryngoscope as a potential source of cross infection. Journal of Hospital Infection 1995; 30: 315–21.

Oldman T Isolated cases. Nursing Times 1998; 94 (11): 67–70.

Perry C, Gore J Now wash your hands please. Nursing Times 19 May 1997; 93: 64–8.

Public Health Laboratory Service. Meningococcal Infections Working Group and Public Health Medicine Environmental Group. Control of meningococcal disease: guidance for consultants in communicable disease control. Communicable Disease Report Review 1995; 5: 189–94.

Public Health Laboratory Service. Invasive fungal infections and contaminated tongue depressors. Communicable Disease Report 1996; 6 (17): 145 and 148.

Rees JC, Allen KD Holy water – a risk factor for hospital-acquired infection. Journal of Hospital Infection 1996; 32: 51–5.

Royal College of Nursing. Hepatitis. London: RCN, 1998.

Sanderson P, Richardson D Do patients with *Clostridium difficile* need to be isolated? Journal of Hospital Infection 1997; 36: 157–8.

Shanson DC Microbiology in Clinical Practice, 2nd Edition. London: Wright, 1989.

Stuart JM, Monk PN, Lewis DA, Constantine C, Kaczmarski EB, Cartwright KAV Management of clusters of meningococcal disease Communicable Disease Report 1997; 7 (1): R3 R5.

Taylor L An evaluation of handwashing techniques 1. Nursing Times January 12 1978a; 74: 54–5.

Taylor L An evaluation of handwashing techniques 2. Nursing Times January 19 1978b; 74: 108–10.

Thompson M, Hempshall P Dirt alert. Nursing Times 1998; 94 (28): 63–4.

UKCC. Standards for Records and Record Keeping. London: UKCC, 1998.

UK Health Departments. Guidance for Clinical Health Care Workers: Protection Against Infection With Blood-borne Viruses. London: HMSO, 1998.

Ward V, Wilson J, Taylor L, Cookson B, Glynn A Clinical Guidelines. London: Public Health Laboratory Service, 1997.

Working Party Report of the Combined Society for Antimicrobial Chemotherapy, the Hospital Infection Society and the Infection Control Nurses Association. Revised guidelines for the control of methicillin-resistant *Staphylococcus aureus* infection in hospitals. Journal of Hospital Infection 1998; 39: 253–90.

Further reading

Benenson AS Control of Communicable Diseases in Man, 15th Edition. Washington: American Public Health Association, 1990.

Finch RG, Ball P Infection. Oxford: Blackwell Scientific Publications, 1991.

Meers P, Sedgwick J, Worsley M The Microbiology and Epidemiology of Infection for Health Science Students. London: Chapman and Hall, 1995.

Wilson J Infection Control in Clinical Practice. London: Bailliere Tindall, 1995.

Appendix 1

Infection Control Audit Checklist
(Reproduced with kind permission of the Journal of Hospital Infection and West Midlands ICNA)

Standard statement: Kitchens will be maintained appropriately to negate the risk of cross-contamination.

		Yes/No or N/A
1	Handwash basin, liquid/bar soap and paper towels are available	
2	Disposable paper towelling is used for cleaning and drying the equipment and surfaces	
3	Cleaning materials used in kitchens are stored separate to other ward cleaning equipment	
4	Cleaning materials are colour coded and the correct colour code is in use	
5	All opened food (e.g. cereal) is stored in pest-proof containers	
6	Patients' food in fridge is labelled with name and date as per policy	
7	Food in the refrigerator is within the expiry date	
8	Milk is stored under refrigerated conditions	
9	The refrigerator is used for food products only (i.e. free from drugs and specimens)	
10	Hands are washed and a clean plastic apron is worn to serve patient meals	
11	The refrigerator temperature is between 0 and 5 °C (by electronic probe)	
12	Freezer temperature is below -18 °C (by electronic probe)	
13	All items of equipment are appropriate for this area	
14	The kitchen is free from infestation	
	Additional comments:	

Standard Statement 2: The clinical environment will be maintained appropriately to negate the risk of cross-infection.

	Yes/No or N/A

Clinical room
1   The room is clean and dust free
2   The room is free from inappropriate items of equipment
3   All sterile products are stored above floor level (excluding recent deliveries of new stock which are to be put away)
4   Items of sterile equipment are in date (randomly select two items and check date)
5   Dressing trolleys are clean and in a good state of repair

Bathroom
6   Bathrooms are clean/free from communal items (multi-use creams, flannels, etc.)
7   The bathroom is free from cork bath mats/cork chairs
8   Anti-slip bath/shower mats are clean and hung over the bath/rail to dry between use
9   All lifting aids are waterproof and easy to clean (e.g. slings, bath seats, etc.)
10 Appropriate cleaning materials are available for staff/patients to clean bath after use
11 The bath has been cleaned following patient use
12 Any ambulift present is clean and in a good state of repair

Toilets
13 Toilet and surrounding area is clean and free from extraneous items
14 Cleaning materials are available for patients/staff to clean the toilet, e.g. sanitizer/wipes where appropriate (e.g. maternity wards)

Sluice/dirty utility room
15 The sluice is clean and free from spillages
16 Wash bowls are stored clean/dry and inverted or patients' own are stored in locker
17 Bedpans/urinals and jugs are stored inverted or on racks
18 Commodes are clean, ready for use
19 Commodes are in a good state of repair
20 Mops/buckets are correctly colour coded and stored as per disinfection policy
21 Used instruments are stored in the sluice in appropriate containers less than two-thirds full
22 Appropriate facilities are available and in working order to ensure correct disposal (or disinfection) of bedpans and urinals (e.g. macerator and/or washer–disinfector)
    Additional comments:

Standard statement 3: Waste will be disposed of safely without risk of cont-amination or injury.

	Yes/No or N/A
1 Waste disposal policy and/or chart is available to staff 2 Correct segregation of glass, clinical and household waste 3 Waste bags are less than two-thirds full, securely sealed and labelled 4 There are foot-operated bins in working order for clinical waste 5 Waste bags are stored safely, away from the public 6 The disposal area is locked and inaccessible to unauthorized persons 7 The storage area is cleaned regularly Additional comments:	

Standard Statement 4: Linen is handled appropriately to prevent cross-infection.

	Yes/No or N/A
1 Linen is segregated in appropriate colour-coded bags 2 Bags are less than two-thirds full, and are capable of being secured 3 Bags are stored in the dirty utility/linen disposal or sluice prior to disposal 4 Clean linen is stored in a clean area (not in the sluice/bathroom) 5 Curtains are visibly clean and in a good state of repair 6 How do you dispose of infected linen? (randomly question a member of staff) Additional comments:	

Standard Statement 5: Sharps are handled safely in order to prevent injury.

	Yes/No or N/A
1 A container as specified by the control of infection committee in use (BS 7320)	
2 Box is less than two-thirds full	
3 Box is free from protruding sharps	
4 Sharps box is available on the crash/arrest trolley	
5 Sharps box is available on the medicine trolley	
6 Sharps box is assembled correctly	
7 Sharps box is labelled/signed according to hospital policy	
8 Sharps are disposed of directly into a sharps box following use of outstationed laboratory equipment, e.g. blood gas analyser, autolet, etc.	
9 What action would you take following a needlestick injury?	
10 Sharps boxes are stored safely, away from the public and out of reach of children Additional comments:	

Standard Statement 6: Equipment is cleaned/decontaminated/stored correctly to negate the risk of infection.

	Yes/No or N/A
1 Chairs, tables and lockers are clean and in a good state of repair	
2 Suction equipment is clean and dry. Catheter not attached (clean cover acceptable in some emergency areas)	
3 Thermometers are stored dry	
4 Bed frames are clean and free from excessive dust	
5 Mattress covers are in a good state of repair. Test: Randomly select bed, examine mattress – no staining should be visible, mattress should be impermeable to fluids. Place paper towel beneath cover, press down on mattress for 10 seconds, pour 50 ml of water on to area, press down for further 30 seconds. Remove and examine paper towel for signs of leakage through cover.	
6 Single-use items used once only (if it is local policy to re-use then mark N/A)	
7 Staff are aware of the need for decontamination and a certificate prior to sending equipment for maintenance/repair	
8 Staff clearly state the procedure for returning biohazard equipment to HSDU (i.e. autoclavable bags, where this is local policy) Additional comments:	

Standard Statement 7: Disinfectants are available and used correctly to prevent cross-infection.

	Yes/No or N/A
1 Appropriate disinfectants (hypchlorite) and dilution charts are available to deal with blood spillages	
2 Correctly diluted disinfectants are used for blood spills (10,000 ppm hypochlorite)	
3 Chemical disinfection is only used for heat-labile equipment, e.g. fibre optic scopes	
4 Data sheets are available for disinfectants used (COSHH) Additional comments:	

Standard Statement 8: Hands will be washed correctly, using a cleansing agent, at the facilities available, to reduce cross-infection.

	Yes/No or N/A
1 Liquid/bar soap is available at all sinks in the clinical area	
2 Paper towels are available at all sinks in clinical areas	
3 Sinks in clinical areas are free from nail brushes	
4 Access to handwash basins is clear	
5 The sinks are free from used equipment, e.g. medicine pots which are soaking	
6 Chlorhexidine and/or alcohol handrub is available for use in at least one clinical area (where this is local policy)	
7 A trained member of staff is observed to carry out the correct handwashing technique (observe throughout audit, mark down if handwashing should have occurred but did not). Criteria: Wet hands prior to using soap, lather and wash for a minimum of 20 seconds, rinse and dry using more than one paper towel.	
8 Untrained staff member observed carrying out correct handwashing technique as above	
9 Hands of staff carrying out patient care are free from jewellery, e.g. watches, stoned rings	
10 A poster demonstrating a good handwashing technique is available by at least one clinical sink or is in the policy manual	
11 Mixer taps are available in sinks in clinical areas	
12 A good handwashing technique is included in new staff induction programmes Additional comments:	

Standard Statement 9: Clinical practices will reflect infection control guidelines and reduce the risk of cross-infection to patients, whilst providing appropriate protection to staff.

	Yes/No or N/A

The following protective clothing is available for use by staff:
 1   Latex non-sterile and sterile gloves
 2   Plastic disposable aprons
 3   Eye protection
 4   Sterile dressings are used to cover intravenous venflon sites
     Criteria: Select one patient at random with an IV and observe site
 	
 Enteral feeding
 5   Feeds are replaced at appropriate time intervals according to
     local recommendations
 6   Aseptic technique is used during all procedures affecting the feed
 	
 Urinary catheter care
 7   Non-sterile latex gloves are worn for emptying urinary catheter bags
 8   A disposable receptacle or heat-disinfected jug is used for emptying
 9   Catheter stands are in use and catheter taps are above floor level
     Tick as appropriate for the above questions in relation to catheter care:
     Observed practice:
     Questioned about practice:
 10 Infected patients are nursed with the appropriate isolation precautions
     and according to hospital policy
 11 Staff can state the procedure when dealing with specimens from
     patients with known infections
 12 Staff can state the procedure when handling deceased patients who have
     not had a known infective condition, e.g. hepatitis B, HIV (i.e. body bags)
 13 A clean plastic apron and gloves are worn for handling body fluids
 14 Staff can locate the infection control policy manual
 15 The policies in the infection control manual are the most up-to-date
     versions
     Additional comments:	

From Millward et al., 1993.

Appendix 2
Summary of specific infections

Infectious agent	Reservoir	Signs and symptoms	Control measures
Bacillus cereus (Food poisoning)	Soil, raw, dried and processed food	Nausea, vomiting, colic, diarrhoea, lasting about 24 hours	Good food hygiene, keeping cooked rice cool and storing safely
Incubation period	**Method of spread**		**Treatment**
1–6 hours if vomiting 6–24 hours if diarrhoea	Ingestion of contaminated food especially cooked rice which has been stored at room temperature		None
Period of infectivity			
N/A			
Infectious agent	**Reservoir**	**Signs and symptoms**	**Control measures**
Bordetella pertussis (Whooping cough)	Humans	Paroxysmal cough lasting some months, inhalation is a high-pitched whoop. Pneumonia and brain damage may result	Immunization
Incubation period	**Method of spread**		**Treatment**
7–10 days	Inhalation of droplets or contact with respiratory discharges		Erythromycin or ampicillin. Treat suspected contacts with erythromycin
Period of infectivity			
Greatest in early catarrhal stage Not infectious at 3 weeks			

Infectious agent	Signs and symptoms	Control measures
Campylobacter jejuni	Profuse, watery, blood-stained diarrhoea and/or vomiting, severe abdominal cramps and fever	Precautions with faeces, good food preparation, storage and cooking; pasteurize milk and water; handwash after handling puppies, kittens and poultry; infected food handlers must stay off work until symptom-free
Incubation period 3 to 5 days	Only a few hundred organisms may cause disease because they multiply within the gut	**Treatment**
Duration of infectivity May be several weeks		Rehydration. Antibiotics e.g. erythromycin only if the disease is severe
Reservoir Bowels of farm and domesticated animals, pets and birds		
Method of spread Ingestion of contaminated food, water, milk, etc.		
Person to person spread is unlikely		
Infectious agent *Clostridium difficile*	**Signs and symptoms** Diarrhoea with a distinctive odour, sometimes mucus. There may be pseudo-membranous colitis	**Control measures** Precautions with faeces, good personal and environmental hygiene, appropriate and prudent use of antibiotics outlined in an Antibiotic Policy
Incubation period Variable		**Treatment** Withdraw causative antibiotics, if symptomatic treat with metronidazole or vancomycin
Duration of infectivity While symptomatic		
Reservoir Human gut, especially of the elderly and young children		
Spores may survive for months on furniture, toilets, etc. Keep clean using detergent and water		
Method of spread Endogenous infection caused by suppression of normal gut flora following broad spectrum antibiotic therapy and cephalosporins		
Person to person spread by ingestion of spores from contaminated hands, equipment or environment		

Infectious agent	Reservoir	Signs and symptoms	Control measures
Clostridium perfringens 1. Gas gangrene 2. Gastroenteritis **Incubation period** 1. Not applicable 2. 6 to 24 hours **Duration of infectivity** 1 and 2 Not applicable	Human intestine, guts of farm animals and fish, also the soil **Method of spread** 1. Endogenous infection by contamination of wounds (surgical and traumatic) or in conditions of ischaemia (necrosis or poor blood supply) 2. Ingestion of contaminated food which has been cooked slowly and eaten much later or person to person spread. Infectious dose = $>10^5$ organisms per gram of food	1. Necrosis of tissue and crepitus, may cause septicaemia 2. Colic, diarrhoea and nausea	1. Wound cleansing, prophylactic antibiotics if wound heavily contaminated, sterilize surgical instruments 2. Good food hygiene **Treatment** 1. Excision of necrotic tissue and penicillin 2. Supportive treatment only
Clostridium tetani **Incubation period** 3–21 days **Duration of infectivity** Not applicable	Intestines of man and animals, soil and fomites **Method of spread** Contamination of wounds by soil or gut organisms. Needs the presence of necrotic tissue or foreign body. Person-to-person spread via contaminated instruments	Muscle spasms leading to paralysis Fatality is 30–90% depending on age	Vaccination Sterilization of instruments **Treatment** Benzylpenicillin, human tetanus immunoglobulin and tetanus toxoid. Wound cleansing or surgical treatment may be needed. Artificial ventilation may also be required in severe cases of prolonged spasm

Infectious agent

Corynebacterium diphtheriae (Diphtheria)

Reservoir

Human nose or throat

Signs and symptoms

Infection of the throat, mucous membranes or skin

Control measures

Vaccination, follow up of close contacts. In hospital, precautions with oro-respiratory secretions

Method of spread

Endogenous infection affecting the larynx, pharynx or skin

Person to person spread via contact is also possible

Treatment

Antitoxin, erythromycin or penicillin

Incubation period

2–5 days

Duration of infectivity

2–4 weeks

Infectious agent

Creutzfeldt-Jakob Disease

Reservoir

Nervous tissue of infected animals and humans. In recent years suggested link between the bovine form (bovine spongiform encephalopathy) and vCJD

Signs and symptoms

Progressive neurological symptoms, dementia, myoclonic jerks, spasticity, wasting, coma. Always fatal

Control measures

Destroy surgical instruments contaminated with the causative prion. Risk assessment prior to surgery involves identifying the likelihood of previous exposure to the organism, and the degree of contamination with nervous tissue during the procedure

Method of spread

Familial or transfer of infected nervous tissue during surgery, cornea, dura mater and pituitary gland transplant, use of human growth hormone

Treatment

None

Incubation period

1 to 20 years

Duration of infectivity

Continuous

Infectious agent	Reservoir	Signs and symptoms	Control measures
Cryptosporidium parvum	Bowels of man and farm or domesticated animals	Profuse watery diarrhoea, and vomiting and anorexia in children	Precautions with faeces, good public health programme, filter raw water, boil water during outbreaks, handwashing after handling animals
Incubation period	**Method of spread**	In the immunocompromised, e.g. AIDS, the disease is protracted and may not respond to treatment. They may be infectious for the rest of their lives	**Treatment**
3 to 10 days	Consumption of contaminated food and water or ingestion of oocysts from infected faeces		None except rehydration
Duration of infectivity			
While symptomatic			
Infectious agent	**Reservoir**	**Signs and symptoms**	**Control measures**
Cytomegalovirus	Humans	Mild glandular fever	There is a high level of human immunity
Incubation period	**Method of spread**	In pregnancy there may be foetal damage involving liver, central nervous system, jaundice, convulsions, death in utero	Body fluid and urine precautions
3–12 weeks	Contact with the virus shed in the urine, saliva, breast milk and other body fluids, kissing, transplacental transmission and transplantation of organs from CMV positive people into CMV negative people.		**Treatment**
Period of infectivity	After primary infection, may reactivate throughout life		Gancyclovir for CMV retinitis in the immunosuppressed
Periodic shedding of virus over many years, plus reactivation			

Infectious agent	Reservoir	Signs and symptoms	Control measures
Ebola-Marburg disease	Unknown	Sudden onset fever, malaise, joint pain, headache, pharyngitis. Progression to vomiting, diarrhoea, maculopapular rash, involvement of the liver and kidneys	Standard precautions with blood and body fluids, restrict sexual contact, strict laboratory precautions
Incubation period	**Method of spread**		**Treatment**
Ebola 2–21 days Marburg 3–9 days	Inoculation of infected blood, secretions, organs, semen, needles and syringes		None other than supportive measures
Period of infectivity			
Prolonged			

Infectious agent	Reservoir	Signs and symptoms	Control measures
Entamoeba histolytica (Amoebic dysentery)	Humans	Often no symptoms. Illness may be mild (abdominal pain, diarrhoea with blood and mucus) or severe (with chills, ulceration of the peri-anal skin and abscesses in the liver, brain or lung)	Food and hand hygiene and enteric precautions
Incubation period	**Method of spread**		**Treatment**
2–4 weeks, may be years	Faecal–oral route, ingestion of contaminated water or food. Also oro-anal sex		Metronidazole followed by iodoquinol to eradicate cyst passage
Period of infectivity			
While excreting cysts			

Infectious agent	Reservoir	Method of spread	Signs and symptoms	Control measures	Treatment
Epstein-Barr virus (Glandular fever) **Incubation period** 4–6 weeks **Period of infectivity** Prolonged	Humans	Direct contact with oro-pharyngeal secretions e.g. kissing	Fever, sore throat, lymphadenopathy. Usually mild and self-limiting	None	None
Escherichia coli (Enterotoxigenic strains) **Incubation period** 24–72 hours **Period of infectivity** Prolonged	Humans and animals	Ingestion of contaminated food or water. Low infective dose	Abdominal cramps, vomiting, profuse watery diarrhoea, dehydration *E. coli* 0157 may lead to renal failure in the elderly and children	Precautions with faeces, good food hygiene, hand and environmental hygiene. Exclude from work affected food handlers and children under 5 from school/nursery. Identify sources of outbreaks and further cases	Supportive measures only

Infectious agent

Giardia lamblia

Incubation period

5–25 days

Period of infectivity

Duration of infection

Reservoir

Humans and wild and domesticated animals

Method of spread

Faecal-oral route, ingestion of cysts from contaminated items and water

Signs and symptoms

Diarrhoea, abdominal cramps, steatorrhoea

Control measures

Treatment of water and sewerage, personal hygiene

Treatment

Metronidazole

Infectious agent

Hepatitis A

Incubation period

28–30 days

Period of infectivity

About a week before, and a few days after, jaundice

Reservoir

Humans

Method of spread

Faecal-oral route, ingestion of contaminated food, water and shellfish, rarely blood transfusion

Signs and symptoms

Sudden onset fever, malaise, anorexia, nausea, abdominal pain, jaundice. Can be asymptomatic, mild or severe and disabling

Control measures

Good food hygiene, exclusion of affected food handlers from work, cooking shellfish thoroughly, surveillance for clusters of cases

Treatment

None except passive immunization of contacts

Infectious agent	Reservoir	Incubation period	Method of spread	Period of infectivity	Signs and symptoms	Control measures	Treatment
Hepatitis B	Humans	60-90 days	Inoculation of blood and body fluid especially semen, vaginal secretions. Also contact with contaminated instruments	Varies	Slow onset with nausea, vomiting, anorexia, abdominal discomfort, fever, joint pain, rash, often jaundice. May go on to develop chronic hepatitis or cirrhosis	Standard precautions with blood and body fluids, safer sex, needle exchange schemes, screening of blood and tissues for transplant, vaccination of health care workers	Follow-up of inoculation injury, sometimes administration of vaccination or immuno-globulin
Hepatitis C	Humans	6–9 weeks	Like hepatitis B but sexual contact is less risky	One week before, some become carriers	Like Hepatitis B but may progress to chronic active hepatitis or cirrhosis years later, with an increased risk of liver cancer	Universal precautions with blood and body fluids, screening of blood and tissues for donation	Follow up by a liver specialist, some centres give interferons

Infectious agent	Reservoir	Signs and symptoms	Control measures
Hepatitis D	Humans	Like Hepatitis B but sudden onset, may become chronic	As for Hepatitis B, but there is no vaccine
Incubation period	**Method of spread**		**Treatment**
Unknown	Infected blood and sexual intercourse. The virus can only replicate within cells previously infected with hepatitis B		As for hepatitis B
Period of infectivity			
Prolonged, very infectious just before acute illness			

Infectious agent	Reservoir	Signs and symptoms	Control measures
Hepatitis E	Humans	Like Hepatitis A but fewer sequelae	If hospitalized take precautions with faeces, good food hygiene, exclude affected food handlers from work
Incubation period	**Method of spread**		**Treatment**
6–8 weeks	Ingestion of contaminated food and water. Epidemics in India, but rare in developed countries		None
Period of infectivity			
Unknown			

Infectious agent	**Reservoir**	**Signs and symptoms**	**Control measures**
Lassa virus (Lassa fever)	Wild rodents in West Africa	Headache, spiking fever, malaise, cough, sore throat, nausea, vomiting, diarrhoea, joint pain, inflamed and exuding pharynx, conjunctivitis, shock, pleural effusion, bleeding, convulsions, swollen face and neck, albuminuria	Standard precautions with blood and body fluids, strict laboratory precautions, surveillance of contacts
Incubation period	**Method of spread**		**Treatment**
6–21 days	Direct and indirect contact with excreta from infected animals also person-to-person via needles, oro-respiratory secretions, urine and sexual intercourse		Ribavirin
Period of infectivity			
While virus is present, about 3–9 weeks			

Infectious agent	**Reservoir**	**Signs and symptoms**	**Control measures**
Legionella pneumophilia (Legionnaires' disease)	Stagnant water	Pneumonia, myalgia, malaise, headache, non-productive cough, temperature, consolidation and petechiae in lungs	Prevention of water stagnation, clean pipework, maintenance programme, heat water to >65°C and <20°C. Infection has occurred in hospital clinical settings when tap water has been used for topping up humidifiers etc.
Incubation period	**Method of spread**		**Treatment**
2–10 days	Inhalation of aerosolized water from air-conditioning, whirlpools, showers etc. There is no evidence of person to person spread. Susceptible people are men aged over 50 with existing chest problems		Erythromycin and/or Rifampicin, ciprofloxacillin
Duration of infectivity			
N/A			

Infectious agent	Reservoir	Signs and symptoms	Control measures
Listeria monocytogenes	Soil, silage and intestines of animals and humans. The organism can survive freezing, drying and cooking	Premature delivery of neonates, neonatal septicaemia and meningitis, 'flu-like symptoms, septicaemia and sometimes lesions on the hands	Pregnant women should avoid eating high-risk foods. Good food hygiene practice
Incubation period			**Treatment**
3–70 days	**Method of spread**		Penicillin and ampicillin, aminoglycosides, tetracycline, chloramphenicol. Ampicillin in pregnant women
Duration of infectivity	Contact with animals and raw meat. Ingestion of contaminated food including fruit, vegetables and soft cheeses. The immuno-suppressed, elderly and pregnant women are also at-risk groups		
7–10 days			

Infectious agent	Reservoir	Signs and symptoms	Control measures
Measles	Humans	Red, blotchy rash starting on the face then becoming generalized. May include conjunctivitis, Koplik spots and cough as prodrome. In developing countries serious complications may develop	Vaccination, exclusion from work or school. If hospitalized take respiratory precautions
Incubation period	**Method of spread**		**Treatment**
10 days	Direct contact with secretions from nose, throat and droplets		None
Period of infectivity			
Just before prodrome to 4 days after rash			

Infectious agent	Reservoir / Method of spread / Incubation period / Period of infectivity	Signs and symptoms	Control measures / Treatment
Infectious agent Meningitis (bacterial causes incl.: *Neisseria meningitidis*, TB, *Streptococcus pneumoniae*. viral causes include: coxsackie, measles, varicella, *Haemophilus influenzae*) **Incubation period** Viral infection 2–4 days Bacterial infection 2–10 days **Period of infectivity** While organisms persist	**Reservoir** Humans **Method of spread** Varies, but usually close contact with infectious secretions (kissing, family contacts)	**Signs and symptoms** Varies depending upon cause. Include: fever, rash, headache, neck stiffness	**Control measures** Identify contacts of cases of meningococcal disease and offer prophylaxis. Reduce overcrowding and improve hygiene **Treatment** Varies depending upon causative organism: *Neisseria meningitidis* – Penicillin *Haemophilus influenzae* – Rifampicin.
Infectious agent *Mycobacterium leprae* (Leprosy) **Incubation period** 9 months to 20 years **Period of infectivity** Until treated for 3 months	**Reservoir** Humans **Method of spread** Contact with lesions and nasal discharges which are thought to contain the bacilli	**Signs and symptoms** May be lepromatous – progressive, leading to nodular skin lesions and nervous involvement or tuberculoid – non-progressive with macular skin lesions and severe asymptomatic nervous involvement. Tissue and nerve damage may be followed by spontaneous healing	**Control measures** No specific isolation precautions, regular monitoring of family contacts and administration of chemoprophylaxis **Treatment** Dapsone or rifampicin

Infectious agent	Reservoir	Signs and symptoms	Control measures
Mumps virus Mumps (infectious parotitis)	Humans	Acute infection, fever, swollen and tender salivary glands, orchitis in some males and oophoritis in some females. Infection in 1st trimester of pregnancy may lead to spontaneous abortion	Vaccination, exclusion from work or school, if hospitalized single room isolation
Incubation period 12–25 days	**Method of spread** Direct contact with saliva and droplets		**Treatment** None
Period of infectivity 1 week before to 9 days after parotitis			

Infectious agent	Reservoir	Signs and symptoms	Control measures
Mycobacterium tuberculosis (Pulmonary TB)	Humans and infected animals	Cough, chest pain, weight loss, haemoptysis, night sweats	Tracing of close contacts and screening for disease. BCG vaccination. If hospitalized single room isolation for 2 weeks of treatment
Incubation period 4–12 weeks, often infection is latent	**Method of spread** Inhalation of droplet nuclei exhaled during cough, singing, sneezing. Usually requires close prolonged contact.		**Treatment** Combined anti-TB therapy for 6 to 24 months or longer. BCG must not be given if the recipient is immunosuppressed
Period of infectivity Until sputum negative	Ingestion of contaminated milk or dairy products		

Infectious agent	Reservoir	Method of spread	Incubation period	Period of infectivity	Signs and symptoms	Control measures	Treatment
Polio virus (Poliomyelitis)	Humans	Faecal-oral route, ingestion of contaminated food and drink, contact with pharyngeal secretions	3–35 days	A few days before and after symptoms begin	Varies from mild viral illness (fever, headache, malaise, nausea and vomiting) to severe illness (muscle pain, stiff neck, paralysis affecting respiration and swallowing)	Vaccination, precautions with oro-respiratory secretions and faeces	None, other than prevention of complications

Infectious agent	Reservoir	Method of spread	Incubation period	Period of infectivity	Signs and symptoms	Control measures	Treatment
Rabies virus (Rabies)	Wild and domesticated animals in North and South America, Canada and Europe	Bite from an infected animal (inoculation of saliva)	2–8 weeks	3–10 days before and during the illness	Headache, fever, malaise, paresis or paralysis, difficulty swallowing, delirium, convulsions, fatal encephalomyelitis	In the UK – quarantine animals which have visited countries with a known rabies problem	Administer rabies immunoglobulin to bitten individuals

Infectious agent

Respiratory Syncytial Virus

Incubation period

1–10 days

Duration of infectivity

Shortly before symptoms and for duration of illness. Children may be infectious for several weeks

Reservoir

Humans

Method of spread

Person to person by airborne route, plus contact with respiratory secretions and contaminated utensils

May cause community or hospital outbreaks

Infected hospital staff should not care for susceptible patients

Signs and symptoms

Chest infection and pneumonia in children and the elderly. Also fever, headaches, malaise, anorexia and, in children, acute gastro-enteritis

Control measures

In hospital, single room isolation. Exclude from school while ill, careful disposal of hankies and heat disinfection of utensils.

Treatment

Usually none, but ribavirin may be administered to compromised individuals

---

Infectious agent

Ascariasis
(Roundworm)

Incubation period

Not applicable

Period of infectivity

1–2 years while female worms live in the gut

Reservoir

Humans and the soil

Method of spread

Ingestion of eggs from contaminated food or the environment

Signs and symptoms

Excretion of eggs or live worms from anus, mouth or nose. Usually symptomless but may develop lung or bowel complications

Control measures

Hand and environmental hygiene, adequate toilet facilities. Identify contacts

Treatment

Mebendazol and albendazol

Infectious agent

Rubella virus (German measles)

Incubation period

16–18 days

Period of infectivity

1 week before rash to 4 days after

Reservoir

Humans

Method of spread

Direct contact with naso-pharyngeal secretions and droplets

Signs and symptoms

Mild illness in children, maculopapular rash. Often no symptoms.
Infection in 1st trimester of pregnancy may lead to congenital rubella syndrome which can result in deafness, cataracts, heart defects, spontaneous abortion or death

Control measures

Vaccination, screening of young women and pregnant women for rubella antibody

Treatment

None

Infectious agent

Salmonella species

Incubation period

12–36 hours

Period of infectivity

Duration of illness, some become chronic carriers

Reservoir

Animals, infected people and carriers

Method of spread

Ingestion of contaminated food include eggs, poultry, unpasteurized milk. Person-to-person e.g. infants' nappies

Signs and symptoms

Often none, sudden onset headache, diarrhoea, abdominal pain, fever and sometimes vomiting

Many types of salmonella are pathogenic, most commonly *S. typhimurium* and *S. enteritidis*

Control measures

Food hygiene and thorough cooking, exclusion from work of affected food handlers, enteric precautions

Treatment

Usually none, antibiotics may prolong the duration of excretion of organisms

Infectious agent	Incubation period	Duration/Period of infectivity	Reservoir	Method of spread	Signs and symptoms	Control measures	Treatment
Salmonella typhi and Salmonella paratyphi (Typhoid, paratyphoid)	1–3 weeks (typhoid) / 1–10 days (paratyphoid)	Duration of infectivity: 7 days to 2 weeks, but carriers are possible	Intestine of humans and, in the case of paratyphoid, domesticated animals	Ingestion of contaminated food, milk, water especially shellfish. Person to person spread by ingestion of food contaminated by infected person	Enteric fever, septicaemia, headache, anorexia, rose spots on the trunk and constipation is more common than diarrhoea. It is possible to excrete the organisms for months	Treatment of water and sewerage, pasteurization of milk and water, control of flies and vaccination to prevent infection. Precautions with faeces and exclusion of food handlers from work in cases of infection	Amoxicillin, co-trimoxazole or chloramphenicol if there is enteric fever
Shigella sonnei (Bacillary dysentery)	12–96 hours	Period of infectivity: Up to 4 weeks, some carriers	Humans	Faecal-oral route, requires ingestion of only 10–100 organisms	Diarrhoea, fever, nausea and vomiting, blood and mucus in the faeces arising from confluent micro-abscesses. Sometimes mild or symptomless, usually self-limiting	Enteric precautions, good food hygiene, exclusion from work of affected food handlers and contacts, identify the source	Usually none, sometimes co-trimoxazole

Infectious agent	Reservoir	Signs and symptoms	Control measures
Small Round Structured Viruses e.g. Rotavirus, Norwalk	Probably humans	Vomiting and/or watery diarrhoea, possibly abdominal pain	Precautions with faeces and vomit
Incubation period	**Method of spread**	Immunity develops after infection but weakens later in life	In outbreaks, closure of wards until 48 hours after last new case, exclude symptomatic cases from ward and school, and catering in particular
24–72 hours	Person to person through ingestion of organisms via the hands, food, environment. Also may be possible to swallow aerosolized organisms which have been inhaled or inoculate them onto mucous membranes	Outbreaks are common and those infected are highly infectious because millions of organisms are excreted in the first few days	**Treatment**
Duration of infectivity			Self limiting illness usually needing no treatment except rehydration in some cases
While symptomatic			

Infectious agent	Reservoir	Signs and symptoms	Control measures
Streptococcus group A	Humans	Range of acute infections include skin lesions, septicaemia, cellulitis, tonsillitis, erysipelas, scarlet fever	Aseptic technique, exclude from work, school/nursery in acute infection
Incubation period	**Method of spread**		**Treatment**
1–3 days	Direct and indirect contact with infected people, nasal carriers and contaminated hands		Penicillin
Period of infectivity			
10–21 days or 48 hours if treated			

Infectious agent	Reservoir	Signs and symptoms	Control measures
Streptococcus group B	Female genital tract	Disease in the new-born include: sepsis, respiratory distress, pneumonia, and meningitis in older babies	Treatment of infected mothers, skin preparation during child-birth
Incubation period First 5 days, but may also be late onset	**Method of spread** Direct and indirect contact with infected people		**Treatment** Penicillin
Period of infectivity N/A			
Infectious agent *Toxoplasma gondii* (Toxoplasmosis)	**Reservoir** Intestines of cats who have eaten birds and small mammals	**Signs and symptoms** Usually mild but infection in early pregnancy may lead to foetal death and brain damage. May also be asymptomatic	**Control measures** Pregnant women should not handle cat litter trays, protect sandpits from cats, cook meat well, wash hands after handing cats and before food preparation
Incubation period 5–23 days	**Method of spread** Ingestion of the eggs of the protozoal parasite, which may be found in sandpits etc. Or ingestion of contaminated raw meat, milk and other foods, also transplacental		**Treatment** None
Duration of infectivity N/A			

Infectious agent	Reservoir	Signs and symptoms	Control measures
Vibrio cholerae (Cholera)	Humans	Usually symptomless, otherwise sudden onset, acute watery diarrhoea. 50% fatality if untreated	Enteric precautions, general hygiene, control of flies, surveillance of contacts, identification of the source
Incubation period	**Method of spread**		**Treatment**
2–3 days	Faecal-oral through ingestion of contaminated water or seafood. Also person-to-person		Rehydration, tetracycline
Period of infectivity			
Few days after recovery, some carriers			

Adapted from: Benenson AS (Ed.) (1995)
Elliot T, Hastings M, Desselberger U (1997)

Index